ENDANGERED LIVES
Public Health
in Victorian Britain

Anthony S. Wohl

ENDANGERED LIVES

Public Health in Victorian Britain

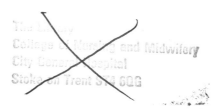

Methuen

To My Parents

First published in 1983 by J. M. Dent & Sons Ltd

First published as a University Paperback in 1984 by
Methuen & Co. Ltd
11 New Fetter Lane, London EC4P 4EE

© 1983 Anthony S. Wohl

Printed in Great Britain at the
University Press, Cambridge

British Library Cataloguing in Publication Data
Wohl, Anthony S.
    Endangered lives.–(University paperback 866).
    1. Public health–Great Britain–History
    19th century
    I. Title
    363′.0941   RA485
    ISBN 0–416–37950–8

Contents

Acknowledgments

Research for this book was undertaken in several libraries and I owe a debt to the librarians of the Vassar College library, Poughkeepsie, New York and the Welch Medical Library of Johns Hopkins University, Baltimore, Maryland, and, in London, of the Wellcome Institute for the History of Medicine, the British Library (British Museum), the Society of Community Medicine, the library of the University of London, and the Guildhall Library. Much of the final manuscript was typed by my Vassar College student assistant, Nancy Richardson, and my thanks are due to her for her cheerfulness and reliability. Throughout the long gestation of the book Peter Shellard at Dent displayed remarkable forbearance and humour and I am enormously grateful to him for his enthusiasm for the project, his continuous encouragement, and shrewd comments. Finally to my wife and daughters, who learned far more about contagion and cesspits, dirt and disease, than I suspect they ever wanted to, and who understandably came to look upon me as something of a 'drain-brain', my loving gratitude.

List of Illustrations

Abbreviations

MOH	Medical Officer(s) of Health
ARMOHPC	Annual Report of the Medical Officer to the Privy Council
ARMOHLGB	Annual Report of the Medical Officer to the Local Government Board
ARLGB	Annual Report of the Local Government Board
PP	Parliamentary Papers
RCNV	Royal Commission on Noxious Vapours
SCSP	Select Committee on Smoke Prevention
RCRP	Royal Commission on the Prevention of the Pollution of Rivers

'Sur, – May we beg and beseach your proteckshion and power, We are Sur, as it may be, livin in a Willderniss, so far as the rest of London knows anything of us or as the rich and great people care about. We live in muck and filthe. We aint go no priviz, no dust bins, no drains, no water-splies, and no drain or suer in the hole place. . . . The Stenche of a Gully-hole is disgustin. We all of us suffer, and numbers are ill, and if the Cholera comes Lord help us . . .

Preaye Sir com and see us, for we are living like piggs, and it aint faire we shoulde be so ill treted.'

Letter to *The Times*, 5 July 1849.

'What do we mean by sanitary science? We mean, I apprehend, that science which deals with the preservation of health and prevention of disease in reference to the entire community, and to classes within that community, as contradistinguished from medical science in the ordinary acceptation of the term, which latter study has for its aim the restoration of health when lost, and deals with the case of each individual separately.'

Lord Stanley, *Transactions of the National Association for the Promotion of Social Science*, 1857, p.41.

1
The Setting

'There is reason to believe that the aggregation of mankind in towns is not inevitably disastrous.'
William Farr, *PP*.XVII (1840), 'Second Annual Report of the Registrar-General, Appendix', p.xi.

Despite its wealth and social prominence the family found that it was unable to isolate itself from the stinks, pollution, and health hazards of the day. As newly-weds they had wanted the latest sanitary appliances, but the inexperience of the workmen putting in the water closet resulted in the waste overflowing into the rainpipe and down the dressing-room window. The cesspools beneath their Thames-side residence were notoriously foul, even by the standards of the day and when, at last, they had a new drainage system installed, the stench from the old cesspools remained and made parts of the dwelling almost uninhabitable. Some twenty years later the sewers blocked up after heavy rains and became 'most offensive and putrid'. Although living by the Thames was certainly most scenic, whenever the river rose their lawns were saturated with the raw sewage, which habitually floated on the surface of the water. Resigned to this inevitability, they simply had the lawns raked and the filth shovelled back into the river. In dry weather, on the other hand, the Thames' muck was left high and dry along the banks and gave off an appalling odour.

Probably as a consequence of the poor drainage system, the father contracted one of the most lethal and dreaded of what the Victorians called 'filth diseases' – 'bowel fever' or typhoid – and after struggling through a crisis on Friday, 13th December, succumbed the following day. The mother had contracted typhoid herself when she was sixteen and quite understandably she dreaded the disease which was a major killer. She was also morbidly superstitious, so one can imagine her horror when her eldest son came down with typhoid and reached a crisis also on 13 December, exactly ten years after the father's. But to her immense relief and amazement, her son pulled through and was miraculously snatched back from, as she put it, 'the very *verge* of the grave . . . hardly anyone had been known to recover who had been so

1

ill as he was.' December 14, the day that had made her, like so many others in that era, a young widow, always filled her with foreboding. Perhaps her superstitious dread was justified, for on that day one of her daughters, Alice, died of a disease, diphtheria, which was as puzzling as it was common (it also carried off her grand-daughter). She no doubt consoled herself with the thought that compared to many mothers she had been fortunate, for of her nine children not one had died in childbirth, but then she had had the best and most experienced doctors and midwives.

In other, considerably smaller ways the family was affected by the environmental abuses and dangers of the day. In 1858 a family 'pleasure cruise' on the Thames was abruptly terminated by the stench from the river. Many years later the bucolic pleasures of their South Coast home were rudely disturbed by the fumes and stench of industrial pollution from a local cement factory. Influential as the family was, its indignant protest to the Local Government Board failed to get results.

This family, with its troubles, tragedies and near-tragedies from bad sewers and filth diseases, forced to live amidst stink, and water and air pollution, was the Royal Family.[1] However remote it might appear to be, entrenched in its great residences in London, Windsor, and Osborne, it could not remain untouched by the forces which played so large and debilitating, and often so deadly a role in the lives of ordinary Victorians.

Countless articles and books have been written on the Victorian mind, but relatively few on the Victorian body.[2] There should surely be no excuse needed for a book which examines the connection between the physical and social environment and the human body in Victorian Britain, yet I must confess that I feel rather like the Rev Charles Girdlestone, who in 1845 had to apologize for giving, in his *Letters on the Unhealthy Condition of the Lower Classes of Dwellings, especially in Large Towns*, what might be considered 'an undue prominence' to the 'outward frame and condition of men'.[3] For public health history is traditionally associated with administrative, professional, and scientific, rather than social, domestic or private matters. Although parliamentary committees of investigation, royal commissions, the Privy Council, the Local Government Board and other administrations, and the contributions of local governments and medical officers are included, as indeed they must be, in this book, the emphasis is less upon central and local reform agencies, public administration, and

2

medical and scientific aspects than upon the social and physical environment and its effects upon the public's health.

Two main emphases of this book should be explained. In two respects the Royal Family was not representative of the families which, however anonymously, are the subject of this book. It was not really *urban* nor, of course, was it *working-class*. The emphasis upon towns in a history of public health is surely justified on the grounds that urban growth created vast problems of sewerage and water supply, multiplied the risk of infectious and contagious diseases, and increased awareness of the need to combat these challenges. Malthus casually included 'great towns' among the 'positive checks' to population such as wars, plagues, famine, extreme poverty and other 'miseries'. It was not that rural conditions were good but that many elements necessary for good public health – cleanliness, uncontaminated water, systems of excrement removal that would not saturate the sub-soil, leach into water supplies, or create diseased breeding grounds for flies, good ventilation, and isolation from diseases – were much more difficult to provide in the congested and burgeoning cities. As the quotation at the head of this chapter suggests, the town was regarded by many as the inevitable nexus of disease and premature death.

The Victorians were forced to adjust, often in a frantic and *ad hoc* manner, to town living in an age of unprecedented urban growth. It is too easy to condemn the Victorians for the pace of their sanitary reforms. Though, as we shall see, it is certainly pertinent to talk in terms of *laissez-faire*, local autonomy, and low rates, the often hesitant or erratic progress was as much due to inexperience and uncertainty bred of ignorance as to any conscious political or economic philosophy. The early and mid-Victorians were, quite simply, pioneers faced with a set of problems that were novel not only in their form but in their magnitude.

The urban development with which they had to cope was not a slow or steady trickle: it was a deluge which demanded large-scale responses. At the beginning of the century roughly 20 per cent of the population of England and Wales lived in towns of over 5,000 residents; by 1851 over half the population (54 per cent) did so and by 1911 almost 80 per cent. By 1801 only London had a population of over 100,000; by 1851 there were ten such towns (with roughly one-quarter of the nation's inhabitants living within them) and by 1911 there were thirty-six towns of that size and 43.8 per cent of the nation dwelt in them (compared to 11.0 per cent in 1801).[4] The movement from the countryside to the towns and the towns' natural growth were relentless throughout the century. In 1851 the nation for the first time had more town than country dwellers. In 1871 there were 14,041,000 urban dwellers and 8,671,000 rural residents; in 1901 the figures were, respectively, 25,058,000 and 7,469,000.[5]

It was the *rapidity* of urban growth, even more than its remorseless nature, which created so many problems. This on-rush of population can best be expressed in tabular form:

Town	1801	1831	1851
Birmingham	71,000	144,000	233,000
Bradford	13,000	44,000	104,000
Liverpool	82,000	202,000	376,000
Manchester	75,000	182,000	303,000
Sheffield	46,000	92,000	135,000
Leeds	53,000	123,000	172,000

[6]

By 1901 Birmingham had a population of 760,000, Liverpool of 685,000, and Manchester, 654,000. Glasgow, which in 1801 had 'only' 77,000 inhabitants, had 904,000 in 1901.[7] By that date there were 6,600,000 people living in the Greater London conurbation, 2,100,000 in the cities of South-Eastern Lancashire, 1,500,000 in the conurbations of the West Midlands and West Riding of Yorkshire, and 1,000,000 and 680,000 people living along the Merseyside and Tyneside respectively.[8]

This urban demographic revolution and its accompanying densities and pressures upon air, water, and space, must be borne in mind throughout the following pages. For what was time-honoured practice in the countryside, or acceptable as barnyard muck, became dangerous to health, indeed a question of very survival, in the densely-packed towns. As Engels commented, 'Dirty habits . . . do no great harm in the countryside where the population is scattered. On the other hand, the dangerous situation which develops when such habits are practised among the crowded population of big cities, must arouse feelings of apprehension and disgust.'[9] It did not take much to observe, either through one's own senses, or from the statistics which were readily available, that the countryside was far healthier than the towns and that towns had become hazardous to human health, regions unfit for human habitation. Hector Gavin, one of the most vigorous of early Victorian social investigators and health reformers, was giving utterance to a widely-held view when he commented in 1847 that it was clearly demonstrable that the countryside was much healthier than the town, that some towns were healthier than others, and that within individual towns there was a wide range of healthiness. Gavin did not deny that factors of climate, elevation, and soil were important, but he thought that 'the causes of the high mortality of towns' were basically man-made and so subject to preventive medicine. These causes, he argued,

> are traceable to the density of population, to the want of ventilation, and consequent impurity of the air; to the defective state of paving, drainage, and sewage; to the filthy state of the dwellings of the poor and of their immediate neighbourhood; to the *concentration* of unhealthy and put-rescent emanations from narrow streets, courts and alleys; to the crowded and unhealthy state of workshops and to the injurious occupations which are carried on in them.[10]

Gavin's concentration upon the poor was certainly justified, for while the more comfortable classes often lived, as the example of the Royal Family suggests, in far from sanitary surroundings, their general standards of nutrition, living conditions, ability to isolate ill children, healthier occupations and working conditions generally guaranteed them greater longevity and some protection from the epidemics which were the scourge of the poor. Early Victorian reformers stressed the remarkable gulf in life expectancy between various classes. The following, extracted from a considerably longer table in the *Lancet* is representative of a comparative statistical technique which was almost a cliché of early Victorian sanitary reform and which was designed to play upon respectable Victorians' feelings of guilt and fear and suggest that much death was preventable:

Longevity of families belonging to various classes: average age at death

District	Gentry & Professional	Farmers & Tradesmen	Labourers & Artisans
Rutland	52	41	38
Bath	55	37	25
Leeds	44	27	19
Bethnal Green	45	26	16
Manchester	38	20	17
Liverpool	35	22	15

[11]

The dramatic impact of such statistics – and the Victorians were bombarded with them – is obvious. That a labouring man's family,

living in Liverpool, could on average expect to have less than one-third
the life-span of that of a professional family in Bath or even in Bethnal
Green in London's East End, was shameful and outrageous. Although
the statistics were inaccurate and misleading (they did not take into
account the age-structure of the various classes or the age-structure of
the migration flows from country to town), it was a marvellously
effective reform technique. And although the differences were exaggerated by the crude statistics, the fact remains that there was, indeed,
a difference in life expectancy between town and country and between
rich and poor.[12]

Dr Buchanan, a prominent medical officer, was fundamentally correct in reminding his fellow medical officers that it was essential for
them to study the condition of the working classes since 'these are the
persons among whom disease is chiefly engendered and perpetuated.'[13] Of that there can be little doubt, and serves I hope as sufficient
justification for my emphasis upon the working-class family in this
book. Sanitary reforms were often initiated by the more comfortable
classes to improve the comfort and value of their own houses or
districts. But the rich knew that if they neglected the poor it would be
at their own peril, for, as Dickens put it, it was certain that 'the air
from Gin Lane will be carried, when the wind is Easterly, into May
Fair', and, he added, 'if you once have a vigorous pestilence raging
furiously in Saint Giles's, no mortal list of Lady Patronesses can keep it
out of Almack's.'[14] Civic duty and social concern coincided, as is often
the case with reform, with self-interest.

One other general theme needs mentioning at the outset. For the
Victorians, public health, like so many other social reforms and
endeavours, took on the form of a moral crusade. To most Victorians,
epidemics were not scourges sent by God to punish man for his sins but
were the consequences of man's sinful neglect of God's earth and of
His injunction to care for the sick and the weak. Sanitary reform,
health care, visiting the poor, slum clearance, education of the poor in
matters of health and hygiene, were all vital causes for a people
inspired by both the evangelical concept of duty and, increasingly, a
new secular concern for the well-ordering of society. Whether the
inspiration was religious or secular, whether it stemmed from a sense
of shame or altruistic duty, from self-interest or fear of the ravages of
epidemics, the most widely held of Victorian social doctrines was that
physical well-being and a pure environment were the essential foundations for all other areas of social progress. In short there could be no
moral, religious, or intellectual improvement without physical

improvement. This essentially environmentalist concept is apparent in the early public health movement and thus pre-dates Darwin, but it gathered strength enormously after Darwin, with his emphasis upon adaptation and survival, had encouraged men to look even more closely at their physical environment.

Public health thus became a kind of *fundamental* reform, an underpinning and *sine qua non* for all other reforms. Chadwick was simply voicing a common attitude of mind when he commented 'how much of rebellion, of moral depravity and of crime has its root in physical disorder and depravity ... The fever nests and seats of physical depravity are also the seats of moral depravity, disorder, and crime with which the police have the most to do.'[15] If the diagnosis was that immorality was rooted in physical impurity then the remedy, the preventive medicine, called for the abolition of evil through abolition of dirt and disease. It was a challenge which could not fail to strike a chord in the bosom of Victorian evangelical Christianity. To Charles Kingsley, who encouraged men and especially women to equate cleanliness with godliness, the formula for social progress was obvious. The social state of a city depended on its moral state and 'the moral state of a city depends ... on the physical state of the city; on the food, water, air and lodgings of the inhabitants.'[16] The leading evangelical layman, Lord Shaftesbury, never tired of presenting this environmentalist and materialist social philosophy:

> It is to no purpose to send out the schoolmaster, it is to no purpose to employ the missionary, it is to no purpose to preach from the pulpit, it is to little or no purpose to visit from house to house and carry with you the precepts and the lessons of the Gospel, so long as you leave the people in this squalid, obscene, filthy, disgusting, and overcrowded state.[17]

When clergymen with some experience in the slums took the same view it carried special weight. Thus Robert Bickersteth declared in disgust:

> There are tens of thousands in this metropolis *whose physical condition is a positive bar to the practice of morality*. Talk of morality amongst people who herd – men, women, and children – together with no regard to age or sex, in one narrow confined apartment! You might as well talk of cleanliness in a sty, or of limpid purity in the contents of a cesspool.[18]

Still something of a controversial statement in the eyes of churchmen when Bickersteth made it in 1855, it had become an orthodoxy by the 1880s.

To those who made it their personal duty to go down into the slums it was simply absurd to expect any lasting good to come from any measure of social reform until the domestic environment had been greatly improved. Charles Dickens, for example, commented that his experiences

> have strengthened me in the conviction that Searching Sanitary Reform must precede all other social remedies, and that even Education and Religion can do nothing where they are most needed, until the way is paved for their ministrations by Cleanliness and Decency.[19]

Gavin, though a little more nervous about questioning the power of the Good Book to bring forth light even in the darkest places, also confessed that his experience compelled the belief that before a man could become 'a good son, husband, or citizen, I almost dare say, or Christian, his home must be made clean, the impurities by which he is surrounded, removed.'[20] Public health was always more than just a movement for social reform – it took on the intensity of a mission. The enthusiasm with which the Victorians threw themselves into this mission was fed by a sense that they would succeed, and that cleanliness and good health, the forces of Light, would triumph over dirt and disease, the forces of Darkness. Typical of that conviction was John Simon, the greatest of the Victorian medical officers who, throughout his career as a public servant, always stressed that public health was concerned with *preventable* disease. Similarly, far from becoming depressed by the immense amount of poverty and premature death he encountered in the slums, Dr Gavin optimistically and fervently insisted that 'all this death, and all this sickness, with their attendant misery, wretchedness, poverty, pauperism, immorality, and crime, are in our power *wholly* and *entirely* to prevent.'[21] Though they did not minimize the magnitude of the challenge, the early- and mid-Victorian sanitary reformers for the most part did indeed think that good health was wholly in their power to achieve.

Not until attention swung away from public to more private, domestic aspects of health, from sewers and drains to living conditions and standards of living did the tone of public health reform take on a more cautious or pessimistic note. For it was not until public health administrations, central and local, were established, and experience gained in the field, that the connection between disease and poverty (obvious to many doctors and social investigators from the 1830s on) became a decisive and dominant element in the public health movement. Public health was never totally removed from broader questions of social engineering and general living standards. But for much of the century the enthusiasm and dedication of public health reformers enabled them to throw themselves into the tasks before them without stopping to ask broader social questions. By the 1880s it was no longer possible to ignore these questions.

As the century drew to a close it was quite clear to nose and eye, and also demonstrable statistically, that the Victorians had made progress against epidemic diseases. In the great year of the Diamond Jubilee, 1897, the official journal of the medical officers of health could rejoice:

> Of all the achievements of the Victorian Era . . . history will find none worthier of record than the efforts made to ameliorate the lives of the poor, to curb the ravages of disease, and to secure for all pure air, food, and water, all of which are connotated by the term 'sanitation'.[22]

It is time now to turn to their efforts and to see to what extent this self-congratulatory estimate is justified.

2

The Massacre of the Innocents

'Grandmother, Grandmother
Tell me the Truth
How many years am I
Going to Live?
One, Two, Three, Four . . . .'

Victorian street game

'The death-rate among infants was the most sensitive hygienic barometer . . . .'

Lyon Playfair, President of the Health Section of the Social Science Association, 1874

'As the twig is bent so grows the tree' is a saying which is particularly relevant to public health, for child-rearing practices and childhood illnesses, and indeed childbirth itself often left their mark upon adults. No nation can hope to be truly healthy unless it nurtures healthy children. Those Victorians – and they were many – who crudely applied Darwin's theory of the survival of the fittest took comfort in the argument that the high mortality rate among infants killed off the weak and so created a nation of the strong. But in reality many who survived the numerous physical hazards of infancy did so in a sickly and weakened form and far from strengthening the nation fell into the ranks of the unemployables and became a burden on the poor rates or eventually succumbed, as a result of their weakened resistance, to illness or death.

This chapter then, is literally the foundation for much that follows. It is appropriate for another reason to start this book with the 'mewling and puking' infant. Public health is concerned with the connection between environmental (both domestic and public) and social factors and health, and Victorian health officials and modern authorities agree that the infant mortality rate[1] is a highly sensitive gauge of this connection and reflects the impact of general living conditions upon the health of the community.[2]

One of the most frustrating and seemingly paradoxical facts confronting Victorians was that while the general death rate declined from an average of 22.2 deaths per thousand living during the decade 1851–1860 to 18.2 in the decade 1891–1900, the infant death rate remained constant, at around 153.[3] The infant death rate was actually higher in the last few years of Victoria's reign than at the beginning and still accounted for fully one-quarter of all the deaths in the nation.[4] In 1904 a government committee of inquiry sadly concluded that 'in the volume of vital statistics, from which so many consolatory reflections are drawn, infant mortality remains a dark page.'[5] Statistics are cold things. What does it mean to say that among children under one year of age there were some 153 deaths for every thousand live births? Today in England the figure is under sixteen. Had the mid-Victorian infant death rate been the same as that immediately after the Second World War some 120,000 fewer babies would have died each year, or roughly 2500 fewer infant deaths every week.[6] Every year well over 100,000 infants died before their first birthday in England. In London, as late as the 1890s, 20,000 infants under one died each year. Most large industrial towns had, to use John Simon's memorable phrase, 'Herodian districts' where the infant death rate was well over 200. Birmingham, Blackburn, Leicester, Liverpool, London, Manchester, Preston, and Salford were among the towns which had large central districts where the infant death rate was 220 or higher in the last decade of the century.[7]

As appalling as these statistics are, they in fact under-represent the true picture. Civil registration of births and deaths commenced in 1837, but it was not until 1874 (1855 in Scotland) that they were made compulsory. William Farr at the Registrar-General's Office estimated that perhaps as many as 40,000 still-births went unrecorded every year in England and Wales and in 1904 the Inter-Departmental Committee on Physical Deterioration was still lamenting the fact that still-births were not being recorded.[8] The statistics for infant mortality in the last quarter of the century are probably more accurate than in the earlier period and that would account, in small measure, for the continued high infant mortality figures. But on the other hand, in the last quarter of the century, illegitimate births constituted a smaller percentage of total births, and since the illegitimate infant death rate was always considerably higher than the legitimate one, there should have been some corresponding decline in the total infant death rate.[9]

One ready explanation for the persistently high infant mortality rates offers itself. As the century progressed, more and more children – and certainly a higher percentage of the total number of children in the nation – were being born in towns. In the early 1890s, when the infant death rate for England and Wales as a whole was around 153, the twenty-eight largest towns had an average infant death rate of 167 and mining towns were almost twice as lethal for infants as completely rural areas.[10] In 1891 the Registrar-General's Office studied 100,000 children born in the three rural counties of Hertfordshire, Wiltshire, and Dorset and 100,000 children born in what were, admittedly, three of the worst towns in England, Blackburn, Leicester, and Preston. Of the former group 90,082 reached their first birthday; of the second, only 78,197.[11] As the century wore on and as the populations of the major towns depended less on migration from the countryside and more on self-generating growth, the fact that a higher percentage of the nation's babies were conceived and carried by mothers who had spent most or all of their lives in the less healthy atmosphere of the towns may also partly explain why infant mortality did not decline together with the general mortality rates.

Certainly the health of the mother was an enormously important influence on the health of the infant and its chances of survival. A great gulf existed between Victorian ideals of 'motherhood' and the working-class reality: thousands of babies were born annually to mothers who were underweight and undernourished, who had contracted pelvises, who worked too hard and perhaps too late during the pregnancy, and who received no sound advice, either from health societies, or from any supporting network of women, about pre- and ante-natal care.

Few working-class women received the extra nutrition which modern authorities have found desirable for pregnant and lactating women. When, as was often the case in a society where seasonal unemployment and under-employment prevailed, there was not enough food to go around, it was the women who got the least. Even in good times it was customary for the men to get the meat and much larger portions in general and the mothers and daughters made do with bread, weak tea, and scraps – a custom which continued well into this century.[12]

Recent studies show that low nutritional standards increase the risk of premature births (which were, as we shall see shortly, one of the principal causes of infant mortality), or make childbirth hazardous. In Maryland, in the United States, a study of women who subsisted on a diet deficient in milk, butter, eggs, green vegetables, and fruit – on a diet, that is, remarkably similar in its omission of vital foodstuffs to that of the Victorian urban working classes – has revealed that seventy per cent of the women were seriously anaemic and that many had contracted pelvises. Similarly, the nutritional inadequacies of the

Victorian working-class diet often led to rickets which could cause contracted pelvises, making childbirth difficult.[13] In Aberdeen in the 1940s it was discovered that the fetal mortality rate of underweight and small (5′ 1″ and under) women was twice that of women over 5′ 4″, and that short women had more still-births and underweight babies. In this connection it becomes extremely significant that anthropometric studies done in the Edwardian period indicated that working-class women were seriously underweight and small in stature. In Manchester just before the First World War thirteen-year-old girls from working-class families were three inches shorter and eight pounds lighter than girls of a 'good class'; they stood seven inches shorter and weighed twenty-three pounds less than girls of a similar age living in the 1950s.[14] Recent studies also indicate that in poor families where the diet is inadequate there is a much greater possibility of premature birth and also of infant deaths after the second or third baby than in families of higher income. The World Health Organization has discovered that 'malnutrition and severe anaemia adversely influence the course and outcome of pregnancy, affect fetal growth and birth weight and hence contribute significantly to perinatal mortality', and that 'a rapid succession of pregnancies may aggravate a pre-existing nutritional anaemia, resulting in infants of low birth weight with early iron deficiency.'[15] Given the large families of the Victorian working classes the connection between diet, general physique, and infant mortality becomes critical.

As with so many other aspects of public health a single factor – poor nutrition or small maternal stature – taken in isolation may not appear to be terribly significant. But when poor nutrition was added to other aspects of working-class lives, arduous labour, damp, cold, and overcrowded dwellings, inadequate sanitary conditions, it could mean the difference between life and death for the mother. In the second half of the nineteenth century maternal deaths in childbirth averaged between four and five for every thousand births. In his early years at the Registrar-General's Office, William Farr recorded over 3,000 deaths of mothers every year: in the last year of Victoria's reign 4,400 mothers died in childbirth.[16] The two principal causes of the continued high maternal death rate, puerperal fever (a streptococcal infection of the uterus immediately after birth) and what were reported and recorded as 'accidents in childbirth' belong more to medical history than to a study of public health. Both, however, indicate generally poor domestic standards of hygiene and low standards of obstetrics and midwifery. Despite the publication in 1843 of

Oliver Wendell Holmes's great plea for cleanliness in childbirth, Semmelweiss's successful demonstration, in 1855, of the importance of cleanliness in combating puerperal fever, and the great work of Pasteur, Lister and Koch, the use of antiseptics by doctors and midwives tended to remain the exception rather than the rule right down until the end of the century. According to Dr W. S. Playfair, Consultant to the General Lying-In Hospital, not one medical man in a hundred in private practice used antiseptics in a systematic manner.[17]

As for childbirth practices, the great wonder is that so many babies survived.[18] The vast majority of deliveries were by midwives, the vast majority of whom in turn were untrained. In 1870 the proportion of deliveries by a midwife to total births varied from between five and ten per cent in small, non-manufacturing towns to over 90 per cent in rural districts and large industrial towns. In Leeds, Sheffield, and Birmingham over half the babies were delivered by midwives, in Glasgow over three-quarters, in Coventry about 90 per cent. Generally the more poverty the more widespread the use of midwives. In the East End of London in the 1870s over half the babies were delivered by midwives, in Wimbledon only five per cent, and in the fashionable West End only two per cent.[19] In the second half of the century at least 70 per cent of all babies were delivered by midwives without any additional assistance from doctors, and it has been estimated that perhaps as many as 90 per cent of all the babies of the poor were delivered by midwives.[20] In 1870 the Registrar-General, analyzing a report from the Obstetrical Society of London, concluded that it was generally assumed that 'midwives were born, not made; their professional training was wholly neglected, or left to chance' and that throughout England midwives suffered not only from 'a want of any special education, but gross ignorance and incompetence, and a complete inability to contend with any difficulty that may occur.'[21] A British Medical Association Committee sourly commented in 1873 that 'in general midwives commenced their business on no more experience than that of having attended one or two labours.'[22] Although there was some improvement towards the end of the century, the majority of babies were still being brought into the world by midwives lacking any formal education and ill-equipped either to diagnose or handle any trouble. Few midwives were as fortunate as Mrs Layton, who, practising as a 'maternity nurse' in Cricklewood, found local doctors who were willing to show her how to deliver with forceps and to take her to a post-mortem of a pregnant woman.[23] As late as 1914 in Wigan, of the 57 midwives in the town, only 23 had any

14

training. Between them the midwives delivered approximately 87 per cent of the babies born in Wigan.[24] At the turn of the century the Local Government Board estimated that roughly two-thirds of the 12,251 midwives in the nation were still totally untrained. Little wonder then that so many infant deaths were recorded as 'still births', or simply 'accidental' deaths or 'deaths in childbirth'.[25]

Both doctors, fearful that highly-qualified midwives might rob them of income and prestige and, rather ironically, feminists who feared that a system of qualifying examinations would rob women, especially widows and deserted wives, of one of the few occupations open to them, opposed examinations and registration for midwives. Despite the advocacy of such a system by Farr and James Stansfeld, President of the Local Government Board, and despite the work of the Female Medical Society in establishing education for midwives, it was not until 1902 that a system of registration was first introduced.[26]

Clearly one cannot make a precise correlation between infant deaths and midwifery, and I do not want to be misunderstood – I am not condemning home births or midwifery in general. When the midwives are qualified, trained to recognize or anticipate irregularities and prepared to call in a doctor immediately, and when they can operate in an hygienic domestic environment, there is a great deal to be said, both from a purely medical and a psychological viewpoint, for home deliveries. But neither the vast majority of midwives nor the homes of the poor met these criteria at any time during the nineteenth century. Probably the majority of doctors delivering babies were not greatly superior in knowledge, nor perhaps even in cleanliness, to experienced midwives, and certainly hospital conditions could be far from sanitary. But the fact remains that while the alternatives might not have been vastly better, the actual practices of the day often meant that the infant was brought into the world by unskilled hands working in dirty and germ-laden surroundings.[27]

If the baby were healthy and the delivery completely uncomplicated then perhaps much of what has been discussed over the past few pages would not be terribly relevant to the analysis of infant mortality. But in the nineteenth century a large number of babies were sickly from birth. Although the registration of infant deaths was far from accurate and coroners were generally unskilled and casual when it came to defining the cause of perinatal deaths (from twenty-eight weeks of gestation to the first week after birth), it is clear that prematurity was a major cause of infant mortality – indeed, perhaps the single most important cause throughout the century.[28]

A modern medical text stresses that 'a premature infant is ill-equipped to deal with any infection, so that respiratory, gastro-intestinal, umbilical and other infections which might not be serious in a mature infant may prove fatal in a premature one', and, it continues, even if the premature baby survives these dangers, 'it still has to face special difficulties of nutrition.'[29] The growth rate of premature babies (especially males) was slow and uncertain and no doubt many of the neo-natal deaths registered as 'fatal convulsions', 'nine-day fits', 'atrophy', or 'debility' were due to prematurity.[30] The causes for about half the babies born prematurely today are unknown, but bad maternal diet is certainly important and recent studies have suggested that a low maternal age, low maternal weight, low social class, and a previous history of low-weight, full-term births increase the risks of prematurity.[31] All these factors may be included as characteristics of a 'culture of poverty': they all existed among the Victorian masses. We have noted that many Victorian working-class mothers were under-nourished and under-weight: a modern study of almost 17,000 births in England, Scotland, and Wales has shown that women who weighed less than eight stone had a premature birth rate some three times higher than women who weighed over nine stone.[32]

Here, then, was a major cause of infant mortality and perinatal deaths, a cause which was rooted in the mother's physique. George Newman, one of the great late-Victorian authorities on preventive medicine, in a survey he undertook at the turn of the century of mothers whose babies died in their first year, claimed that 39 per cent had poor physiques or a history of ill-health, and that 44 per cent had had a previous history of miscarriages, abortion, or premature birth. Newman was tempted to sympathize with the goals of the eugenicists who wanted controls on 'unfit' parents, and he concluded that 'infant mortality is a social problem concerning maternity'.[33] A similar study by a member of the City of Westminster Health Society in 1907 of some 1,237 families revealed the infant death rate of babies born to mothers in 'delicate' health to be almost three times that of babies born to 'strong' mothers. For infant deaths during the first month it was some five and a half times higher.[34]

II

At this stage one might well ask what, if anything, could have been done by health officials to help reduce infant mortality from the causes so far discussed. Victorian literature is full of descriptions of the frail and worn-out bodies of working-class women, and the MOH could hardly have been unaware of their under-nourished physiques. Why, then, did they not raise the issue? Perhaps they were caught up in the *laissez-faire* credo and hoped that free trade would continue to lower food prices and that, consequently, higher real wages would result in better nutrition. Certainly they knew full well that interference in the way the family chose to divide up its food among its members was well outside the accepted sphere of government activity. It is true that when, in the Edwardian period, it was discovered that there was widespread malnutrition among school-children, the government moved quickly to establish a system of subsidized school-meals. But the diet of mothers and girls was a far more private, domestic matter than that of school-children, and, as we shall shortly see, Parliament had a horror of interfering with the sanctity of the family.

Victorian MOH did give vent occasionally to their frustration and complain that the problems they were called upon to handle stemmed from broader social ills (see Chapter 7), but for the most part they realized that they would only antagonize their local authorities if they questioned the distribution of wealth and extent of poverty in society, or suggested remedies which would require state or local subsidies to the poor. The connection between healthy mothers and healthy babies can be tenuous and doubtless the thought of trying to raise the standard of nutrition of an entire nation of mothers was a deterrent to any discussion, but it is perhaps strange that the Privy Council and later the Local Government Board (the two principal government agencies for public health) were willing to examine the connection between working mothers and infant mortality but were unwilling to conduct a similar survey in the nineteenth century of the connection between unhealthy or impoverished mothers and prematurity, still-births, and perinatal deaths. In this regard public health officials were hardly more backward than the medical profession in general. The standard text, W. S. Playfair's *Science and Practice of Midwifery* (1898), made no mention whatsoever of ante-natal examinations, and ante-natal diet and care were not taught to medical students.[35] While motherhood was praised endlessly in the abstract and the Victorians developed what amounted to a cult of motherhood, it must be said that in practice motherhood and the nutritional standards and physiques of mothers failed to excite the interest or compassionate concern of either the government or of the medical profession as a whole. In that sense the Victorians may be criticized for failing to trace infant mortality back to its source – the mother.

Among the many causes of infant mortality beyond the immediate control of public health authorities perhaps the most important was the attitude of parents towards infant diseases. Reluctance to incur medical costs, fear and awe of the doctors' often overbearing and condescending manner, distrust of doctors, reliance on traditional folk medicines and home remedies, and a certain fatalism, all combined to make the poor unwilling to call in the doctor to attend infant maladies. 'It is quite common for women to defer sending for medical aid, when the children are ill', wrote one observer in Sheffield, 'until it is too late. They do this quite consciously, and say to the doctor, "Little un's very bad; you can't do no good, but we want you to see un in case aught should happen, so as you may give us a paper".'[36] Even the most ardent of reformers often regarded infant deaths as inevitable: young infants, in Farr's view, were 'feeble; they are unfinished; the molecules and fibres of brain, muscle, bone are loosely strung together; the heart and the blood, on which life depends, have undergone a complete revolution; the lungs are only just called into play. The baby is helpless. . . . It is not surprising that a certain number of infants should die.'[37] If medical men and health reformers felt this way, small wonder that the poor, with evidence of the 'inevitability' of infant death all around them, were often resigned to their children's fate. It was the 'culpable indifference' and 'gross ignorance' of parents which, according to one leading MOH, helped to spread whooping cough and measles. When medical officers discussed measles with parents they found that parents generally had a common philosophy – 'childers like to 'ave it', 'it's a sickness as come to 'em natural like', 'they all 'as to 'ave it', 'sickness will come, its no use goin' agen it'.[38] The MOH for Sunderland told the Sanitary Institute in 1882 that he commonly encountered among the poor the attitude that 'children must die – you can't prevent them'. Mothers took their children with them when visiting a neighbouring house where there was infectious disease, and they often placed healthy children in bed with sick siblings so that they could get the nursing over and done with all at once. Ignorance, necessity (lack of separate bedrooms and even beds), or fatalism, or a combination of these, made the poor resistant to doctors' pleas to isolate the sick children from the healthy.[39]

These attitudes of mind and habits died hard. So did the reliance upon folk medicine and traditional remedies. In East Anglia a common remedy for whooping cough was to give the sick child a fried mouse to eat.[40] At the end of the century a medical officer encountered a typical folk remedy when he asked a mother why her son, suffering from whooping cough, was allowed to play in the gutter. 'I let him play in the gutter', the mother replied, 'because they say as how the dirt draws out the whooping cough.'[41] Throughout Britain, and right down until the end of the century, parents would seek out the owners of donkeys (which were believed to have miraculous powers from their association with Christ) and would pay to have their ill children walk seven times around the donkey, or go through other mystical practices – 'proprietors of donkeys, who worked the fairs and beaches during the summer, travelled the whooping cough circuits through the winter.'[42]

The medical profession, given its inability to prevent or cure many diseases (see Chapter 5), should have understood the appeal of these folk practices. But it could, of course, hardly condone them, and they served to reinforce the impression that the poor were superstitious and primitive. In other ways the doctors thought that the working classes had a disregard for the health of their offspring that amounted to criminal negligence. Just as doctors criticized the wealthier classes for keeping their babies in over-heated rooms and swaddled in too much clothing or bedding, so they roundly condemned the working classes for needlessly exposing their babies to the cold. Life in the slums was, perforce, lived in the streets and courtyards, and Victorian photographs and illustrations in the graphic journals suggest that working-class mothers spent time gossiping at their doors, with ill-clad babies in their arms. As with so many aspects of working-class life, there was a gulf between what was considered ideal by the upper and middle classes and the realities of working-class domestic existence. If the babies were ill-clad that was due as much to the mother's poverty as to her neglect, and if the baby was exposed to the cold air and winds of the slum courtyard it was not the indifference of the mother to her baby's health so much as her desire to get out of the damp and often foetid atmosphere of the slum dwelling or the belief that the brisk air was healthy for the baby. One medical officer remonstrated with some mothers for gossiping in the cold with their 'bawns' in their arms; he was indignantly told that 'it makes the child hardy.'[43]

Doctors considered that 60° was a healthy domestic temperature for babies.[44] No doubt the poor would have loved to heat their flats to this temperature, but fuel was very expensive. Writing in 1893 the MOH for Birmingham held that exposure to the cold was 'a prolific cause of infantile mortality'.[45] In 1903 some 27,000 infants died of pneumonia, bronchitis, and other lung ailments, accounting for 22 per cent of all infant deaths.[46] Even today, infant death rates in England are higher in the winter months and death rates from respiratory illnesses linked to the cold are twice as high among infants from the poorest homes as among infants belonging to families from the upper two social classes.[47] In the nineteenth century, when perhaps one-third of the population of major industrial towns was living in poverty, hypothermia and respiratory ailments took their toll over the winter months. Once again, apart from offering advice and admonitions, there was very little that public health officials could do about this cause of infant mortality.

Given the strained budgets and traditional eating habits of the poor, the same applies to yet another cause of infant deaths – feeding of infants. A vicious circle was established where undernourishment weakened the child's resistance to infection and infectious disease often resulted in a weakened digestive system, leading to further malnutrition at a time when protein was being destroyed during the illness.[48] The World Health Organization concluded some years ago that a high infant mortality rate can in part 'be attributed to the synergism between malnutrition and infectious diseases' and that malnutrition in infants lowered their resistance to tuberculosis, measles, acute diarrhoeal diseases, typhus, and whooping cough.[49] In Victorian Britain, as in much of the Third World today, poverty was the hand-maiden of infection and lay behind much of the infant mortality of the age.

When one reads what working-class babies were fed the wonder is that so many survived. Liebig's baby food was introduced in 1867, followed by Allenbury's, Nestlé's, Berger's, and other brands, but these were too expensive for the very poor, and as soon as the baby was taken off the breast it was fed the most indigestible mixtures imaginable.[50] The most popular weaning food was a mixture of arrowroot, oatmeal, sago, corn flour and baked flour, but it was a common practice to feed the baby on 'whatever was going'.[51] By the end of its first year the baby was getting a taste of whatever its parents ate – beer, cheese, onions, heavy breads.[52] As late as 1904 the government learned that it was still a common practice to feed young infants off the parents' plates – 'They live as we do.' The unbalanced and indigestible food forced into the baby's mouth often resulted in deaths by 'projectile vomiting' and 'convulsions': more generally it led to serious malnutrition.[53]

A far greater cause of infant mortality was the alternatives to breast-milk which were widely used. From the 1860s onwards medical men thought that too many women who could nurse were turning to bottle-feeding and that bottle-feeding killed babies.[54] That artificial feeding could be very harmful in the nineteenth century there can be little doubt. Even today, when the artificial milk is generally nutritional and pure, the World Health Organization, War on Want, and other organizations opposed to artificial feeding in the Third World, have found that there simply is no satisfactory and healthy substitute for mother's milk when certain conditions prevail. And all these conditions – general ignorance about personal hygiene, inadequate domestic sanitary facilities, and poverty – existed among the Victorian poor.

Mother's milk provides the infant with immunity to microorganisms to which the mother has already been exposed and which the infant is likely to encounter, and modern research has shown that 'feeding infants with human milk reduces the incidence of gastrointestinal infections', infections which, as we shall shortly see, were a major cause of infant mortality throughout the nineteenth century.[55] Cow's milk, on the other hand, was perhaps the most widely adulterated food in Victorian Britain. In 1877 a quarter of all the milk examined by the Local Government Board was seriously adulterated; in 1882 one-fifth of the 20,000 milk analyses made by the 52 county and 172 borough analysts was adulterated. Not until 1894 was the Local Government Board able to report that adulterated milk accounted for less than ten per cent of all samples.[56] Until very late in the century, with the increased use of milk trains, most of the milk consumed in large cities came from cows kept in stalls right in the town.[57] Medical officers of health were empowered by a variety of acts to inspect cowsheds, but they had inadequate staffs and it was easy for owners to evade the vague sanitary requirements. Thus the Inter-Departmental Committee on Physical Deterioration was told in 1904 that in urban cowsheds:

> the cows are in the most filthy condition, standing in manure, and the cowsheds, the stalls, are covered with manure, and outside the yards are heaped up with it. There is no proper ventilation, the milkers are filthy, their hands and clothes are dirty, and their vessels very often are dirty.[58]

It was common practice for milk churns to be left uncovered and exposed to the flies from the stables.[59] At the beginning of the century in Lambeth the local MOH reported that almost three-quarters of the milk vendors failed to keep their milk covered and over half the milk shops had one or more sanitary defects. In addition, the milk was often three or four days old before it reached the consumers. In Finsbury, in

1903, 32 per cent of the milk contained pus and 40 per cent dirt. As if these general conditions were not bad enough, it was estimated in 1901 that ten per cent of all milk cows produced tubercular milk.[60]

Given the atrociously low standard of cheap milk it is perhaps just as well that the working classes did not drink much of it; but they did buy it for their infants, and ignorance and poverty led to further adulteration with water and so the milk's nutritional value was even lower by the time it reached the baby. The most widely used substitute for cow's milk among the poor was condensed milk, which was cheap. In the early part of the present century nearly half of the working-class families in Finsbury depended solely on condensed milk for their milk supply. Yet it was lacking in essential nutrients, especially fat and vitamins A and D; although the *Lancet* questioned the nutritional value of tinned milk much earlier, it was not until 1894 that it became compulsory for manufacturers to put a label on the tin stating that the contents were unsuitable for infants.[61]

Even if cow's milk and condensed milk had been more nutritional and pure than they were, they would still have been harmful to infants, for by the time the baby actually drank the milk it could have sat around for hours, or even days, in unhygienic containers. Health authorities might advise mothers not to use opened tins of condensed milk over several days, but budgetary constraints dictated otherwise. As for cow's milk, it was often a lethal potion as served to the baby. India-rubber teats had begun to replace teats made of softened parchment or wash-leather in the mid-1850s, but the poor classes could not afford them and so old rags or cloths continued to be used. As these became warm and wet they served as a perfect nexus for germs.[62] Old ginger-beer bottles and other containers were pressed into use and since the homes of the poor, even in the final quarter of the century, generally lacked running water, inevitably the bottles were not washed as frequently as they should have been, or were washed in water that had already been used for other purposes.[63]

When Victorian doctors condemned artificial feeding, with its unhealthy dilution of milk with water and its bottles of questionable cleanliness, they were unaware of the special benefits conferred by mother's milk and were basing their criticism, just like those who criticize artificial feeding in the Third World today, upon the connection between unhealthy and unnourishing milk and gastro-intestinal diseases, especially diarrhoea. In the 1880s the Local Government Board undertook an extensive examination of diarrhoea throughout England and concluded that it was among the most fatal of infant ailments.[64] Diarrhoea, or 'English cholera', 'cholera nostras', or 'infantile cholera', was a gastro-intestinal disease closely linked to insanitary domestic conditions. In Victorian parlance it was a classic 'filth disease'. In the summer months 75 per cent of all deaths from it were of children under one year old, and in 1899 it accounted for approximately a quarter of all infant deaths, and was the single largest cause of infant mortality.[65] Even in the early years of Edward VII's reign, when deaths from diarrhoea declined sharply, it was the second largest killer of infants, accounting in 1903 for over 17,000 deaths of children under one.[66] Just as important as the number of deaths was the distressing and bewildering fact that despite sanitary improvements and a general rise in the standard of living the infant death rate from diarrhoeal diseases sharply *increased* after 1885; just before the century ended it was twice as high as it had been in 1885.[67]

The causes of gastro-intestinal diseases are complex – the baby's general condition and its resistance to disease, dentition, and feeding during the teething period, summer temperatures, excrement removal, and general sanitary conditions are among the factors involved – but to many medical men the major cause was clear, and mothers who bottle-fed their babies, especially those who did so in order to go out to work, were held guilty of virtual infanticide. It is perhaps natural that with infant death rates continuing to run high and deaths from diarrhoeal diseases actually increasing, contemporaries would look for a simple explanation or seek a scapegoat. Considerable prejudice coloured the late Victorian discussion on bottle-feeding, for medical authorities shared the common view that mothers should be true to their natural function – a mother's 'first duty' was in the home.[68]

The bias of doctors must be borne in mind when reading their statistical correlations between bottle-feeding and infant mortality. Evidence of such correlations poured in from all over England. Dr Howarth, MOH for Derby, argued that in his town the death rate in 1903 among bottle-fed babies was almost three times higher than among breast-fed. Even more startling was the difference between breast-fed and bottle-fed babies for deaths from diarrhoea – some six times higher for the latter group. In Finsbury at the same time, Dr Newman discovered from a four-year study he conducted that over half the infant deaths from diarrhoea were of babies who were wholly bottle-fed babies; babies who were wholly breast-fed accounted for only 18.3 per cent of the deaths.[69] In 1900 the journal of the MOH, *Public Health*, bluntly stated that only three per cent of all infant deaths from gastro-enteritis were of breast-fed babies.[70] In Preston the infant death rate among the poor Irish, was lower than among the English because, it was claimed, the Irish women suckled their babies. In Birmingham the MOH pointed out that deaths from diseases of the digestive organs accounted for 41 per cent of all infant deaths but in Norway, where almost all women breast-fed their babies, the corresponding figure was only 12.5 per cent. In Liverpool, the MOH, Dr Hope, produced figures demonstrating that the death rate of babies under three months and wholly or partially bottle-fed was fifteen times that of babies wholly nursed, and memories were revived of the great cotton famine there during the American Civil War, when, despite widespread distress, the infant mortality actually declined when unemployed mothers stayed at home and presumably nursed their infants. In Brighton breast-fed babies constituted only 6.5 per cent of all babies dying from diarrhoea – babies raised on cow's milk accounted for 36 per cent, and babies fed condensed milk accounted for a little over 30 per cent. In Leeds it was claimed that, between the ages of six and nine months, thirty times as many bottle-fed babies died as those wholly nursed.[71]

Local Government Board investigations tended to support these findings. Just before the First World War the Local Government Board carried out an exhaustive survey of infant mortality in Lancashire. Among the towns it examined was Farnworth, which had an infant mortality rate almost twice the national average, and where 98 per cent of the babies surveyed were bottle-fed. While infant deaths in Farnworth from prematurity were approximately the same as for the twenty-four urban areas used for comparative purposes, and from bronchitis and pneumonia actually less, deaths from atrophy, debility, and marasmus (a wasting disease associated with poor nutrition) were twice as numerous and deaths from diarrhoeal diseases were three times as high.[72]

These statistics are very crude and it would be misleading to take them literally. They leave unanswered many essential questions – was the socio-economic status of the families of breast- and bottle-fed babies similar, or did those mothers who bottle-fed their babies belong to poorer families and were they bottle-feeding so that they could go out to work? If so, was it general neglect rather than artificial feeding which was to blame for the high incidence of infant mortality? Were domestic sanitary conditions and diet the same for the two groups? Did those mothers who told medical authorities that they nursed their babies really do so? Were mothers who nursed more aware of health and hygiene in general and so more open to the advice of visiting health officers in a whole range of things that would affect the health of the baby? We simply cannot answer these questions from the evidence given by the local MOH and the Local Government Board.

In one other respect the great differential in mortality between bottle- and breast-fed babies is suspect. Breast-fed babies were, just like bottle-fed ones, given pacifiers or dummies that were nothing short of lethal. In the words of George Newman, the 'comforters'

> are dipped in sugary messes or dirty milk to give them a more palatable taste. They fall on the floor and so collect dust. Flies settle upon them. They are never cleaned except, perhaps, on a dirty apron. They are nearly always moist and warm owing to contact with the child's mouth, and therefore afford an ideal nidus for the multiplication and development of germ life.[73]

Thus even breast-fed babies were exposed to noxious substances from an early age, although the breast-milk doubtless conferred immunities. Similarly, breast-fed babies were also victims of the harmful weaning practices of the age. In the north 'pobs' or 'pobbies', a soggy mixture of bread, water, sugar, perhaps some treacle, and milk, was a commonly used weanling food and was also given to the baby to quieten it whenever it cried from hunger, colic, or indigestion pains.[74] The Privy Council's Medical Department discovered that along the east coast sugar sop, a similar mixture, 'is either given cold, or is left on the fire hob in a cup, seldom or never changed or cleansed, whence the unfermented and sooty mass is heaped into the infant's mouth . . .'[75] In Victorian England, as today in poor countries which have inadequate sanitary facilities, 'weaning diarrhoea' was a major cause of infant mortality.[76]

But, bearing these cautions and caveats in mind, it is clear that there was some connection between the high infant mortality rate from gastro-intestinal diseases and bottle feeding. Certainly late-Victorian medical officers had little doubt that such a connection existed and that it was a cause of mortality that had to be tackled and destroyed before any significant improvement in infant mortality could be accomplished. The question was, since feeding of babies was for the most part such a *domestic* matter what could *public* health officials do about it? Apart from railing against bottle feeding in their various journals many MOH considered that they could be most helpful by attacking what they held to be the underlying cause – the employment of mothers of young babies. The controversy over the effect of working wives on the health of their babies was an acrimonious one. This is not the place to go into all its details, but since so many MOH did devote their energies to the campaign against working wives and thought that by so doing they were combating infant mortality, we must spend some time on it.

As early as 1859 John Simon was attacking female labour; 'The extensive factory employment of female labour is', he wrote to the Privy Council,

> a sure source of very large infantile mortality, both diarrhoeal and convulsive; that where mothers are engaged in factories, infants who should be at the breast are commonly ill-fed or starved, and have their cries of hunger and distress quieted by those various fatal opiates which are in such request at the centre of our manufacturing industry.

It was a view from which Simon never wavered throughout his long career at the centre of state medicine. In his Fourth Annual Report to the Privy Council in 1862 he expressed concern that working mothers were becoming 'to a grievous extent denaturalised towards their offspring', and as late as 1890 he was still arguing

> that in proportion as adult women were taking part in factory labour or agriculture, the mortality of their infants rapidly increased; that in various registration districts which had such employment in them the district death-rate of infants under one year of age has been from two and a quarter to nearly three times as high as in our standard districts; and that in some of the districts more than a few of the infants were dying of ill-treatment which was almost murderous.[77]

Here then was the indictment against the mother — she withheld breast-milk from her baby and left it in the care of baby-minders who neglected or drugged it. More than just an unnatural dereliction of maternal duty, it was positively criminal — the mother, by wilful neglect, had become a murderess, and stood accused of infanticide!

As is commonly the case in emotional debates more heat than light was generated, and many essential questions went unasked. Was it only working wives who bottle-fed their babies? Apparently not, for in Farnworth, where, as we have seen, almost all the babies surveyed were bottle-fed, only half the mothers worked. Was it only working wives who weaned their babies at too early an age, or neglected them? Can we assume that if working mothers had stayed at home they would have nursed their babies? And would they have totally breast-fed them or would they have given them artificial milk as well?[78]

But to many local MOH the connection between working mothers and infant mortality was so blindingly clear that it required no such detailed analysis. Thus the hard-pressed MOH for Blackburn confidently asserted in 1891 that the reason for the high infant mortality in his town 'is not hard to find. It is the necessary consequence of female factory life.' This easy equation was also made by Dr Greenhow, one of Simon's staff at the Privy Council. 'Going into a house in Sheffield', he wrote, 'we saw a haggard infant, and asked what was the matter with it. A woman gave it a glance and said "t' mother works"; a disease with which I was sufficiently familiar, but for which the name was new.'[79] Typical of the arguments presented by the medical world were those of the *Lancet*, which while acknowledging the complexities of the issue seemed predisposed to focus on the mother going out to work as the most important. In October 1875 it called for a thorough official analysis of the question, but two weeks later it could assert: 'in all centres of industry where it is the custom to employ women in manufactories, maternal neglect *of course* ranks high as one of the causes of the waste of infant life.' Yet in the same breath it continued that the death rate was highest where 'the houses are of the worst construction, dirtiest, and most closely packed together – in effect, to bad sanitary conditions is due a large amount of the extra mortality prevailing.'[80]

More cautious medical men were, like the *Lancet*, aware that the causes of infant mortality were complex. Arthur Newsholme, the MOH of the Local Government Board, was still uncertain after years of studying the question how much one could hold working mothers accountable for infant mortality. In 1913 he concluded that many other factors were important: 'poverty, uncleanliness, overcrowding, alcoholic indulgence, and disease are closely inter-related . . .'[81] But even where there was an awareness of other factors there was still a predisposition to condemn the working wife. That is partly because it was held that female employment cut into the labour market for men and created idle husbands and thus did not add to the family income. The Inter-Departmental Committee on Physical Deterioration stated that when wives went out to work it encouraged 'men to loaf while their wives earn the wages, and actually to cut men out of work . . .'[82] According to Dr Vernon, the author of *Why Little Children Die*, a pamphlet put out by the Manchester and Salford Sanitary Association, the issue was clear: 'Fathers should be the bread winners and mothers the nurses and caretakers of their suckling children', and to Lord Shaftesbury the employment of mothers put an end to 'domestic life and domestic discipline . . . Society will consist of individuals no longer grouped into families.' Many female social reformers shared this view. Mrs Ranyard, whose Bible women did so much social good, told the Social Science Association in no uncertain terms that 'the wife or mother going abroad to work is, with few exceptions, a waste of time, a waste of property, a waste of morals, and a waste of health, and life, and ought in every way to be prevented.'[83]

The general indictments received considerable support from numerous statistical surveys. In a much publicised report, Dr Reid, the Staffordshire County MOH, produced figures showing that in the decade 1871–80 the infant death rate in the northern part of his county (where women were engaged in the pottery industry) was 182, while in the southern region (where a few women were employed in the coal and iron industries) the infant death rate was 152. When Reid branched out from his own county to generalize about England as a whole he claimed a direct correlation between the proportion of women employed outside the home and the infant mortality rate.[84] In 1898 *Public Health* published the following table:[85]

Town	Sub-registration to district	Infant death rate 1889–1893	Percentage of married women employed, 1891
Preston	Trinity	266	45.0
Preston	Walton-le-Dale	186	32.7
Liverpool	Dale Street	225	17.7
Liverpool	St. George	200	14.0
Rochdale	Whitworth	177	28.2
Rochdale	Wardleworth	171	26.7
Rochdale	Blatchinworth	133	23.4

When Rochdale is compared with Liverpool it will readily be seen that there is no absolute correlation between the proportion of women employed and infant mortality and that it would be absurd to argue that in *all* cases where many married women were employed a high infant mortality rate *automatically* results. Sunderland, for example, had only 6.5 per cent of its married women employed, yet had an infant death rate of 223 (1889–93). In the exhaustive study undertaken by the Local Government Board in 1913 it was discovered that infant mortality was higher in mining families, where the mother was not employed (160) than in families in textile operatives where she was (148).[86] The author of this study, Dr Newsholme, rightly concluded:

> The inference from this comparison is not that the industrial employment of married women is without effect on child life, but rather that

other detrimental influences of greater gravity in their total effect prevail to a greater extent in the centres of mining industry than in the
textile centres.[87]

Newsholme went on to explore these 'other detrimental influences',
and in a comparison, rare in its close and cautious analysis, between two
cotton towns, just a few miles apart, Burnley and Nelson, showed that
these influences could be crucial. Burnley (population of 106,000) and
Nelson (40,000) had a similar proportion of married women working
in the mills (45.8 per cent and 39.4 per cent of all married women,
respectively). Both towns were relatively free from poverty, and Burnley was only slightly dirtier and more backward in its sanitary
arrangements. Yet Burnley had an infant death rate of 210 while
Nelson's was only 77. Newsholme concluded that 'the influences
appearing to be influential in keeping down the infant mortality in
Nelson are its wide area, its high altitude and slope, its heavy rainfall,
and consequently low temperature.' Perhaps just as important, Nelson's female work force was composed of many immigrants from the
Keighley area, girls who were apparently very healthy and who
breast-fed their babies.[88]

To arrive at a definite conclusion one needs more information than
is available. Was it the practice in Nelson to go home to breast-feed the
babies at lunch time? Did daughters, grandmothers, or baby-minders
bring the babies to the mills to be nursed by their mothers? Were
feeding customs the same in both towns? Were wet-nurses employed?
Were the milk supplies of equal quality? We really have little way of
knowing if Burnley, with all its disadvantages, would in fact have had
a lower rate of infant mortality even if fewer wives had worked. In
other words, Nelson, with its natural advantages, could afford working mothers, but Burnley, less favourably situated, could not.

It is clear that while working wives (and hence bottle feeding) *may*
have been a contributing factor to infant deaths from diarrhoeal
diseases, inefficient excrement removal *certainly* was. Towns with
exceptionally high infant mortality rates, such as Farnworth, Wigan,
and Leicester, had rudimentary forms of excrement removal which, as
we shall see in Chapter 4, encouraged the contamination of food both
by soiled hands and by flies. This in turn encouraged diarrhoea.[89]
Unfortunately, the agitation over infant mortality in the 1890s, rather
than focusing on the connection between bottle feeding and sanitation, focused more on that between bottle feeding and factory employment of women, and pressure built up to ban women in their late
pregnancy and right after childbirth from working. In fact mothers did

not generally rush back to work after the baby was born. Dr Holt, the MOH for Burnley, discovered that only 56 per cent of the mothers returned to work in the first six months and this suggested that, whatever the economic pressures, many working-class mothers were determined to give their babies a good start in life.[90] Similarly it would seem that mill and factory women generally left work well before childbirth. Dr Holt found that, of 878 working mothers, only 30 worked up to the week before their confinement and only another 64 worked in the last month before the delivery. Two hundred and eighty five mothers left at least four months before the confinement, and the rest left between one and four months before.[91]

This interest in the mother's work before and after childbirth was motivated more by an interest in the welfare of the baby than in that of the mother. Throughout the nineteenth century there was no careful analysis of the effect of long hours, a damp and unventilated atmosphere, often physically exhausting work, and long walks to and from the mills, upon the physiques of the expectant mother, or of the relationship between hard industrial work and prematurity or still-births. Throughout Britain there must have been many mothers like Mrs Wrigley who, as soon as she realized that she was pregnant, took in more home work and exhausted herself sewing to put aside a little money for the baby. The effects of hard domestic labour and of work in sweatshops and factories right through pregnancy did not, unfortunately, excite the curiosity of health officials until the very end of the century. Not until 1915 did the Local Government Board relate maternal deaths to factory employment prior to confinement when it pointed out that, of the six towns with the highest maternal death rates, all but Merthyr Tydfil were textile towns where large numbers of women were employed.[92]

Part of the indictment against working mothers was that their infants suffered greatly at the hands of the baby-minders with whom they were entrusted. The abuses of baby farming had become a national scandal during the trial and subsequent hanging of Mrs Walters, a baby farmer, for the murder of her charges, in 1870. But the Better Protection of Infant Life Act of 1872 left untouched the day-nurseries where mothers working in factories and mills placed their children.[93] It was argued that the baby-minders gave their charges opiates and skimped on food and milk and that the very fact that mothers took their babies to the nurseries in the early morning cold (most mills began at 6.30 or 7.00 am) was in itself harmful to the infants, especially those who were ailing.[94]

One might imagine that here was a legitimate area for government intervention, but nothing was done, partly because (as in the controversy over the registration of midwives) it was held that the regulation and licensing of day-nurseries would take work away from experienced baby-minders who might fear examinations and inspections and thus rob women of work. In any case, there were simply too many babies being left with siblings, grandparents, or neighbours to make any form of government inspection practicable or worthwhile.[95]

Faced with the situation of working mothers and the known perils of both baby-minding and bottle-feeding, the most practicable solution would have been for the Local Government Board and local sanitary officials to encourage the establishment of nurseries in the mills and factories.[96] In the general discussion at the 1893 annual meeting of the Royal Sanitary Institute, following the presentation by Dr Reid of his paper, 'Infant Mortality and Female Labour ...', Annesley Kenealy stated the needs of the day with considerable passion. 'If a woman was to be a wage earner', she protested 'she must in some way or other be relieved of the active responsibility of motherhood; if she was to be a good and true mother she must in some way be relieved of the active responsibility of wage earner.' Her outburst was greeted with stony silence.[97] Although well-run crèches existed by the 1880s in several industrial towns they failed to stimulate a general movement.[98] Any talk of municipal crèches was met by bitter opposition. When, for example, the issue was raised in Manchester it was angrily argued that municipalities should not encourage women to leave the home: 'a woman's function is to produce and rear children'.[99]

If the late Victorian controversy over working wives did not stimulate municipal or factory-run nurseries it did produce both national legislation and local efforts which improved the health of mothers and babies. The 1891 Factory Act prohibited the owner of a factory or workshop from 'knowingly' employing a woman 'within four weeks after she has given birth to a child'. The Act seems to have been drafted and passed with little commitment or enthusiasm; there was no machinery for making it effective and since no doctors' letters were required giving the date of birth and there was no legal precision to the phrase 'knowingly', it remained a dead-letter.

The Act lacked teeth because it was generally considered inappropriate for the state to cross the threshold and probe into family affairs. To dictate to the mother what was best for her and her baby struck many as 'a tyrannical interference with the freedom of private life' in the words of one leading factory inspector, and an 'intolerable Government meddling with individual liberty, personal dignity, and social propriety.' He freely admitted to the Social Science Association in 1874 that

> I would far rather see even a higher rate of infant mortality . . . than intrude one iota farther on the sanctity of the domestic hearth and the decent seclusion of private life. . . . That unit, the Family, is the unit upon which a constitutional Government has been raised which is the admiration and envy of mankind. Hitherto, whatsoever else the laws have touched, they have not dared to invade this sacred precinct . . . let the State step in between the mother and her child and . . . Domestic confidence is destroyed, family privacy invaded, and maternal responsibility assailed. For the tender care of the mother is substituted the tender mercies of the State; for the security of natural affection, the securities of an unnatural law!

He concluded, 'Better by far that many another infant should perish in its innocence and unconsciousness, than live to be the victim of such a state of things.' At least one woman agreed with these general views, arguing that the Act 'gave enormous publicity in matters which ought not to be made public . . . it interfered with the home life of one particular class, and involved inspections and details which concerned the women alone.'[100] On the other hand, the government's factory medical inspectors and many MOH, men who might have been able to make the Act more effective, felt that the four-week period was insufficient, and they agitated for three months, without success.[101] The Act does mark the tentative beginnings of state action in infant welfare (and to a lesser extent post-natal maternal care), but its timing, coming before any full discussion of maternity benefits, guaranteed minimum wages, or family support from husbands who had deserted their families, suggests that the Victorians simply slotted the problem of working mothers into the accepted pattern of factory legislation rather than taking a fresh, vigorous approach.

More immediately important, and certainly much more significant in helping to bring down the infant death rate so dramatically in the Edwardian period was the municipal movement to improve milk supplies, and to distribute specially formulated milk for babies. It was a movement which drew strength from the controversy over bottle feeding and its inspiration from French and American examples. Led by its MOH, Dr Harris, St Helens was the first town to establish a milk depot, when, in 1899, it made available sterilized milk at 2d a day; at the milk depots babies could also be inspected and weighed. Liverpool followed in 1901 and by 1905 was supplying 3,000 bottles of baby milk daily and by 1917, 17,000.[102] In London the Battersea Council opened a milk depot where 'humanised milk' (made by adding water, cream, and lactose to milk and boiling for fifteen minutes) was issued. The depot gave advice to mothers on how to keep the bottles clean and one bottle per feeding was handed out. Along similar lines, Dr Sykes, the MOH for St Pancras, opened the first council-run school for mothers in 1907. It offered instruction on baby care and provided dinners for undernourished and nursing mothers from two to three months before childbirth and up to nine months after.[103]

These efforts, accompanied by the growing practice of pasteurizing milk in the 1890s, the closer supervision of milk supplies provided by the Dairies, Cowsheds and Milkshops Order of 1899, and higher standards for milk established by the Board of Agriculture in 1901, marked a significant improvement in infant welfare.[104] There were also improvements in other areas. Earlier in the century public health officials had urged that infanticide was partly responsible for the high neo-natal death rate. Coroners' reports in the early- and mid-Victorian period are full of grisly accounts of babies found dead under bridges, in parks or fields, in cemeteries, canals, and even privies. Suspicion of infanticide by suffocation or starvation, or what Dr Hunter, one of Simon's team at the Privy Council, called 'wilful neglect with the hope of death', were aroused by the immense popularity of infant burial clubs.[105] These clubs paid out between 30s and £5 on a baby's death, and since the insurance could be bought for as little as 1d a week and the funeral of a child rarely cost more than 30s at the outside, a handsome sum could be made for the parents, especially as there was nothing, other than the cost of the policies, to prevent parents joining more than one club.[106] The unregulated use and sale of many poisons and narcotics, the vagueness of the coroners' reports and the unwillingness of juries to find parents or midwives guilty of wilful murder all fed the flames of suspicion that infanticide was not uncommon. In 1854 an eminent judge told the Select Committee on Friendly Societies that 'child murder for the sake of burial money prevailed to a fearful extent.' The *Lancet* cited the case of one father who received £34.3.0d by belonging to various burial clubs.[107]

The Friendly Societies Act (1846) banned the insurance of any child under six in any club established after the Act, but life insurance on children continued unabated, and it was estimated at the end of the century that probably 80 per cent of the nation's children were insured.[108] In 1904 a government committee called for a complete study of infant insurance schemes and a limitation of insurance to actual burial costs, but the men in the best position to know, the insurance men themselves, were convinced that talk of infanticide was wildly exaggerated. In 1895 the manager of the North British Insurance Company maintained that 'the class who insured their children were, almost to a man, the most provident and best workers; and that the idle and intemperate men and the class that would be most likely to insure with felonious motive, did not insure their children at all' – an argument which surely has much to commend it.[109] In any case, infanticide, about which public health officials could certainly do very little, was never a major cause of infant mortality, and while it certainly did exist, accounts of it were probably exaggerated by the tendency of the more comfortable Victorians to believe the very worst of the masses.

It was widely believed, for example, that parents deliberately killed their children by 'overlaying' them or suffocating them. In 1880 1,282 infant deaths were recorded from suffocation; in 1895 over 2,000, in 1900, 1,550, and in 1904, 899 (584 of them in London). At the end of the century one of every fourteen coroners' inquests in London involved cases of overlaying.[110] But the fact that over half the cases were reported on Sundays suggests that the deaths may have been the accidental consequences of what the Battersea MOH called 'excessive indulgence on Saturday night'.[111] The deaths may also have been due to what we now call 'crib deaths', the mysterious Sudden Infant Death Syndrome.[112]

Medical officers were convinced that one of the major causes of infant mortality was the widespread practice of giving children narcotics, especially opium, to quieten them. At 1d an ounce laudanum was cheap enough – about the price of a pint of beer – and its sale was totally unregulated until late in the century. The use of opium was widespread both in town and country. In Manchester, according to one account, five out of six working-class families used it habitually. One Manchester druggist admitted selling a half gallon of Godfrey's Cordial (the most popular mixture, it contained opium, treacle, water, and spices) and between five and six gallons of what was euphemistically called 'quietness' every week.[113] In Nottingham one member of the Town Council, a druggist, sold four hundred gallons of laudanum annually.[114] At mid-century there were at least ten proprietary brands, with Godfrey's Cordial, Steedman's Powder, and the grandly named Atkinson's Royal Infants Preservative among the most popular.[115] In East Anglia opium in pills and penny sticks was widely sold and opium-taking was described as a way of life there – 'there is not a little village shop . . . that sells anything that does not sell its own Godfrey's.'[116] Throughout the Fens it was used in 'poppy tea', and doctors there reported how the infants were wasted from it – 'shrank up into little old men', 'wizened like little monkeys' is the way they were described.[117] Far from being an underground drug, opium and opium mixtures were widely and openly sold for a variety of ailments – rheumatism (hence their popularity in the damp Fenlands), diabetes, consumption, syphilis, cholera, diarrhoea, constipation, and as a sedative. Engels casually mentioned that it was commonly held that opium strengthened the heart. It was widely enough used for Mrs Beeton to offer advice on how overdoses should be treated.[118]

We can certainly sympathize with the need, among the working classes, to have a sedative to quieten the baby in their overcrowded flats; the Privy Council was informed that without opium to give the baby the rest of the family would never get a night's sleep.[119] Coroners tended to regard parental ignorance, rather than design, as the cause of infant deaths from overdoses of drugs, and they generally recorded these deaths as 'natural causes', 'convulsions', or 'accidental deaths'.[120]

Opium killed far more infants through starvation than directly through overdoses. Dr Greenhow, investigating for the Privy Council, noted how children 'kept in a state of continued narcotism will be thereby disinclined for food, and be but imperfectly nourished.'[121] Marasmus, or inanitition, and death from severe malnutrition would result, but the coroner was likely to record the death as 'debility from birth', or 'lack of breast milk', or simply 'starvation'.[122] The Privy Council's Medical Department was convinced that opium usage was a significant cause of infant mortality and in 1868, several years after it had first drawn attention to its widespread usage, a Pharmacy Act was passed which permitted the sale of opium only by qualified pharmacists and legally registered chemists. But no restrictions were placed on the amounts sold and the purchaser did not have to give his name. More important, patent medicines were exempt.[123] Like the failure to register midwives or to improve the standard of milk, this might be seen as a terrible example of the ineffectiveness of the public health movement to agitate successfully for measures which would lower the infant death rate. But the Privy Council was unable to convince the governments of the day that Parliament was a more appropriate body than the Pharmaceutical Society to control the flow of drugs. Vested interests combined with the fear that controls would lead to a black market in opium guaranteed that opium would remain freely available down to the end of the century.[124]

In the early years of the present century Robert Roberts remembers opium being sold in his native Salford as 'Mother's Friend', or, more familiarly, 'knock out drops' – 'it relieves your child from pain', ran the advertisements, 'and the little cherub awakes bright as a button.'[125] But as the general standard of living improved, so opium-taking declined. Ironically, had not opium been adulterated (with, among other substances, pea-meal, water, honey, sugar and flour), probably more infants would have died.[126] As it is, it is impossible to calculate how many children died from the effects, direct or indirect, of opium. In the manufacturing districts, where the infant mortality rate was so very high, its use was widespread, and unskilled daily baby-minders would reduce their weekly charge by 3d or even 6d if the mother provided 'quietening mixture'.[127] Given the low nutritional standards of the day and the physical weakness of so many of the new-born infants, opium-taking must be regarded, as it was by the Privy Council, as a serious and important aggravating factor in the continued high level of infant mortality. As such, the Victorians must be criticized for not taking more vigorous measures to prohibit it.

To many Victorians a much more pressing need existed – to tackle 'the ignorance of mothers of the way in which their children should be managed, and their carelessness of the welfare of their off-spring . . .'[128] Among those convinced that infant mortality would decline once working-class mothers were educated to the manifold duties of motherhood was the Ladies' National Association for the Diffusion of Sanitary Knowledge (the Ladies' Sanitary Association), founded in 1857. By 1865 the Association had branches in Brighton, Aberdeen, Oxford, Bath, Reading, Dublin, Dundee, Glasgow, Leeds, Bristol, and Manchester, and between 1857 and 1881 had distributed a million and a half tracts.[129] Most of these tracts were aimed, rather uneasily, at the artisan and lower middle class, rather than the poorest working classes who most needed them. Titles included *Health of Mothers* (this contained sound advice on pre-natal matters, food, exercise, and tight corsets, which, it said, cause 'miscarriage, and falling of the womb, piles, varicose veins, sore breasts, flattened nipples. . .') *How to Rear Healthy Children*, *How to Manage a Baby*, *The Evils of Wet-Nursing*, *On the Evils Resulting from Rising too Early after Childbirth*, *Measles*, *A Tract for Mothers*. Occasionally the Association would resort to doggerel verse to get across its message:

mothers were told that when baby 'by sounds and signs' asks to be fed from the table:

> Remember, he can't chew
> And solid food is bad for him
> Tho' very good for you.[130]

Other voluntary associations which hoped to improve standards of domestic hygiene and child care were the Manchester and Salford Sanitary Association (founded in 1852 by an obstetrician who was convinced that maternal ignorance lay at the root of high infant mortality), the Liverpool Ladies' Sanitary Association (founded in 1891 to train day-care nurses), and the Ladies' Committee of the Yorkshire Board of Education (1870).[131] The Manchester and Salford Sanitary Association published its own tracts on child care, and it had salaried workers, which was unusual among these volunteer organizations. These sanitary societies were an outgrowth of Bible mission societies and, like them, they stressed house visits. Their workers were well versed in the rudiments of domestic hygiene and, as we shall see in the next chapter, did much to bring the gospel of soap and water into the homes of the masses. The movement was infused with enthusiasm and compassion and brought a fund of good common sense to the poor on a whole range of matters, from covering food to protect it from flies, to boiling milk, to washing hands after going to the privy or w.c. While the patronising and interfering home missionaries, like the infamous Mrs Jellyby in *Bleak House*, were often thoroughly disliked by the poor, there is evidence that the poor were receptive in the late-Victorian period to the volunteers who visited their homes with the goal of improving their health.[132] Without the hard work performed on a daily basis by these societies the municipal milk depots would have had only a limited success.

In one other respect the sanitary associations were significant: they enabled the lady health visitors to develop considerable expertise in matters which were of vital concern to public health and thus provided a bridge to the professional employment of lady health visitors by local authorities.[133] By 1905 the Royal Sanitary Institute was offering lectures on child care as a course for lady sanitary inspectors, and the Liverpool Ladies' Sanitary Society and other societies had formed schools to train health visitors. Though a Victorian concept, the system of lady health visitors did not really catch fire until the Edwardian period.[134] Similarly, classes in child-care and domestic science and hygiene grew in popularity only slowly in the late-Victorian period. In

1898 only two per cent of the girls in elementary schools were taking such classes and only 15 of the 55 teacher-training colleges offered courses in hygiene and domestic economy at the end of the century.[135]

But it was a beginning, and together with the numerous schools which were started in mothercare, such as Mrs Petty's St Pancras School for Mothers, founded in 1910 to give mothers lessons in cooking and child-care, it marked the start of a new era.[136] At the first Annual Meeting of the Ladies' Sanitary Association the hope was expressed that the society would help to bring down the infant mortality rate by 40 per cent.[137] It must have seemed like a vain hope to many present. Yet between 1900 and 1914 the infant death rate, which had been so frustratingly immutable for so long, suddenly declined, and declined sharply, consistently, and dramatically, from 156 to 105 – a decline of some 33 per cent. There are many reasons for this decline, but Newsholme was certainly correct in stressing in his 1913 report to the Local Government Board that, *inter alia*, 'education in hygiene' and 'the widespread awakening to the national importance of child mortality, with concentration on efforts of child welfare such as had never previously occurred', were vital.[138] Though belated, the effort had immediate effect and, as in so many other areas of Victorian public health, demonstrates the felicitous marriage between municipal enterprise and private philanthropic endeavour.

This chapter began with the statement that infant mortality rates are a very sensitive barometer of environmental conditions. As such they can respond dramatically to just small changes. The factors we have so far studied – milk supply, for example, or drug usage – were in themselves not examples of dramatic improvement. But taken together with a rising standard of living and of domestic sanitation, along with other factors, they become significant. Among the other factors the most important was the declining birth rate. The middle classes had been practising birth control from at least the 1860s onwards, but the working classes did not begin to do so on a large enough scale to influence the general birth rate until the end of the century. Obviously, with fewer children the mother could devote more care (and give more food) to each. More important, before the use of contraceptives, Victorian women had to face the dangers of pregnancy and childbirth right into late middle age. The more children she had already given birth to, the more likely it was that her uterus was exhausted. Somewhat ironically, in view of the bitter opposition to working wives, the attraction of mill and factory work for women might have encouraged them to practice birth control and thus help

38

bring down the infant birth rate. Certainly since so much infant mortality was related to poverty the supplemental income of the working wife was important and birth control enabled the wife to work continuously. If, as was increasingly possible in the last years of Victoria's reign, the additional wages went to purchase wholesome milk in hygienic bottles for the baby, it certainly helped rather than harmed the baby's health and the family's general welfare.[139]

If the period covered in this book went to the First World War we could end on a positive note with the decline in infant mortality. But for the Victorian period no such 'happy ending' is possible. Compared with infant death rates of over 270 for Russia, almost 200 for Prussia, and over 170 for Italy, England's 156 cannot be considered high, especially in view of her massive urbanization (more rural Scotland and Ireland had significantly lower infant mortality rates).[140] That there was little cause for rejoicing, however, was clear to contemporaries when they looked at the figures for healthier countries such as Norway (with an infant death rate of only 93) and New Zealand (80).[141] While rising medical standards and improvements in the environment and general standards of living helped to bring down the death rate for children between one and five, the continuing high level of deaths of infants from prematurity and diarrhoeal diseases indicated that low standards of maternal health and nutrition and, as one Local Government Board doctor expressed it, 'domestic darkness and general dirtiness of dwellings' still prevailed at the end of Victoria's reign.[142]

The infant death rate in 1900 serves as a sobering reminder of the fact that whatever vast strides the Victorians had made in sanitary reform, there was still a long way to go. Nothing serves as a better indicator of this than the variation in infant death rates between various classes. In England and Wales as a whole just before the First World War, infant mortality in families of unskilled labour was double that in families belonging to the upper two social classes.[143] Similarly, in London in 1891, the infant death rate in a poor and crowded district such as the Strand (229) was approximately double that of a solidly middle-class area such as Plumstead (115). As the accompanying map indicates, though infant death rates had declined steeply by the end of the Edwardian period, the London borough with the highest infant mortality was *twice* as lethal for children as the healthiest area (Shoreditch and Hampstead, 145.1 and 71.5, respectively). To be born to poor parents at the beginning of the century

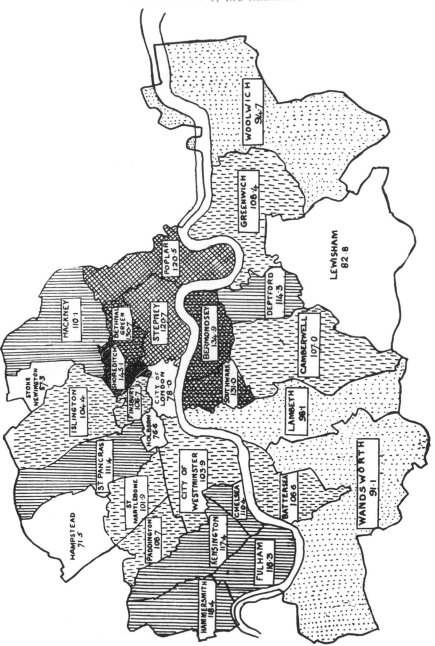

1. Map showing comparative infant death rates in London, 1907–10 (deaths per thousand live births). The concentration of poverty in the East End and south of the Thames is reflected in the infant mortality statistics.

Source: Parliamentary Paper XXXII (1913), 'Forty-Second ARGLB, 1912–13. Supplement . . .', p. 18

meant that one was twice as likely to die before reaching one's first birthday.[144]

In some ways it would doubtless be comforting to end this chapter by agreeing with those members of the more comfortable classes who argued that while the high infant mortality rate among the poor was distressing, it was (rather like other unavoidable features of poverty, stench, say, or dirt) *less* distressing to the poor than to social reformers and explorers and those with heightened sensibilities. Deaths of babies, the argument went, were so common, so *expected*, that working-class parents accepted them stoically and passively, without much pain or remorse. A class which could stoop to infanticide and which, generation after generation, had come to accept the inevitability of losing one or more children in infancy could hardly, it was held, be expected to feel sorrow at the passing of a baby. Dr Greenhow unquestioningly accepted the evidence of local doctors in Nottingham that working mothers were quite indifferent to the deaths of their babies, and his superior at the Privy Council, John Simon, wrote that the more degraded working-class mothers were 'more or less careless and indifferent' about their babies

> and as so many of those children die, the mothers become familiarised with the fact, and speak of the deaths of their children with a degree of nonchalance rarely met with among women who devote themselves mainly to the care of their off-spring.[145]

But both Greenhow and Simon drew their examples from mothers who went out to work to bolster their argument against the practice, and they were careful to exclude the working class as a whole. Stoicism was, perhaps, a 'front' put on by the working classes. They were unlikely to display inner emotions when confronted with local bureaucracy in the form of the MOH. From the scattered evidence we have a very different picture emerges, one of sorrow and sadness. The following scene, recorded by Mrs John Brown (who, influenced by Charles Kingsley, did social work among the poor of Burnley), has the ring of authenticity to it. She had been asked to investigate the case of a young collier with a wife and two children, and she set out on a bitter, damp, and frosty day:

> All the furniture they possessed was in a room below, a bed, a chair, a rickety chest of drawers, and a small, round three-legged table – not a vestige of comfort. There was no fire – only a handful of burnt-out cinders and ash in the grate. . . In the bed was a young woman, about twenty-three. She was white and wan and looked dazed. She was holding a week-old baby to her empty breast. Over her cotton

nightdress was her husband's waistcoat, and over her knees his coat –
these were the only coverings of any warmth.

It was so pitiful I did not know what to say. 'I've come to help you,
but I thought there were two children'. 'There was three days ago', the
woman said, 'Show her, Jem.' The man got up heavily, and went and
opened the bottom drawer of the rickety chest, and there lay a little dead
child of about two or three years old, her tiny hands folded on her breast
over her tiny striped nightie, and a look of infinite calm and pathos on
the worn little face – it seemed to illuminate that dingy drawer – 'Oh', I
gasped, 'Why is she here?' The man said 'We be waiting for the parish to
coom and bury her'. And the mother said, 'We couldn't find it in our
hearts to put her upstairs alone in th' empty room'.

I stood still, the tears pouring down my cheeks, and a sob choking me;
but the parents shed no tears, nor said a word, except when Jim closed
the drawer he said, 'She war a nice little lass, she war.'[146]

It is easy to see how, when the 'parish' did come it might mistake the
passivity and poverty-induced fatigue for callous indifference. A. S.
Jasper, in his autobiographical *A Hoxton Childhood*, recounts a
similar scene of sorrow when a baby, just a few weeks old, died in his
large family.[147] And the death of a child haunts the memories of the
wife of the Devon fisherman in Stephen Reynolds's vividly evocative
A Poor Man's House:

> Nothing would please me for months after but to go up to the cementry
> [*sic*] to her little grave. Most every evening I walked up after tea – didn'
> feel as if I could go to bed an' sleep wi' out . . . . it did ease me, like, to go
> up there, an' it heartened me a little for next day's work.

The baby died 'of convulsions from teething' and the doctor filling in
for the regular doctor refused to look at the child. The husband
stoically commented that while the rich could always get medical
attention, the poor could not: 'Us can't do nort an' that's the way o' it.
Rose did' never ought to ha' died.'[148]

It is impossible for the historian to say with any accuracy whether
these scenes of grief and quiet sadness are typical. If they are, the lives
of the poor parents and of the siblings of the dead baby were pro-
foundly touched by the high infant mortality, and as much sadness and
sorrow tinged their lives at the end of Victoria's reign as at the
beginning.

3
'Tolerable Human Types'

'The greatest foe to health and long life is poverty. Not only do all
epidemic visitations fall with tenfold severity upon the poorer classes of
society, but all descriptions of disease find in them their chief victims'.
Lancet, 1 April 1843, p. 9, a lecture by Dr George Gregory.

Poverty and the culture to which poverty gave rise greatly aggravated
the problems of public health. Poverty affected the spread and direction of diseases, nurtured contagion and infection, transformed
endemic into epidemic diseases, and frustrated the efforts of central
and local health authorities. Though other factors were also involved,
poverty lay behind the overcrowding and slums, the poor sanitation,
inadequate diet, and feeble bodies which encouraged illness. Public
health must be placed within the context of a nation in which approximately one-third of the population at the beginning of the present
century lived in poverty – that is, an absolute lack of surplus after they
had provided for the basic needs of food, shelter, fuel and clothing.
This chapter concentrates on the poverty (and its meaning in terms of
diet, physique, and personal hygiene) of the great mass of the unskilled
labour force, the 'great unwashed' who presented so formidable a
challenge to health officials.

The controversy over the impact of the industrial revolution on the
standard of living has raged, often with as much emotion as reason,
among historians for over half a century now. Although in general
terms one might agree that

> there was a negligible improvement in the Napoleonic war years, an
> upward trend in the immediate post-war years (though this may have
> been outweighed by post-war unemployment), an unprecedentedly
> rapid improvement in the second quarter (which may also be modified
> on the basis of unemployment data), and an indisputable rise in the third
> and fourth quarters. This had begun to lose speed before the century
> ended.[1]

national wage and consumer price indices are very misleading. Only local
studies provide an accurate picture and those that have recently been
undertaken indicate that whatever progress there was was from such

43

a low base that poverty continued to be the norm for vast numbers throughout the reign of Victoria. Even the assumption that the second half of the century witnessed an 'indisputable rise' in living standards must now be modified. A recent study of the miners in the Black Country stresses that between 1851 and 1900 there were only twenty-three years of full employment. With ever steeper food prices there until the 1870s and rents rising throughout the entire century, very little improvement in living standards occurred and in only ten years between 1850 and 1889 did real wages climb back to the 1850 level.[2] Other local studies similarly qualify the picture presented by national figures. Agricultural labourers in Kent, if fortunate enough to be in regular employment, enjoyed at the most a five per cent rise in the standard of living over the first forty years of the century, but for the large numbers who were hit by the seasonal and cyclical unemployment which was a feature of southern agriculture there was a 'catastrophic fall in real wages for almost the whole of the period 1790–1840'.[3] In Exeter there was little improvement between 1850 and 1870. Prices there were rising at least as fast as wages, and there was widespread intermittent unemployment.[4] In the high-density area of the Merseyside in Lancashire it would seem that the mid-Victorian years were by no means as prosperous for labour as was once assumed, and although money wages were rising there the sharp increase in food prices held back whatever progress would otherwise have been made. Taking Liverpool specifically, food prices soared in the third quarter of the century, running over 40 per cent higher than the 1850 level by the early 1870s, and still 27 per cent higher as late as 1875. When the increasing cost of housing is taken into account it is clear that the mid-Victorian years did not bring a significantly higher standard of living to either skilled or unskilled labour in Lancashire.[5]

Thus, though over the nation as a whole living standards rose in the second half of the nineteenth century, there was also much lingering poverty. In London, where the steep rise in rents did much to nullify the rising wages, approximately one-third of all Londoners lived in poverty in the 1880s, and in Holborn, Stepney, Bethnal Green and Southwark the figure approached a half. In many densely packed districts, each with a population equal to a good-sized provincial town, 60 per cent or more of the inhabitants were living beneath the poverty line.[6] For the casual labourers – and one family in ten in London was connected with casual labour – earnings at around £1 a week after mid-century left no surplus after basic necessities had been paid for, and even fully employed, casual labourers were rarely more than a week's wages away from destitution. But full employment was beyond the wildest expectations of thousands of labourers, both in London and in the other major towns. In his 1887 survey of some 30,000 men in various parts of London, William Ogle discovered that 89 per cent had recently been unemployed.[7] In York the extensive survey conducted by Seebohm Rowntree at the turn of the century disclosed the dismal fact that almost half the working-class families earned wages which were 'insufficient to provide food, shelter, and clothing adequate to maintain a family of moderate size in a state of bare physical efficiency'. Rowntree sadly wrote that almost all labourers with three or more children would inevitably pass through a period of poverty when their families would be underfed.[8] At the outbreak of the First World War approximately one-third of the regularly employed adult male work force earned less than the twenty-five shillings a week widely regarded as necessary to rise above poverty and to maintain minimum bodily efficiency. To talk to these men of national prosperity or rising standards of living would have been a mockery.[9]

This is not to say that the general improvement in living standards had no effect on the nation's health, but, rather, to offer a revision to optimistic interpretations and to suggest that the high infant death and the persistence of several infectious and contagious fatal diseases at the end of the century reflect a perilously low standard of living for the masses. This living standard not only virtually condemned many to death but acted as a brake on the progress which sanitary reformers made in so many areas of preventive medicine.

It was impossible, in early Victorian England, to be unaware of the connection between poverty and disease, if only for the obvious reason that death rates were higher in the poorer neighbourhoods: 'slums' and 'fever dens' were used interchangeably. As early as 1832 the *Lancet* printed a letter which offered a simple economic solution to the problem of cholera: 'Give food to the hungry, clothe the naked, remove the filth from the habitations of the poor, and the cholera will quickly disappear.'[10] The link between poverty and illness found official expression in England in 1839 when Edwin Chadwick at the Poor Law Board commissioned three doctors, Kay, Arnott, and Southwood Smith to investigate the connection between disease and poverty. Their findings stressed the vicious circle — poverty contributed to disease and disease often turned poverty into pauperism. Dr Southwood Smith, for example, maintained that as much as one-fifth of all pauperism in London stemmed from fever, and he argued that the best means of holding down the poor rates lay in the control of fever.

45

Although only four per cent of the population were paupers – a figure which remained more or less constant throughout the nineteenth century – the problems of pauperism remained a major concern of the Victorians, and the fact, reiterated by poor law officials, that roughly 80 per cent of all pauperism was the consequence of ill-health, did much to underscore the urgency for public health reform.[11] Towards the end of the century Booth concluded that, in the area he investigated, roughly ten per cent of the poverty was the direct product of illness; Rowntree in York placed the figure at 20 per cent. But the Royal Commission on the Poor Laws concluded in 1909 that 'It is probably little if any exaggeration to say that, to the extent to which we can eliminate or diminish sickness among the poor, we shall eliminate or diminish one-half of the existing amount of pauperism.'[12] Almost from the inception of the Poor Law Commission, paupers who were suffering from ill-health were given medical treatment outside the workhouses or in dispensaries within the poor law system.[13]

But it was far easier for Poor Law doctors to tackle the problem of pauperism by treating illnesses than it was for doctors and sanitary officials to tackle the problems of public health by drawing attention to poverty. Of course in England, and perhaps to an even greater extent in Scotland, they tried to raise the question of poverty as a root cause of widespread diseases.[14] 'Turn which way we will', wrote Professor Cowan, referring to his experiences in Glasgow, 'in seeking the main causes of these epidemics of fever. Destitution stares us in the face – the main cause of all.'[15] 'The greatest foe to health and long life is poverty', Dr Gregory wrote in the *Lancet* (1843), and Dr Julian Hunter, one of the most knowledgeable social investigators within medical ranks observed in 1849 that, 'If other causes have slain their thousands, poverty has slain its tens of thousands'. Hunter wryly added that 'The relation of poverty to disease is so great and inseparable that it is astonishing legislators should not ere now have acknowledged it.'[16] The *Lancet* and the general periodical press were full of such statements: indeed, they amounted to something approaching a commonplace or truism. But while those attending the Social Science Association's annual meeting in 1858 might listen solemnly to a paper on 'The Influence of Poverty and Privation on Public Health', it was far easier for them to agree with the connection than to suggest what could be done about it. Political philosophies, a conviction that the poor, through indolence, self-indulgence, and immorality were themselves responsible for their condition, lack of specific knowledge about the extent and depth of poverty, all stood in the way of a close analysis of the causes of poverty and of the formulation of sweeping social policies to alleviate it. Not until the 1880s was there a coherent attempt to evaluate poverty not in terms of personal failings and moral crusades, but in terms of the supply of and demand for labour and goods, and the distribution of wealth in society. By the 1880s a half-century of sanitary and social reform had made it clear that sound housing, pure water, and even personal hygiene were often beyond the means of the poor; to preach self-help amid such poverty was absurd: 'Just as well tell the blind to see, the deaf to hear, the lame to walk', Sir Robert Rawlinson, the President of the Royal Sanitary Institute of Great Britain told the Institute in 1884, 'as to tell these people to be well-housed, well-clothed, and well-fed.'[17] Rawlinson's speech had been preceded by a tour of the slums of Dublin, those 'seed-beds of disease and revolution', in Rawlinson's phrase, and his address was full of solemn warnings:

> Sanitation . . . is an all-round question, and the improvements con-nected with it cannot come from below – they must come from above. . . . if the highest classes will not voluntarily forego some of the wealth they accumulate and give some attention to enabling these people to be healthier, happier, and live better, then you may depend upon it there is a stratum of vice and misery now existent, which if made desperate by famine and neglect, would be quite sufficient to overturn all that is above, and if this state of things should continue for any length of time you may have social disturbances like the French Revolution of the past century, which upset society from top to bottom.[18]

Rawlinson's was just one of many voices raised at this time in warning against possible revolution. The alarm, whether genuine or calculat-ing, served to accelerate concern for the health and well-being of the masses. Fear and self-interest were powerful forces in the complex phenomenon of the public health movement.[19]

Of the many aspects of poverty, inadequate diet, heating, clothing, and housing, it was housing which aroused the most widespread concern (see Chapter 11). As for fuel and clothing, although they attracted the attention of health officials there was surprisingly little concentrated analysis of the effects of either upon the general health of the nation. Apart from random comments there was little that the public health officers thought they could, or should, do about either. That mill and factory hands often walked miles to work in the rain and had to work in drenched clothing (which in the humid atmosphere of the cotton mill never dried out), was pointed out as a contributing cause of illness, as was the fact that the very poor did not wash their clothes partly because they had no replacement to wear.[20] Inadequate clothing and fuel probably proved fatal only to the very young or very old. Rural cottages were notoriously damp and poorly insulated, but at least fuel, in the form of sod and peat and scraps of timber, was cheaper in the country than in town. Working-class budgets indicate that coal for a single-roomed flat could cost up to one-third of the rent, or 1s a week.[21] For those earning under £1 a week this was a considerable outlay, all the more burdensome since it fell in winter when so many casual labourers were laid off. The empty hearth, the grate with a single smouldering stick, served both artists and novelists as symbols of poverty and despair, and they were symbols based on reality. One MOH, strangely oblivious to the realities of working-class life, argued that 'for a man neither very old nor ill a fire is a luxury, not a necessity', and he clinched his argument, at least in his own opinion, by adding 'I speak from experience of winters spent in rooms at Oxford and in London.'[22] Similarly social workers were always telling the poor to throw open their windows. But the poor, with their undernourished bodies and damp dwellings needed all the warmth they could get. Fresh air might well ventilate the home, but it also struck chill into the bones of the poor. Health inspectors, often reeling with nausea from the filth accumulated indoors, rushed to open windows which, no doubt, were immediately closed on their departure.

The consequences of poverty are most apparent in the diets of the poor. It takes a considerable leap of the imagination to recapture the Victorian working-class diet, for we have preconceived notions of the 'good old days' before the onslaught of pre-packaged, processed, artificially coloured, 'convenience' foods, and we have, perhaps, an image of John Bull, contentedly overweight from all the benefits of free trade and the beef and ale diet which distinguished the English from unfortunate foreigners. But to enter the world of the Victorian working man's diet is to enter the world of the savage – it was uncertain in supply, primitive in content, and unhealthy in effect. Few of the poor had ovens and had to rely either on open-fire pan cooking, buy their hot food out, or make do with cold meals. Even at the turn of the century social workers entering the homes of the poor to teach wives how to cook were aghast to discover that the family possessed only one pot, and that before their lesson in economy stews and soups could begin the pot would have to be cleaned of the baby's bath-water, or worse.[23] As late as 1904 an official committee of inquiry was distressed to learn how few of the poor had sufficient utensils and appliances to cook at home.[24] Primitive or non-existent cooking facilities, lack of cheap fuel, poverty, ignorance, and adulterated foods combined to produce a nation, not of John Bulls but, by today's standards, of pygmies, who were undernourished, anaemic, feeble and literally rickety. Today's well-fed teenage schoolgirl would have little trouble looking over the head of the average Victorian workman.

The foodstuffs which we associate today with rural living – fresh eggs and milk, game, meat, and fowl, locally raised fruit and vegetables – were all valuable cash crops and most rural labourers saw as little of them on their table as did their city counterparts. If the rural labourer did have a small allotment for himself he had to augment his income from it.[25] The exigencies and pressures of his budget hardly allowed him to raise for the family table crops which could be turned into cash. It is rash to generalize about the rural diet – consumption of meat in 1863 varied, for example, from less than 7 oz per head per week in Salop, Essex, Somerset, Wiltshire, and Norfolk to between 24 oz and 30 oz in Durham, Lancashire, Northampton, Surrey, and Yorkshire.[26] Yet one may agree with a recent judgment that 'The agricultural labourer was, in fact, the worst fed of all workers in the nineteenth century.'[27] Esther Copley's *Cottage Cookery* (1849) suggests the poverty of the rural diet, for her recipes were for potato pie, stirabout, stewed ox-cheek, and mutton chitterlings.[28] In Wiltshire, admittedly one of the poorer counties, the Poor Law Commission found that the standard fare consisted of bread, butter, potatoes, beer, and tea, with some bacon for those earning higher wages. We should not be surprised then that according to a Wiltshire doctor the vast majority of female patients suffered from complaints directly attributable to a diet which was 'insufficient in quantity and not good enough in quality'.[29]

'Slow but sustained improvement in the [rural] labourer's diet' was 'first noticeable in the 1870s' and it was not until the last quarter of the century that meat became a regular part of the rural labourer's diet. Thirty per cent of the labourers visited by Dr Edward Smith in 1863, on behalf of the Privy Council, had never eaten butcher's meat, only bacon. In many cases the meat which was eaten was the flesh of sick sheep given in lieu of wages![30] Oral history, though it tends to transform an exceptional and memorable event into a regular occurrence, confirms that the agricultural labourer's diet was indeed sparse. Several farm hands remember eating sparrows and the aptly named Mrs Jay remembered how in Suffolk they would net sparrows, skin them, and stew the breasts or make a pie from them. Her husband recalls,

'I'd trap as many as forty and bring 'em home and skin 'em. We used to boil them up in a saucepan or a boiler; we'd make a soup out of them.' Another recalled eating sparrow dumplings, adding simply, 'A lot o' people never tasted meat, and that was better than no meat at all.'[31] Between 1814 and 1871 potato acreage in England and Wales rose from 160,000 to 513,000 acres and the daily consumption of potatoes rose over the same period to about a pound for every man, woman, and child. This represented a 'potato standard', for potatoes were a substitute, rather than a supplement, for bread.[32]

As in the country, so in the town, the staples were bread, potatoes, and tea. The major difference discovered by Smith in his survey was that the rural labourer ate more bread and cheese.[33] If the rural poor ate birds then the urban poor ate pairings of tripe, slink (prematurely born calves), or broxy (diseased sheep).[34] Edgar Wallace recollects working-class families along the Old Kent Road shopping for 'tainted' pieces of meat and 'those odds and ends of meat, the by-products of the butchering business'.[35] Sheep's heads at 3d each and American bacon at between 4d and 6d a pound (half the price of the native product) were too expensive for the irregularly-employed casual labourer to have frequently. In Macclesfield 23 per cent of the silk workers and in Coventry 17 per cent of the labourers had never tasted meat. Stocking weavers, shoe makers, needle women and silk weavers ate less than one pound of meat a week and less than eight ounces of fats. Bread formed the mainstay of their diet with a weekly consumption which varied from almost eight pounds a head in the case of the needlewomen to over twelve pounds per adult among the 2,000 or so agricultural labourers in Smith's survey. Large numbers of workmen were getting their carbohydrates and calories mainly in bread – over two pounds of it daily![36] Dr Buchanan, another of John Simon's team at the Privy Council's medical department, sadly concluded that there were 'multitudes of people . . . whose daily food consists at every meal of tea and bread, bread and tea.'[37]

It was not until the last quarter of the century that the working man's diet improved significantly. Between 1877 and 1889 the cost of the average national weekly food basket of butter, bread, tea, milk and meat fell by some 30 per cent, and it was in this period that the first really appreciable nutritional improvement (aided by a greater variety of foods and new methods of retailing), occurred.[38] The cheaper food products which came in with the refrigerator – and then freezer – ships, the development of inexpensive margarine, the fall in price of most consumer items, all served to increase both the variety and quantity of the workmen's diet in this period.[39] By the end of the century a significant fall in weekly bread consumption had taken place to under seven pounds per family, and consumption of sugar, meat, and milk had all increased. We should note, however, that a leading historian of diet, basing his conclusion on seventeen separate surveys covering some 2,500 family budgets, does not date this improvement much before the final decade of the century.[40] Three separate surveys conducted between 1889 and 1895 revealed that over 50,000 school children in London were underfed, and in 1904 the government committee looking into national physical deterioration was shocked at the continuing low standard of nutrition among the masses. Roughly one in six London schoolchildren was underfed and suffered physically from a 'systematic course of malnutrition'. Estimates for Manchester were similar and the committee was informed that there the standard diet was 'tea and bread and butter for breakfast, potato and herrings perhaps, for dinner, and tea and bread and butter for tea.'[41] Budgets for the nineteenth century reveal that in those families earning between 20s and 35s a week every extra penny earned was spent on food rather than on clothing, fuel, or extra accommodation. It was hardly a question of priorities in allocation of disposable income: rather it was a question of fulfilling the basic human instinct of self-preservation. Roughly 60 per cent of the working-class income was spent on food at the turn of the century.[42]

While the total calorific intake might have been generally adequate, the Victorian working-class diet was heavy in carbohydrates and fats, low in protein, and deficient in several vitamins, notably C and D. Nearly all the diets investigated reveal a serious lack of fresh green vegetables, a low protein intake, and very little fresh milk. Although such estimates are bound to be only rough indications, it is interesting that a modern study places the Victorian diet at the end of the century at only 2,099 calories *per capita* for the working-class family: as we shall shortly see the menfolk would get considerably more than this average, the womenfolk correspondingly significantly less, but in either case it means that the Victorian working classes were getting far less than the recommended standards of the Council of Nutrition today (3,580 calories for men and 2,930 for women). The same study concludes that for approximately one-third of the entire population there would be a ten-year period or so when the children were too young to contribute significantly to the family income, during which the family would be underfed.[43] This must be put within the context of Victorian life – long working hours, often arduous physical labour, and long walks to and from work. Modern nutritional studies show that adults walking a distance to work and engaged in strenuous activity may use 3,700 or more calories a day, and that the body uses up far more calories when recovering from sickness.[44]

Two important points must be borne in mind in assessing the nutritional value of the diet of the Victorian working classes. First, as we have just mentioned, much of the family's food was consumed by the father and after him the other male bread-winners. Dr Smith found that the common attitude of mind was that 'the husband wins the bread, and must have the best food'. Smith commented that, in families where the husband had a little meat or bacon every day, 'the wife and children may eat it but once a week, and that both himself and his household believe that course to be necessary to enable him to perform his labour'.[45] Robert Roberts in his splendidly evocative memoir, *The Classic Slum: Salford Life in the First Quarter of the Century*, recalls how his father's corner shop sold 'relishes' and tidbits, but only for the head of the family:

> brawn, corned beef, boiled mutton, cheese, bacon (as little as two ounces of these), eggs, saveloys, tripe, pig's trotters, sausage, cow's heels, herrings, bloaters and kippers, or 'digbies' and finnan haddock . . . These were the protein foods vital to sustain a man arriving home at night, worked often to near exhaustion.[46]

The nutritional cost to the women and therefore to the next generation, and to children, was considerable.

The second point is that much of the food consumed by the working-class family was contaminated and positively detrimental to health. One is reminded of the old joke of the two women in conversation at a resort hotel. 'The food here is dreadful', complains one. 'I know', replies the other, 'and the portions are so small.' Perhaps in view of the quality, it was just as well that the quantity of so many family diets was so small. Adulteration of food was not unique to the nineteenth century, but the mass production and marketing techniques developed in the period, the anonymity afforded in the urban setting, and the scale of operations called for by the large, densely-packed urban populations, combined to increase the scale and range of adulteration. The ingenuity of those involved in adulteration outstripped the ability of authorities to check the process, and as the century wore on so the list of adulterated foodstuffs grew longer. To look back nostalgically and assume, for example, that the bread which formed the staff of life was home-baked, or, if bought, was wholesome and nutritional, is romantic nonsense. By the 1840s home baking had died out among the rural poor; in the small tenements of the urban masses, unequipped as these were with ovens, it never existed. In 1872 Dr Hassall, the pioneer investigator into food adulteration and the principal reformer in this vital area of health, demonstrated that half of the bread he examined had considerable quantities of alum. Alum, while not in itself poisonous, by inhibiting the digestion could lower the nutritional value of other foods.[47]

The list of poisonous additives reads like the stock list of some mad and malevolent chemist: strychnine, cocculus indicus (both are hallucinogens) and copperas in rum and beer; sulphate of copper in pickles, bottled fruit, wine, and preserves; lead chromate in mustard and snuff; sulphate of iron in tea and beer; ferric ferrocyanide, lime sulphate and turmeric in chinese tea; copper carbonate, lead sulphate, bisulphate of mercury, and Venetian lead in sugar confectionery and chocolate; lead in wine and cider; all were extensively used and were accumulative in effect, resulting, over a long period, in chronic gastritis, and indeed, often fatal food poisoning. Red lead gave Gloucester cheese its 'healthy' red hue, flour and arrowroot a rich thickness to cream, and tea leaves were 'dried, dyed, recycled again and again'.[48] As late as 1877 the Local Government Board found that approximately a quarter of the milk it examined contained excessive water, or chalk, and ten per cent of all the butter, over eight per cent of the bread, and over 50 per cent of all the gin had copper in them to heighten the colour.[49] As we saw in the previous chapter milk adulteration (which first became on offence in 1860) continued down to the end of the century. In the major cities between one-quarter and one-half of all samples collected were contaminated.[50]

It will be seen from the preceding list of adulterated foods that all social classes could be victims and that all food, from basic necessities to luxuries, was affected. For example, ice cream, which became increasingly available and popular (some 2,000 Italians plied the trade in London alone) could contain, as the London County Council's MOH was horrified to discover, 'cocci, bacilli, torulae, cotton fibre, lice, bed bugs, bugs' legs, fleas, straw, human hair, cat and dog hair'. The high incidence of diphtheria, scarlet fever, diarrhoea, and enteric fever was attributed in part to ice cream and severe warnings concerning its adulteration and unhygienic production were issued and posted in English and Italian.[51] The Privy Council estimated in 1862 that one-fifth of all butcher's meat in England and Wales came from animals which were 'considerably diseased' or had died of pleuro-pneumonia, and anthracid or anthracoid diseases. 'Carcasses too obviously ill-conditioned for exposure in the butcher's shop', the Privy Council remarked, 'are abundantly sent to the sausage-makers, or sometimes pickled and dried'. Given the consumption of such 'measly' meat, it comes as no surprise that tape-worm was common among the working-classes.[52]

For much of the century, even though so much was at stake, little was done. The comment of the *Lancet* (which led the demand for more stringent food controls) in 1831 that due to the 'caprice and neglect of the community . . . the people are allowed to poison themselves with adulterated food, without the slightest concern being manifested by the rulers of the land', was unfortunately equally applicable twenty years later.[53] It was not until Dr Hassall published his *Food and its Adulteration* in 1855 that a government committee on this subject was appointed.[54] The first of several food and drug acts was passed in 1860, enabling local authorities to appoint analysts, but it was an adoptive, not a compulsory, act, and remained practically a dead letter. Up to 1872 only seven analysts were appointed, and of these only Dr Charles Cameron in Dublin appears to have implemented the act enthusiastically. The analysts could examine food only on receipt of a complaint, and those bringing the complaint had to pay the analyst's fees. Although the Adulteration of Food, Drink and Drugs Act, 1872, still made optional the appointment of public analysts, local medical officers could now initiate analyses without waiting for public complaints, and another Food and Drug Act in 1875 defined pure food more precisely. As part of the growing professionalism of local government in England, the Society of Public Analysts was formed in 1874 and in the 1880s the Local Government Board put pressures upon local administrations to appoint analysts. Liverpool had appointed the first public analyst in 1872 and Manchester had followed in 1873. By 1877 there were 126 analysts operating in England and Wales, with almost a third of them working within London. In 1882 there were 52 county and 172 borough analysts, but there were still many parts of England where there was no analyst, or where, if he did exist, he did little work. In 1882 in Berkshire, Dorset, Hereford, Hertford, and Suffolk not a single sample was taken. The uneven administration of the food and drug acts continued throughout the remainder of the century and fines when applied were absurdly small — the average fine for the 4,319 cases of adulterated food which were prosecuted in 1899 was a mere £1.16.8d.[55] In York vendors guilty of adulterating their milk by 30 per cent with water faced only a ten-shilling fine.[56]

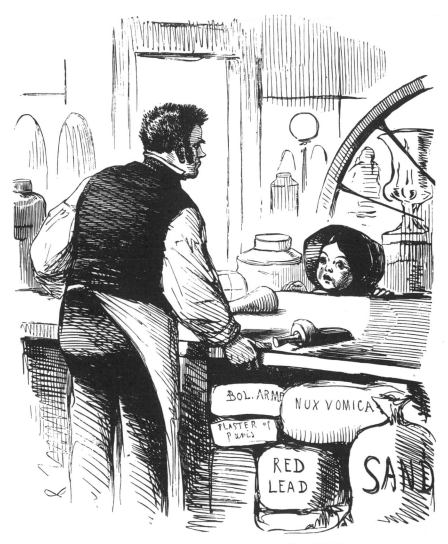

THE USE OF ADULTERATION.

Little Girl. "IF YOU PLEASE, SIR, MOTHER SAYS, WILL YOU LET HER HAVE A QUARTER OF A POUND OF YOUR BEST TEA TO KILL THE RATS WITH, AND A OUNCE OF CHOCOLATE AS WOULD GET RID OF THE BLACK BEADLES!"

2. *Punch*'s comment on the lethal ingredients in commonly consumed food and drink was part of a campaign it waged on behalf of pure food and drugs.
Source: Punch, 4 August 1855

It is a commonplace of modern medical opinion that nutrition plays a crucial role in the body's ability to resist disease and the experience of the World Health Organization indicates that where sanitary conditions are rudimentary and disease is endemic (that is, where nineteenth-century conditions prevail, so to speak), diet may be *the* crucial factor in infection.[57] This point clearly and sadly emerges in the case of nineteenth-century Ireland, where typhus deaths jumped from just over 7,000 in the year before the famine occurred to over 17,000 in the first year of the famine, and to over 57,000 deaths as the famine deepened.[58] The continued virulence and variety of infectious diseases down to the end of Victoria's reign, despite all the sanitary improvements, suggest how precarious was the balance between micro-organism and host and how marginal, in medical terms, was the improvement in diet. That death rates did decline is the result, among other things, of an improved diet; that they did not decline as sharply as the remarkable sanitary engineering of the Victorians merited was due to the low nutritional standards which, despite general improvement, still prevailed.

One of the more obvious external signs of malnutrition among the labouring classes was rickets. As we noted in the last chapter, rickets, a Vitamin D deficiency disease, could result in a narrowing of the pelvis, which in turn could make childbirth difficult and lead to complications. It could thus stunt children from birth, and it continued to be a scourge throughout life for thousands of people. Samuel Gee of the Great Ormond Street Hospital (one of the few specialist hospitals for children) discovered in 1867 that roughly one-third of the sick children under two years of age was suffering from rickets. In 1884 *every* child examined on Clydeside was found to be rachitic.[59] By the late 1880s the British Medical Association was sufficiently alarmed to undertake an exhaustive geographical analysis of the distribution of rickets throughout the nation. It concluded that though it existed everywhere, there were five main areas of concentration – the Tyneside and Tees towns; the towns of Durham, industrial Lancashire, Yorkshire, Cheshire, Derbyshire and Nottingham; the Black Country; the mining and industrial region of South Wales; and London. Although it stressed that rickets 'is mainly a disease of towns, and industrial regions and especially of large industrial towns', the only rural areas which were found to be relatively free of the disease were in Scotland, North England, North Wales, and Ireland (with the exception of Ulster County), and it was exceptionally prevalent in Cornwall, Kent, and Essex.[60] What is of interest in this study is that while rickets is caused by both lack of sunlight and a dietary deficiency of vitamin D, its geological distribution would appear to be related far more to the latter than the former.[61]

Although cod liver oil was known from the 1840s as a cure for rickets, there was no attempt to give it systematically to the poor, and rickets continued to be accepted as the normal, if unfortunate, condition of the masses – the 'English disease', as it has been called.[62] As a consequence it would not be an exaggeration to say that the *majority* of English children grew up ill-formed and ill-equipped to lead vigorous lives or to sustain the heavy labour which was their lot. Modern nutritionists have concluded that though rickets does not kill, the deformities it leads to 'may persist into adult life, at which time the shrunken chest may predispose to lung diseases . . .'[63]

Victorian urban society was overcrowded, subject to desperately low sanitary conditions both at home and at work, and was more exposed, as a transient mass, to the dissemination of viruses and bacteria. Amid such conditions an adequate diet could mean the difference between life and death, strength or debility. When the Millbank penitentiary cut the diet of its inmates from 3,500 calories to 2,644 (still well *above* the per capita national average), there was far more scurvy and dysentery, and the death rate went up.[64] It is important to note in this context that while the workhouses budgeted 3s per week per capita for food, Mrs Pember Reeves, in her study *Family Life on a Pound a Week* (1912), found that more than 2s per head was rarely spent on food by the London families she surveyed.[65] The lank-haired, hollow-chested creatures who stare out at us from the illustrations of Doré, or from the pages of *Punch*, the *Illustrated London News*, or *The Graphic*, were no exaggeration, no artist's licence, no mere rhetorical device. They graphically illustrate a race condemned by poor nutrition.

The effects of heredity and diet were apparent in the difference in stature between classes. Rowntree discovered in York that thirteen-year-old boys from the better-paid working-class families stood some 3½ inches taller and were 11¼ lbs heavier than those from poorer families. Somewhat subjectively, Rowntree considered that over half the boys from the poorer districts of York were in bad health, and he commented that they 'presented a pathetic spectacle'. Their diseased and under-developed physiques were a sad indication, he wrote, of both poverty and parental neglect. To Rowntree and other observers, the physical consequences of malnutrition, poverty and wasting diseases were only too apparent among working-class children.[66]

An extensive anthropometrical study undertaken between 1878 and 1883 by the British Association into the height, weight, and measurements of some 53,000 children revealed that eleven- and twelve-year-old boys from industrial schools were almost five inches shorter than boys of similar age from public schools.[67]

Caught up in the general concern over the nation's physical well-being in the aftermath of the set-backs of the Boer War, the Edinburgh Charity Organization Society conducted a survey of some 1,400 children in that city. It discovered that over two inches in height separated five-year-old boys from one-roomed flats from those who lived in four-roomed flats. By age thirteen this height difference had stretched to almost three inches and there was a weight difference of over eight pounds. For thirteen-year-old girls the difference in height amounted to four inches.[68] These are cold figures: Charles Booth evoked the reality behind them when he described the underfed schoolchildren he came across in his London survey:

> Puny, pale-faced, scantily clad and badly shod, these small and feeble folk may be found sitting limp and chill on the school benches in all the poorer parts of London. They swell the bills of mortality as want and sickness thin them off, or survive to be the needy and enfeebled adults whose burden of helplessness the next generation will have to bear.[69]

It was not until the twentieth century that general concern arose over the effects of poor nutrition upon the health of the masses. Well before that, however, it was argued that in one particular item and its misuse the poor were damaging their physiques. That item, was, of course, alcohol. In the second annual report of the Registrar-General (1840) William Farr wrote heatedly that

> Spirit drinking almost always ends in impairing the health; it takes away the appetite, wastes the limited means of the artizan, deprives his family of food, firing, clothing, and clean, ventilated lodgings, leads to dissoluteness of every kind and must, therefore, be considered one of the indirect, but certain causes of fevers, and other diseases.[70]

Temperance advocates stressed the damage done by alcohol to the body, but they received little sustained support from the medical profession. In its annual report for 1869–70 the National Temperance League bitterly complained that:

> amongst the numerous obstacles that have impeded the progress of the Temperance Reformation, none, perhaps, have been more powerful and perplexing than those which have sprung from the attitude generally

assumed by the medical profession in regard to the use of intoxicating drinks. Under the influence of medical sanction and recommendation, the erroneous opinions everywhere prevalent respecting the value of alcohol in health and disease have been strengthened and extended, and the results, moral as well as physical, have, in thousands of instances, been of the most ruinous and disastrous character.

Most doctors, accustomed to recommending heavy doses of brandy and port for a variety of ailments, would agree with Dr Richard Todd, who insisted that 'it is far more dangerous to life to diminish or withdraw alcohol than to give too much'. The British Medical Temperance Association of teetotal doctors was founded in 1876, but had only 235 members in 1880; the *Temperance Lancet*, founded in 1841, folded after just a few months.[71] For much of the century there was a running debate over the physical effects of alcohol on the body. The feats of the great walker, E. P. Weston, who walked 55 miles in twelve hours on beef tea, gruel and grapes, and who walked 5000 miles in 100 days (starting out from the offices of the Church of England Temperance Society), were produced as evidence on one side. They were hardly convincing to the confirmed advocates of the therapeutic value of liquor, who could always produce the counter-evidence of the beer-drinking winner of the London to Brighton walking race, or, even more impressively, W. G. Grace, who greatly enjoyed his glass of wine.[72]

At the end of the nineteenth century consumption was still as high both for beer and spirits as it had been at mid-century. It may be argued that this reflected the growing affluence of the middle classes and artisans, but there was general agreement at the time that the poorest classes were continuing to spend a disproportionate amount of their wages on drink.[73]

A survey by the British Association for the Advancement of Science in 1881 reported that drink was the largest single item of expenditure on food in the working-class budget (about 14 per cent of the total budget), followed closely by meat (11.4 per cent), and bread (8.8 per cent).[74] The accuracy of this finding must be questioned, for few workmen voluntarily offered correct information and few social workers or investigators were in a position to get it. Perhaps in some odd cases the wives, embittered by their husbands' drinking, might exaggerate the amount, but generally the working classes would deliberately underestimate their expenditure on drink. Charles Booth thought that the working man spent one-quarter of his salary on drink; so, too, did George Sims, the popular writer and journalist, who was well acquainted with working-class customs. One authority places the amount at one-third and estimates that as a consequence the working-class family suffered a loss of 17.6 per cent in their calorific intake![75] Higher wages often went into increased drinking and it was not until the rise in real wages due to falling consumer prices that the family as a whole began to share in the higher living standards. Not until the variety of food increased in the last two decades, and housewives managed to keep a steady sum for house-keeping in a period of generally falling food prices, is it likely that domestic living standards went up significantly.[76] Well-established patterns of behaviour – the payment of wages in pubs, the continuation of 'Saint Monday' on which to recover from the weekend's drinking, the stimulus to drink of overheated and unventilated workplaces, the attractiveness of pubs as refuges from slum flats – all combined to keep the level of drinking high enough to affect the nation's health.[77]

Although MOH consistently argued throughout the second half of the nineteenth century that better housing conditions and water supplies were the prerequisites for a reform of drinking habits, the problem of drink 'missed the main current of public health policy'.[78] The teetotal movement was always more of a moral crusade than an integral part of the public health movement. It was not until the end of the century, when concern mounted for England's international position and the supposed physical deterioration of her population, that closer attention was paid by authorities to the connection between drink and ill-health. Much to the alarm of the Inter-Departmental Committee on Physical Deterioration many qualified witnesses thought that drinking among women was on the rise, and it was pointed out, with considerable alarm, that, 'If the mother as well as the father is given to drink, the progeny will deteriorate in every way and the future of the race is imperilled.' The Committee concluded that the 'abuse of alcoholic stimulants is a most potent and deadly agent of physical deterioration.' Although the Committee was not prepared to go so far as to suggest that established drinking patterns were resulting in the physical deterioration of the nation, that connection was part of temperance propaganda. A prize-winning essay in a competition for children stated with youthful moral fervour that, 'Before so much alcohol was taken, the British were sturdy, strong, square-shouldered men', but now they were 'thin, puny, round-shouldered.'[79] The connection between drunken mothers and infant mortality began to attract some attention in the Edwardian period, and, rather too late to have any social effect in the Victorian period, medical authorities in the late Victorian period at last began to stress (in the words of the Birmingham MOH) that 'the drink question has a public health aspect of the greatest importance.'[80]

Like the diet, drink and drugs which all weakened the body's resistance to disease, dirt and dismally low hygienic standards were an integral part of the Victorian culture of poverty. Lack of cleanliness was an inevitable consequence of the woefully inadequate water supply of the day. It was all very well for the prescriptive literature of the day to preach to the poor, as did *The Labourers' Friend Magazine* in 1840 that 'The number of deaths in proportion to the number of people, is always found to be according to the cleanliness of their habits', but cleanliness was, quite literally, beyond the reach of large numbers of working-class families.[81] Well-meaning Victorians might associate cleanliness with Godliness, but church and chapel were far more accessible than bathing or washing facilities.

For most of the nineteenth century it took far more effort than just turning on a tap to keep clean. It involved hauling in water, perhaps a quarter of a mile or more, and carrying it, perhaps, up several flights of

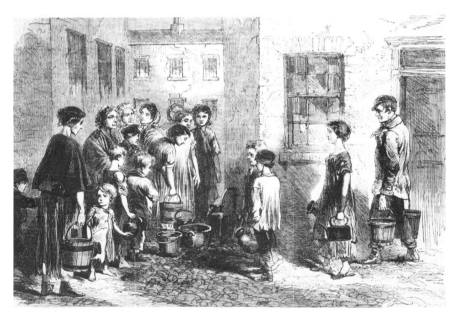

3. A street plug, Bethnal Green. Queuing for water in all weathers and carrying it back home were part of the daily round of working-class life and imposed a considerable physical burden, especially on women and children.

stairs. It is easy to dismiss this as a minor inconvenience; even Octavia Hill, the eminent housing reformer, who ought to have known better, thought that a water supply on each floor of a large tenement block, was unnecessary. Yet, for most labourers' families, lack of running water meant queuing up at the local street pump or tap, in foul weather as well as fine, carrying heavy pails through muddy and uneven streets and courtyards, an endless round of drudgery, day in, day out. Perhaps, like filth and noise, smells and overcrowding, the poor got used to it, although no doubt children would grumble when given the task. Even if it was simply yet another of the many accepted chores of working-class life, it was one which acted as a deterrent to cleanliness and thus to health.

Water was by no means universally laid on even at the end of the century. In the 1840s only about 20 per cent of the houses in Birmingham had piped-in water; in Newcastle only ten per cent.[82] In London at that time some 30,000 inhabitants were without piped water, even from communal street taps.[83] Even where water was laid on the service was often erratic; in Wolverhampton, for example, the waterworks company turned off the supply between 7.00 pm and 5.00 am. In Hanley, the largest of the North Staffordshire pottery towns, it was standard practice to turn off the water every night to build up pressure in the mains; in parts of Etruria there was no supply for weeks on end. The East London Waterworks Company did not supply any water on Sundays and in several densely-packed courts the dwellings were supplied from 4.35 am to 4.55 am only, or from 7.10 am to 7.25 am. In Bristol it was actually an offence to draw water on a Sunday.[84] In many towns the poor had to rely on unfiltered rain water butts for their water supply, and gruesome stories abounded of the consequences. In Darlington one rainwater butt was so offensive that it was eventually drained, to reveal the decomposing body of a baby which had lain there for a month.[85]

In Edinburgh in 1872 well under half the houses below a rateable value of £5 had water; in West Bromwich in the same period only 16 per cent of all the houses were supplied.[86] In 1879 over one quarter of all the local authorities in Great Britain still had no piped water whatsoever.[87] When in 1875 the Local Government Board conducted an investigation of urban water supplies it found that there were still huge concentrations of population without easy or cheap access to water. Kingston-on-Thames, Gravesend, Deal, and Uxbridge were all without a constant supply.[88] Even as late as 1904 a survey of Manchester revealed that only one water tap had been provided, on average, for every fourteen houses, and in one district the average was one for every forty houses.[89] In 1909 Gravesend was still without any piped-in water.[90]

It is significant that although water was widely sold at the street tap, or pump, it is rarely mentioned in the budgets of the poor. It was estimated in Burton-on-Trent that hand-carried water (at 1d for three buckets) cost upper-class families 11½d a week, middle-class families 5½d, and working-class families about 3d. The difference is suggestive.[91] Bearing in mind that these costs included water for cooking as well as for cleaning, the level of cleanliness among the working classes of Burton-on-Trent can be imagined. They purchased an average of nine buckets of water a week for a family of five or more for *all* purposes.

The improvements which were made in the municipal supply of water are discussed in the next chapter. The purpose of this present brief discussion of water supply is to suggest that for much of the nineteenth century domestic realities tipped the scale in favour of dirtiness over cleanliness. As late as 1894 only five per cent of the houses of Northern industrial towns had baths, for example, and as late as 1930 the figure was still under one-third; in 1940 one-third of all dwellings in country districts had no fixed bath, and 16 per cent had no bathtub of any description.[92] A bath was still something of a rarity, an object of curiosity, in Edwardian England, and later. Robert Roberts recalls that:

> When in 1910 on my mother's insistence, the landlord installed a cast iron bath (one shilling a week on the rent) several customers [of his father's corner shop] asked to be allowed to inspect it. My father took them on a conducted tour, pointing out the hot and cold water taps and the purposes of plug, chain, and overflow pipe. Till then some had never seen a bath, much less used one.

Similarly, in his marvellously evocative autobiography, *Whatever Happened to Tom Mix?*, Ted Willis describes the excitement and keen anticipation when his mother finally realized her dream and moved into a house 'which actually had a bathroom':

> My mother and I went in to look at this marvel together and my heart sank to my boots at what I saw. The walls were covered with thick, brown paper which was peeling and discoloured; the taps were rusted in and would not turn; the bath itself was chipped, stained, and filthy. Yet my mother turned to me with tears in her eyes and she bore the look of someone who had reached the end of a long journey. Within a week the taps were polished and working, and the bath clean if not shining.[93]

Among the curious neighbours there were doubtless many who thought that Roberts's and Willis's families were reaching above their station in life. In the opinion of the Chairman of the Crewe Water Committee baths were 'a great luxury' for the working classes and absolutely unnecessary.[94]

For late-Victorian working-class families bath night might entail a succession of quick dips and a hasty scrub in a long metal tub, the water of which would be replenished, but not renewed, for each new member, from a cauldron kept on the stove. Occasionally there would be lighter moments: during one such Friday night ritual one father unfortunately confused, in the dim candlelight, the two cauldrons on the stove and topped up his lukewarm bath with mutton-stew rather than hot water – 'We were most upset', recalls his daughter, 'but poor old Dad didn't seem to mind as the water must have always been polluted by the time he used it.'[95]

When managers of railway companies objected to workmen's trains, it was partly because it was the smell of the workmen themselves, not just their clay pipes, which upset the other travellers. For similar reasons, many churches made the poor unwelcome, and the poor themselves, coming into contact with the higher classes, were made acutely aware of the differences. Smell, as much as anything, separated the classes. John Liddle, the industrious and perceptive MOH for Whitechapel, thought that one of the worst smells he had ever encountered in his house-to-house inspections was when he chanced upon the poor washing their clothing:

> They merely pass dirty linen through very dirty water. The smell of the linen itself, when so washed, is very offensive, and must have an injurious effect on the health of the occupants. The filth of their dwellings is excessive, so is their personal filth. When they attend my surgery, I am always obliged to have the door open. When I am coming down stairs from the parlour, I know at a distance of a flight of stairs whether there are any poor patients in the surgery.[96]

Hard chairs, rather than upholstered ones, were kept by doctors for their working-class patients. It is possible that what Dr Liddle called 'dirty water' was actually 'wash', that is, urine kept in stone bottles until very strong and then used in washing clothes.[97] According to Louis C. Parkes, Chelsea's MOH, and a man who was compassionate towards the poor, wherever they gathered in large numbers, the working classes formed a kind of human air pollution. 'The air of a London police court', he wrote, 'furnishes a striking example of such air pollution.' Indeed, one London magistrate was forced by the odour to adjourn the court, put on his hat, and continue the hearing in the back yard.[98] 'Strong stomachs and weak noses' were two essential requirements for slum-school teachers.[99]

Given the lack of good washing facilities it is hardly surprising that the poor were both dirty and smelly. What *is* remarkable, however, is that so many of them would work so hard to keep themselves and their possessions clean in such depressing surroundings. In some working-class budgets as much was spent on soap and washing materials as on fuel, or tea and milk.[100] Hard, impervious surfaces, varnished woods, brown paint and whitewash, linoleum and oil-cloth, these were the products which helped the poor to give their dwellings an air of cleanliness, and some status thereby among their neighbours. In her autobiography, Elizabeth Flint recalls that, for her mother, the brightness and polish of an iron stove was the 'sole way of assessing another woman's ability as a housewife', and she commented drily that 'any slut could win praises from my mother if she happened to have polished up her range.'[101] For many, cleanliness became more than desirable; it became an obsession. Robert Roberts has described how some people were driven mad by it:

> Few who were young then will ever forget the great Friday night scouring ritual in which all the females of a house took part. . . . Women wore their lives away washing clothes in heavy, iron-hooped tubs, scrubbing wood and stone, polishing furniture and fire-irons. There were housewives who finally lost real interest in anything save dirt removing. Almost every working hour of the week they devoted to cleanliness and re-cleaning the same objects so that their family, drilled into slavish tidiness, could sit in state, newspaper covers removed, for a few hours each Sunday evening. On Monday the purification began all over again. Two of these compulsives left us for the 'lunatic asylum', one of them, I remember vividly, passing with a man in uniform through a group of us watching children to a van, still washing her hands like a poor Lady Macbeth.[102]

Whether they resisted or accepted it, noticed it or were unaware of it, most of the working classes lived in barnyard conditions amid stench and filth which we today would find intolerable. Body lice, nits (the eggs of lice), and bugs were inescapable. Bedding of straw was a haven for bed-bugs and so acted as a vehicle for the transmission of typhus and other infectious diseases. 'You could tell a child as come from a flee-pit,' said a contemporary, ''cos its neck 'ould all be spotted all over like a plum pudding.'[103] Bed-bugs were prominent in Roberts' memories:

And the bed bugs! With the warm days they appeared in battalions, first in the hovels, then in the better-class houses, where people waged campaigns against their sweet-odoured, sickening presence. They lime-washed bedrooms ('bug-binding' was the delicate term for this) and drenched them with 'kleenzit kleener' disinfectant. The blue flames of blowlamps licked spring mattresses, floorboards, cracked walls, and ceilings; but still they came, creeping along joists and through party walls until even the valiant cleanly housewife gave up in despair and prayed for cold weather. Through summer days one saw the 'fever van' carrying off some child who only too often would be seen no more. In school, inspection showed whole classes of children infested with head vermin; many had body lice. The worst would sit isolated from the rest in a small sanitary cordon of humiliation. They would later be kept at home, their heads shaven, reeking of some rubbed-in disinfectant. Their status did not suffer from this treatment: they had already reached rock-bottom.[104]

Every single child at one of the three Manchester voluntary day nurseries was 'infested with lice', and the nursery had to debug them every day.[105] At the turn of the century almost 70 per cent of the children examined in Edinburgh had some form of skin trouble – half the cases were from fleas or lice, and a quarter of the children had either lice or nits. Girls with long hair were the most affected.[106] Charles Booth described how the inhabitants of the slums would stay up all night fighting off the bed-bugs:

Not a room would be free from vermin, and in many life at night was unbearable. Several occupants have said that in hot weather they don't go to bed but sit in their clothes in the least infected part of the room. What good is it, they said, to go to bed when you can't get a wink of sleep for bugs and fleas.[107]

The insects were, of course, more than a mere irritant: they were the carriers of fatal diseases (see Chapter 5).

Throughout the century the working man was bombarded with advice on all sides on how to keep clean. If sanitary engineering associated with Chadwick represents the public face of the public health movement, the less well-known private aspect is represented in the efforts of the voluntary health visitors and sanitary workers who, entering the homes of the poor, tried to scour the inhabitants as well as their flats. As *The Times* sourly commented, it was a 'perpetual Saturday night', and 'Master John Bull was scrubbed and rubbed and small tooth-combed till the tears ran down his eyes, and his teeth chattered, and his fists clenched themselves with worry and pain.'[108] The cult of cleanliness swept the middle classes and was carried with religious fervour down to the masses. 'For the cult of religion and pedigree', wrote one late Victorian, 'we have substituted the cult of soap and water ...'[109] It is perhaps only natural that, since the evangelicals placed such emphasis upon Bible-reading and spiritual uplift within the bosom of the family, the England of the Evangelical revival should set about cleansing and purifying the domestic temple.

At mid-century Charles Kingsley had urged women to undertake the good work of sanitary reform, since, he argued, good public health called for vigorous house inspections, and while it was unthinkable to have government officials entering private homes, there was a special appropriateness in women doing so. Similar exhortations were made throughout the century.[110] The Ladies' Sanitary Association, which was directly inspired by such exhortations, and which in turn inspired others, believed that much disease could be prevented if only the working classes became educated in the basic laws of personal hygiene. As we saw in the last chapter they had special advice for mothers of young babies, but they arrived on the doorsteps of the working man with bundles of advice for the entire family. Behind this domestic sanitary movement was the conviction that sanitary legislation and sanitary engineering would be effective only if accompanied by changes in personal habits. 'The best-framed Acts of Parliament', wrote L. C. Parkes in the *English Woman's Journal* in 1859, 'will only result in partial reforms, until the habits of the people, engendered amidst bad conditions, and rendered careless by hopelessness, be also changed.'[111]

Public health officials of the stature of Farr, Parkes, Ransome, Roberts and Lankester, gave lectures to, or wrote pamphlets for the Association, and thus the Association served to disseminate their thinking and to bring it down to the masses. This was achieved partly through a series of penny pamphlets, such as *On Healthy and Unhealthy Homes, On Water, On Common Sense applied to Cooking, On Health of Infants, Air, Warmth, Light, The Power of Soap and Water*. Running through these tracts was a certain piety. 'I am no preacher', wrote Dr Challice (MOH, Bermondsey) in his *How People Hasten Death! Plain Words for Plain Folks*, 'but I do not hesitate to declare that hereditary diseases of the body are almost always, if not invariably, the consequence of sin, or departure from God's natural laws.' The tone was often didactic: 'I am sure, wife', promises the husband in *The Power of Soap and Water*, '... if you keep a comfortable home over my head, I am not the man to go to the public house. I

would rather come home and sit with you and the children any day.'
Doggerel was frequently used to get the message across:

> Do you wish to be healthy?—
> Then keep the house sweet;
> As soon as you're up
> Shake each blanket and sheet.[112]

Cleanliness and ventilation were the goals and one of the Association's foremost propagandists, Miss Rayney, pointed out that 'NASTY AIR' was an anagram of 'SANITARY' – 'Who'd have thought it?', she mused, 'And yet, after all, that nasty air is the breeze that has kindled the Sanitary Association into life.'[113] One Association pamphlet warned, 'the bad smell [of body and clothing] is a hint from nature of the presence of something injurious to health', and unwashed clothing 'makes the wearers offensive to all with whom they come in contact, unless it be to those whose habits have accustomed them to the sickening smell which it produces; and it becomes also a cause of disease.'[114] Thus the poor were told to employ self-help in the cause of health; they should use the 'three inspectors of nuisances – your two eyes and nose.'[115] By 1859 the Association had issued 32,000 tracts; by 1861, some 138,500, and between 1857 and 1881 it had issued 1,500,000 and had seen them adopted throughout the world and translated into all the major European languages and Japanese.[116] In a sense it must be regarded as more influential than that other great tractarian movement of the day, the Oxford Movement.

It is difficult to gauge the effectiveness of these pamphlets in raising the standards of hygiene in Victorian Britain. Read today, they preach the obvious in patronising terms, but to many they must have offered the first initiation into cleanliness. For those working-class families intent on 'bettering themselves' by adopting middle-class mores they were useful, but it is doubtful if they did reach down to the most impoverished and dirtiest families, to those who were, in any case, without easy access to water.

But the Ladies' Sanitary Association realized the limits of relying on their tracts alone. 'Tracts, however good, suitable, and well-received', the Association's Secretary admitted, 'must in a very large number of cases, remain unread, or be read so imperfectly, as to convey little information, and it is in vain to depend on their distribution only, or even principally in the work of sanitary instruction.'[117] The Association, therefore, sent out a veritable army of women workers into the homes of the poor, lending brooms and cooking utensils, brushes, whitewash, and syringes, giving coal and soap, and disinfectants. In Aberdeen in 1880 the Ladies' Sanitary Association distributed 1,228 supplies of soap, 203 washing powders, thirty bottles of disinfecting powder, and twelve limewashing brushes. In Manchester by the end of the century health visitors were making almost 36,000 house visits and in Salford, over 23,000. The object, as one lady visitor put it, was to 'go about amongst the people as *friends*, not as Nuisance Inspectors in petticoats.'[118]

To some families these house visitors armed with all the paraphernalia of bourgeois cleanliness no doubt constituted yet another intolerable invasion of privacy, an example of the penchant of the comfortable classes for interfering in their lives, a case of the way the sanctity of the workmen's home was violated in order to carry into it the disciplines of self-help and correct conduct. One clergyman claimed that the visitors were 'regarded a little as faddists' and as 'crochet-mongers, disturbers of the peace, and so forth.'[119] To many workmen cleanliness, after all, represented a surrender to middle-class pressures, to 'bourgeoisification' – 'anything savouring of moderate cleanliness', wrote Arthur Morrison in his classic novel of East End slum life, *A Child of the Jago* (1896), 'was resented in the Jago as an assumption of superiority'. The 'Great Unwashed' were by no means scrubbed out of existence. 'I am afraid there is no denying the fact', lamented the Birkenhead MOH in 1895, 'that by far the greater proportion of our lower working-class population pass their lives from year to year without washing their hands or faces directly.' The wife of one well-paid artisan admitted that she had last taken a bath some fourteen years previously, and the Birkenhead MOH maintained that a house-to-house visitation would reveal a similar sanitary state for 80 per cent of the population. Dr James Kerr, the first MOH for schools, discovered in 1894 that one-third of the school-children he examined had not taken off their clothes for at least six months![120]

The washing of hands after going to the toilet, the covering of food from flies (carriers of the deadly 'summer diarrhoea') the changing of mattress straw and bedding, the washing of underwear, the disinfecting of lousy clothing, the washing of plates and cooking utensils – all these things are difficult, if not impossible, to document, but the decline in typhus deaths before the completion of sweeping sanitary improvements suggests that the new standards of personal hygiene did occur shortly after mid-century and that the very worst personal uncleanliness was becoming somewhat rarer.[121] The work of the

Ladies' Sanitary Association was supplemented partly at the urging of the MOH by municipal effort – by the late 1890s several London boroughs, Nottingham, Birmingham, Norwich, Glasgow, Brighton, Bradford, Manchester, St Helens, Leicester, and Liverpool were employing paid female sanitary inspectors or health visitors. By 1900 women sanitary visitors were so much a part of local government that the Ladies' Sanitary Association had outlived its original purpose and was dissolved.[122] In Dublin in the 1870s the authorities gave out free disinfectant and established disinfecting stations where clothing could be treated free, blankets disinfected for only one penny and carpets for 3d. Infected beds and linens were burned and new bedding given without charge.[123] In Ipswich public disinfecting stations were also established in the 1870s, and in 1877 1,630 beds and articles of clothing were removed from the homes of the poor, disinfected and returned. An incentive to use the centres was that the owners of contaminated articles which were seized and destroyed by health officials were rarely compensated.[124]

That the poor welcomed (or were intimidated into using) these disinfectants is clear from the annual reports of the MOH. To Dorothy Scannell, writing her recollections of an Edwardian childhood in Poplar, the local disinfecting service formed a vivid memory. Every Saturday the Poplar Borough Council would hand out free disinfectant. Miss Scannell's father 'used the disinfectant as though he was attacking the devil', and on Saturday mornings Poplar High Street was a 'human ant colony' of children returning the empty bottles of disinfectant.[125] This do-it-yourself disinfecting was no doubt encouraged by fear of the methods which local authorities employed when they did the job themselves – methods which, after the mid-1880s resembled modern science fiction warfare: 'The house was closed. The wallpaper was stripped and burnt. Then either steam at 260°F was applied for 30 minutes to furniture, clothes, bedding, etc., heaped in an iron "steam chamber", or hot air at 230°F was applied in the chamber for five hours, while the rest of the house was suffused with chlorine and sulphurous acid gas for 12 hours.' The local authorities, when they employed such drastic measures, were responsible neither for the destruction of property (unless proven negligent) nor for sheltering the family during fumigation.[126] When, under the Cleansing of Persons Act, 1897, known throughout its passage more directly as 'the verminous persons bill', St Marylebone established a small bathroom with two hot water baths and disinfecting room for clothing, almost 2,000 people used the facilities during the first six months. The users were not tramps, but labouring men, and interestingly several of them had been turned down by the local railway company as too dirty to be employed. The local MOH was so delighted with the results that he wanted the Act to be made compulsory.[127]

Though art critics might have a different and less kindly interpretation, there is for the social historian of public health perhaps a special appropriateness, even symbolism, in the purchase of Sir Everett Millais's 'Bubbles' by the Pears soap company, for use as an advertisement. For the Victorians approached cleanliness in a spirit of idealism. Purity and bodily cleanliness were one. The Crystal Palace Exhibition of 1851 displayed the wares of some 727 soap and perfume manufacturers, half of them English, and by mid-century the English were well on their way to that standard which drove Treitschke to observe that, for the British, soap was civilization. In 1853 the excise on soap was removed and between 1841 and 1861 consumption of soap *per capita* doubled. By 1891 it had doubled again.[128]

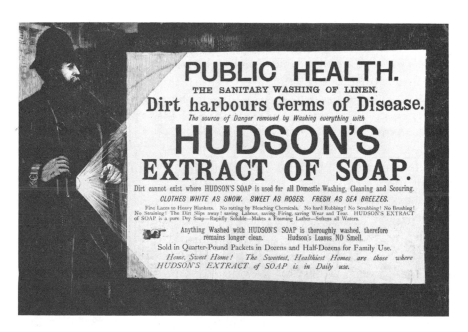

4. A Hudson's soap advertisement. The policeman, with his lantern casting light on darkness was a popular symbol for health reformers. Here *public* health is associated with *domestic* cleanliness.

Source: The Graphic, 1 August 1891

The empiricism of English science stressed the eradication of disease through the preventive approach of cleansing and scouring, rather than through the purer scientific approach of bacteriology. The miasma or effluvia theory of disease, with its belief that, wherever bad smells and noxious effluvia existed, there too were to be found the seed-beds of disease, had as its corollary the avoidance of dirt and the importance of cleanliness. Late in the century English bacteriologists made remarkable contributions to science, but one would have to say that the most characteristic attitude prevailing in the medical profession was one of almost anti-intellectual pragmatism. Typical was the intensely English utopia of Sir Benjamin Ward Richardson. His *Hygeia: A City of Health* (1875) contrasted the immediate benefits of cleanliness with the dubious benefits of pure science:

> Let us cleanse our outward garments, our bodies, our food, our drink and keep them cleansed. Let us cleanse our minds, as well as our garments, and keep them clean . . . Then all elaborate experiments for the prevention of disease will appear, as they are, mysterious additions to evil, which ought not to exist, and which of themselves might re-introduce death into a death-less paradise.

The ideal housewife, to Richardson, was one who 'would make the very act of cleaning and cleansing clean; she would make the very places for cleaning and cleansing – the scullery, the landing, the bathroom, the laundry – the cynosures of the household.'[129] As expressed by Richardson and others, the emphasis placed upon personal hygiene as a central tenet of preventive medicine amounted to far more than a merely practical approach. It was piety, a crusade of puritanical zeal against the sin of dirt.

One manifestation of this crusade was the public baths and wash-house movement. From the first it was imbued with emotion: to Charles Kingsley it was the cornerstone of the whole edifice of social reform: 'with a clean skin in healthy action and nerves and muscles braced by sudden shock [a cold bath], men do not crave for artificial stimulants. I have found that a man's sobriety is in direct proportion to his cleanliness.'[130] It was also a form of social reform which appealed to a broad spectrum of the public and which attracted the support and patronage of Prince Albert, the Bishop of London and several members of the aristocracy.[131] In 1844 the Royal Commission on the Sanitary State of Large Towns had discovered that no public baths cost less than 6d, and that there were no municipally-owned wash-houses. Even worse, most large industrial towns banned public bathing in rivers, pools, and canals.[132] Two years after the Royal

Commission presented its report, the Association for the Establishment of Baths and Washhouses for the Labouring Poor was founded. The Association was not without its critics, for it was argued that washhouses would remain empty since the poor were too debased to use them – and besides they *liked* dirt; their clothes would wear out if washed; subsidized baths would rob the poor of their 'independence'; public baths were likely to become scenes of debauchery and 'sinks of corruption', where virtuous housewives would be forced to mingle with the less virtuous; and, above all, bathing was not essential to good health.[133] But strong arguments could be mustered in support of public washhouses. Above all, paternalistic concern and self-interest combined, as is suggested in this petition to the government from the physicians and surgeons of Southampton for legislation enabling local authorities to establish washhouses:

> That disease is constantly occasioned and aggravated among the labouring classes and the poor by their want of personal and domestic cleanliness; and the overcrowding of their dwellings in very many cases renders their cultivation of habits of cleanliness almost impossible – That the rich are deeply interested in the health of the poor, not only on economic grounds, but also because many infectious disorders, which eventually attack individuals of all ranks, originate in and spread from the densely-crowded quarters inhabited by those who are poorest . . .[134]

Although the Association managed to raise sufficient funds to build a bathhouse in St Pancras (opened in 1846), it regarded itself more as a pressure group for general legislation enabling local authorities to erect washhouses. In this it was successful, for two Acts were passed (in 1846 and 1847). Local authorities, if they chose to employ the Acts, had to provide two classes of bath, and could not charge more than 1d for a cold bath and 2d for a warm one; prices for washhouses were 1d an hour or a maximum of 3d for two hours, including both washing and drying facilities.[135]

Even before this general, permissive legislation, Liverpool, one of the unhealthiest cities in Great Britain, but also a pioneer in public health (in 1846 it appointed the first MOH in Britain), had taken the initiative and built a municipal washhouse in 1841. During the cholera epidemic of 1832 an Irish immigrant, Kitty Wilkinson, the wife of a labourer, had encouraged her neighbours to use her house to wash their clothes, and her yard for drying them, and she had shown them how to disinfect them with chloride of lime. She was aided in this by the District Provident Society and by William Rathbone, a leading Nonconformist in the city. Her efforts were sufficiently popular and successful for Liverpool to follow her example; in 1846 she was appointed superintendent of the second set of baths which the city erected.[136] From this beginning the movement spread throughout the country. By 1865 there were municipal baths and washhouses in Birmingham, Bradford, Chester, Coventry, Derby (where the Board of Health had its offices in the same building as the baths), Durham, Exeter, Gateshead, Mansfield, Maidstone, Newcastle, Nottingham, Oldham, Plymouth, Preston, Stockport, Sunderland, Tynemouth, and several other towns, including, of course, London and Liverpool.[137] But at that date many large towns were still without any facilities, including Berwick, Blackburn, Bolton, Burnley, Cardiff, Carlisle, Dover, Halifax, Ipswich, Leeds, Leicester, Macclesfield, Manchester, Northampton, Rochdale, Sheffield, Swansea, Walsall, Wigan, Wolverhampton, York, and Dublin.[138] The comment of the MOH for Ipswich in 1875: 'With the exception of the few favoured ones, who have a bath fitted up in their own houses, the inhabitants of Ipswich have no means of indulging in the luxury of immersing the whole body in water', was unfortunately applicable throughout much of Britain.[139]

No town took greater pride in its municipal baths than the capital city, where, in 1865, there were public baths in Poplar, St Marylebone, St Pancras, Westminster, Bermondsey, Bloomsbury, Hanover Square, and St Martin's-in-the-Fields.[140] In the first two years that the St Pancras baths were opened (1846–8) they attracted over 280,000 bathers, and over 90,000 people used the laundry facilities.[141] The volume of traffic at the end of the century was just as heavy and indicates how few of the working-class families had adequate bathing facilities in their flats. In the first complete year of the baths in Bow (1892–3), over 73,000 people used the baths or washrooms. In Westminister the new public laundry facilities (opened in 1896) attracted some 300 customers every Saturday.[142] A penny-halfpenny was charged for the first hour and a penny for each succeeding hour; soap and starch were not provided. In the women's section of the Westminster baths there was a changing room where women could remove their under-clothing to wash them. According to Thomas Wright, the author of *The Great Unwashed*, it was a common practice for those 'within easy reach of public baths' to 'take their clean suits to the bath, and put them on after they have bathed, bringing away their [old] suits tied up in a bundle.'[143]

Most of the municipal public baths provided more facilities for men than for women. The Woolwich baths, for example, had fifty-one baths for men, but only twelve for women; in Shoreditch there were twenty first-class baths and thirty-six second-class ones for men, but only five and fifteen baths, respectively, for women. It is understandable, therefore, that according to one estimate at the end of the century only 18 per cent of all baths taken in London's public facilities were by women.[144]

Though the subject of much self-congratulation, the great municipal baths also came in for much criticism. They were rightly criticized for being much too ornate and lavish in construction. Shoreditch's baths, for example, were made of porcelain, slate, and teak. Other baths had slate walls and marble floors. Borough councils throughout London vied with one another in building public baths that began to rival provincial town halls in size and magnificence. The Wandsworth baths, described as 'English Renaissance' in style, had a frontage of seventy-five feet and cost £20,000. When Lambeth opened its baths in 1897, it could rest content that its three swimming baths, ninety-six slipper baths, and sixty-four washing compartments were the largest in the land.[145] The sums spent on the municipal baths and the style of architecture and interior fittings, suggest that by the 1890s the concept of cleanliness for the masses had so permeated national consciousness that it was an ideal which called for appropriate municipal monuments. Normally rate-conscious local authorities voted for the outlay perhaps aware of the fact that they were erecting monuments to their participation in the 'sanitary idea'. The baths and washhouses of Victorian England were, therefore, magnificent brick and stone symbols, metaphors for the progress of the age in public health.

There was also considerable debate on the relative merits of showers (douche baths) and baths (slipper, or reclining baths). At the end of the century the superintendent of Liverpool's six central baths called for the adoption of showers ('rain baths', he called them), arguing that they consumed only one-fifth as much water, encouraged more rapid usage, and 'there is no danger of drowning'. Showers were, he said, 'from a cleansing point of view undoubtedly the baths of the future'.[146] The preponderance of baths over showers also drew the criticism of the President of the Institute of British Architects; 'our idea of cleanliness', he wrote, 'seems to be to first wash our dirt off into something and then to wash ourselves in it.'[147] The debate, of course, is by no means over, and furnishes the subject for much transatlantic banter.

By 1912 well over 5,000,000 visits were being paid annually (over 3,000,000 of them in London alone) to the public baths throughout

Britain.[148] Unfortunately we know little about these users. It would be fascinating to see the way in which the separate first- and second-class bathing facilities in essentially homogeneous districts such as Deptford or Shoreditch were used. In the opinion of the superintendent of the Liverpool central baths few members of the poorest classes showed up. Not only were they embarrassed, he thought, to come into contact with artisans, but 'to many of the uneducated the word "bath" seems to strike them with terror, and taking a bath is looked upon by them as a punishment.'[149] For thousands of men and women however a visit to the public baths became a regular part of their lives. One of the few first-hand accounts we have is Dorothy Scannell's:

> When we were too old for mother to bathe in the little tin bath, we would join the older ones every Friday and go to the public baths. We would have to go early for a large crowd collected in the waiting-room when the young people came home from work. It was impossible for a girl to pop into the baths before a dance, etc. for sometimes it was necessary to wait over two hours for one's bath. We always took a book to read and always saw the local brides there the night before their wedding.

For someone as timid as the young Miss Scannell, the baths could be something of an ordeal, for she could not screw up enough courage to call out ' "more hot, or cold, in number . . . please", even though the baths rang out with the sound of such requests', and she recalls 'when the attendant said "Hurry along in number . . . please", I thought how brave the girl in that numbered bath was, to have to be asked to hurry. I wish I could just lie in the warm water with no one outside waiting for the bath.'[150] '

All these efforts in the second half of the century – the earnest administrations of sanitary workers and health visitors, the improved water supply, and the public baths movement undoubtedly resulted in a working class that was cleaner than in the first half of the century. But to contemporaries it was still a class that was grimy and which smelled both body and in clothing. Indeed, to Reynolds, the Victorian cult of cleanliness had actually served to separate and divide the classes even further. Cleanliness, he wrote, has become 'our greatest class symbol', and 'the bathroom is the inmost, the strongest fortress of our English snobbery.' Thus it was that 'the greatest and most abusive and pejorative term for the masses was *"THE GREAT UNWASHED"* '.[151] With pardonable exaggeration Reynolds concluded that 'there is today a greater social gulf fixed between the man who takes his morning tub and him who does not, than between the man of wealth and family and him who has neither.'[152] Cartoons in *Punch* leave little doubt as to who had not taken his morning bath and the poor are depicted, like the Irish, as a race apart, creatures of different stature, certainly, but also of a strange physiognomy, stunted, coarse, filthy, with matted, unkempt hair, wan, ill-formed features, weak eyes, running noses, spindly and rickety legs, hollow chests and round shoulders. The total effect was to reinforce class prejudices, to maintain and widen the social and psychological gap (which philanthropists were trying so hard to bridge) separating classes, and to make inevitable a certain distance between paternalistic reformers, however well-intentioned and compassionate, and the recipients of their charity or reforms. The urban masses were, literally, 'untouchables'.

It is difficult to say how painful the poor themselves found their filthy surroundings. While many of the slum-dwellers escaped at the first opportunity to the fresh air of the suburbs and others wore themselves out with constant scrubbing, the majority, it seems, accepted filth and smell as parts of their world, as unremarkable and unnoticeable, perhaps, as peeling paint or smog-laden air. The son of Irish immigrants to Leicester, recalling his 'poor, cooped-up vermin-infested' youth, commented:

> I am suffering much more now probably in simply remembering our state than I actually suffered then. We did not feel the dimness and squalor and foul smells – the horror of the bugs and lice and black beetles – as I now, many years after feel them: we had no other life, no other sensations and feelings. This was my life, and we knew no other to contrast it with.[153]

The picture which emerges from a sensitive work such as George Hollingshead's classic of social reportage, *Ragged London in 1861*, is of a race of men and women who were tired, beaten down, compliant. The 'deferential' nature of the Victorian working classes, which gave such social and political stability to the century, should be placed within this physical context. The slums, of course, had their colour and movement, but the human element was probably more lethargic than the bustle and irrepressible energy Dickens's cockneys would suggest. One of Dickens's writers in fact complained that Dickens insisted that his writers for *Household Words* eschew the drab and downtrodden and concentrate upon 'brilliant buoyant things'.[154] Foreigners, like Doré in his illustrations for Jerrold's *London Pilgrimage*, Flora Tristan in her *London Journal* and Taine in his *Notes Sur L'Angleterre*, focused on the capitulation to the physical environment of the slum. Flora Tristan, writing in 1840, was appalled at the condition of the working classes – 'the wretches are all sickly, rachitic, debilitated . . . thin and stooped, with weak limbs, pale complexions, and lifeless eyes; it is as if', she added, 'they were all suffering from consumption.' Taine described, with some horror, the 'thin, shrill, cracked' voices of the working-class women, 'like that of a sick owl', and drew attention to the 'pale, stringy hair, the cheeks of flabby flesh encrusted with old filth.'[155] It was not cockney vitality which the remarkable graphic artists of *Punch*, the *Illustrated London News*, the *Pictorial World*, and *The Graphic* saw in the urban masses, so much as defeat and exhaustion – a people as decayed and seedy as their dwellings.[156]

The dull resignation or mute acceptance was commented on by medical officers. 'Amidst the greatest destitution and want of domestic comfort', wrote the MOH for the West Derby Union, 'I have never heard, during the course of twelve years' practice a complaint of inconvenient accommodation.' To Dr Southwood Smith, 'there is a kind of satisfaction in the thought' that 'the wretchedness being greater than humanity can bear, annihilates the mental faculties – the faculties distinctive of the human being', and so diminishes the suffering of the poor![157] Southwood Smith was a compassionate man and an earnest sanitary reformer; there were others who, with less charity, interpreted the insensitivity of the poor to their own filth as a clear sign of their animalistic and brutal natures. Dickens captures this well in *David Copperfield* when Rosa Dartle asks, 'Are they really animals and clods and beings of another order? I want to know *so* much', to which Steerforth answers, 'with indifference,

> Why there's a pretty wide separation between them and us. . . . They are not to be expected to be as sensitive as we are . . . they have not very fine natures, and they may be thankful that, like their coarse rough skins, they are not easily wounded.[158]

Visitors to the slums, slum doctors, sanitary workers, philanthropists, journalists, 'slummers' could not help but be aghast at the sight of the poor. 'They never learn to blow their noses', wrote one venturer into their midst:

> and grow content to breathe through their mouth, and sniffle all their school days. They become so subject to sore places and abscesses as to seem rarely free from a rag or bandage on some limb or another. Countless physical deformities exist among them, which grow daily worse under such conditions; any tendency to tubercular weakness gains a great start through lack of fresh milk, and air, and sleep. Eyes, mouth, and ears are often sore and inflamed through want of cleanliness and care.[159]

As this quotation indicates, even the way of breathing marked the poor apart from those above them. Forty-four per cent of the Glasgow children inspected at the turn of the century were found to be habitual 'mouth breathers'.[160] Even sympathetic and experienced slum doctors found it difficult to accept the poor as members of the same species: one doctor wrote that he had to 'rouse up all the strength of my previous reasonings and convictions, in order to convince myself that these were really fellow-beings'.[161] As reformers, journalists, and doctors crossed social boundaries into working-class districts their sense of adventure and discovery was heightened by the very real shock that this was, after all, a common humanity. Mrs Humphry Ward, for example, in her novel, *Marcella*, described how visitors to the 'filthy gutters and broken pavements' of a 'sickening and decaying' Drury Lane slum came upon 'children squatting and playing amid the garbage of the street [who] were further than most of their kind from any tolerable human type.'[162]

It was the barely 'tolerable human type' which Rowntree, too, dwelt upon in his description of the 'pathetic spectacle' of boys from the poorer districts of York:

all bore some mark of the hard conditions against which they were struggling. Puny and feeble bodies, dirty and often sadly insufficient clothing, sore eyes, in many cases acutely inflamed through want of attention, filthy heads, cases of hip disease, swollen glands – all these and other signs told the same tale of privation and neglect.[163]

It was in this physical, as well as in the broader, social sense that there were 'two Englands' of the rich and poor. Clothing, physique, accents, smell, breathing, bone structure, posture, skin colouring – everything conspired to accentuate the differences, to exaggerate the gulf, between classes and to make contact and understanding more difficult.

If the poor smelled and looked different from the rich, even more so did their streets and dwellings, for sewering and methods of excrement removal proceeded at a different pace and according to a different timetable in the richer and poorer parts of most towns. While the more comfortable classes were beginning to enjoy the benefits of modern sewer and water systems the poorer classes often remained 'mirred in their own filth', which encouraged even further the comparison with animals. It is to the enormous problem of excrement removal, and the related topic of adequate provision of water, that the next chapter is devoted.

79

4

The Valleys of the Shadow of Death

'The next subject I desire to bring before you, namely excrement removal, I approach with some trepidation . . .'

Edward Sergeant, MOH for Bolton, *Transactions of the Sanitary Institute of Great Britain*, IX (1887–8), p. 104.

'When Good Queen Victoria came to the throne
Very little of 'germs' and 'bacilli' was known.
And a cesspool lay lurking beneath every stone.
Oh! The old smells of old London
And oh! The old London old smells.

We rejoice in a hundred most eminent firms,
Who will 'drain' us and 'trap' us on moderate terms
And secure each man's rights to his own household 'germs'.
Oh! The new smells of new London.
But oh! The new London new smells.'

sung to the tune of 'Roast Beef of Old England', *ibid.*, X (1888–9), p. 350

The urbanization of England meant that there were more jobs, a wider range of social contacts, broader cultural diversity, and infinitely greater colour and excitement in the lives of the masses. But it also threatened to return England to a more primitive age of plagues. Among the many problems which urban densities exacerbated none was greater than the accumulation of excrement, both human and animal, which was the unavoidable by-product of urban growth. 'Scavenging', as one MOH confessed, 'is not, generally speaking, a popular subject.'[1] But it was one of the greatest challenges facing Victorian society and for urban dwellers it was, quite literally, a matter of life or death. The recent books of Victorian and Edwardian photographs recapture the architectural mass above ground, but unless the mass deposits on the ground, and the pools of muck beneath, are borne in mind, the realities of the Victorian town evade us. The amassed filth, growing ever larger with the population, was part of the Victorian topography which was immediately evident to nose and eye. Though an unpleasant, indeed scatological subject, excrement removal deserves far greater attention than historians have given it.

80

To stand close to a defective sewer today is to recapture the essence of early- and mid-Victorian towns. The following pages ought to be 'read' with the nose as well as the eye, for if we were to be transported back to a nineteenth-century town it is probable that we would first be struck, not by its sights but by its smells and, like many health inspectors, we would be able to proceed only at the risk of heaving stomach and nausea. The smell of the city, a compound of broken or inadequate sewers, overflowing cesspools, poorly-drained cowsheds, abbatoirs, domestic pigsties, exposed dung-heaps, and industrial waste — 'The unmistakeable and most disgusting odour of living miasm' — was sufficiently overpowering to have a direct effect upon health.[2] In the opinion of George Buchanan, one of the MOH at the Local Government Board, 'the influence of stink as stink' was not inconsiderable. To it he attributed 'loss of appetite, nausea, sometimes actual vomiting, sometimes diarrhoea, headache, giddiness, faintness, and a general sense of depression or malaise.'[3] Occasionally as in the Great Stink of 1858 it could become a scandal, but generally what Simon described as 'the foetid gases of organic decomposition' were simply accepted as one of the disagreeable features of city life.[4]

Street refuse was made infinitely worse by the accumulations of horse manure and by the droppings of animals driven through the streets to the abbattoirs or market-place. In dry weather these droppings became caked and were blown about in air-borne particles, in wet weather they were converted into a muddy morass. Street scavengers and the crossing sweepers (these latter so prominent in the pages of Dickens and *Punch* cartoons) could only scrape and brush ineffectually at the problem, and protective clothing, especially raised wooden pattens, was necessary. In 1850 the General Board of Health commented that 'strangers coming from the country frequently described the streets as smelling of dung like a stable yard', and in that statistics-conscious age it was estimated that some 20,000 tons of animal manure were deposited on the streets of London every year.[5] In summer, when the accumulations of street and stable were most offensive, and dangerous to health, the local farmers and market gardeners were too eager to return from market to their farms to harvest or load another crop to waste time in town picking up manure, and the railway companies, busy with summer passengers, were understandably not as keen to carry manure as they were in the off-season.[6] When they did the stench was terrible: Swanley Junction, on the London, Chatham and Dover Railway, received 40–60,000 tons of manure each year, and the Local Government Board agreed with one complaint that the 'nuisance from manure [was] terrible at times; such a stench as you never smelled before; it seemed to get right into you'. Walworth in South London had at any given moment 4–5,000 tons of manure in storage, and London was ringed with such depots laden with manure for local farmers. People along the line complained that they could never open their windows, that their houses were infested with flies, and that they suffered from nausea and diarrhoea.[7]

For much of the year early-Victorian town streets were smelly, muddy rivulets. Although the Victorians often lamented the loss of rusticity, the Victorian town would strike us as an incongruous mixture of urbanity and barnyard setting, with town-houses interspersed with stables, pigsties, and slaughter-houses, and where sheep and cows jostled with horse-traffic, and pigs and chickens dwelt in close proximity to human inhabitants. Thus the town, as artifact, symbolized a rural society in rapid and uncontrolled transition. Thomas Blashill, the London County Council's architect, complained bitterly in 1901 about the combined effect of horse-drawn traffic and the Englishman's love of dogs: the horse-droppings were 'worked up into slush in wet weather and ground into dust in dry' and 'the London dog is getting either more numerous or dirtier in its habits.'[8] The continuing tradition of keeping pigs in pens or sties right in the house together with the occupants, added to the agrarian smell of the city. While sanitary inspectors saw only disease in domestic pig-keeping, the working man saw only cheap meat, and he accordingly opposed all attempts to separate him from his swine as an attack upon the 'poor man's pig'.[9] Few towns were without their piggeries tucked away among the close courts of the poorter districts, but many of the poor could not afford pens or sties, and so pigs and people jostled for living space to a degree which made the habitations of the one indistinguishable from the other. Matters were made considerably worse by the value which was put on 'pigwash' as manure.[10]

In the popular mind domestic pig-keeping, like other sanitary nuisances, was associated mainly with the Irish. According to Engels it was the Irish who brought with them the habit of living adjacent to, or with, pigs:

> the Irishman allows the pig to share his own sleeping quarters. This new, abnormal method of rearing livestock in the large towns is entirely of Irish origin. The Irishman loves his pig as much as the Arab loves his horse. The only difference is that the Irishman sells his pig when it is fat enough for slaughter. The Irishman eats and sleeps with his pig, the

children play with the pig, ride on its back, and roll about in the filth with it. Thousands of examples of this may be seen in all the big cities of England.[11]

But pig-keeping was a common practice throughout much of Britain and by no means confined to Irishmen. Its disappearance probably owed as much to the advent of cheap American and Canadian bacon as to the increasingly persistent strictures of the health authorities. In the western suburbs of London, in the 'Potteries' of Notting Hill, according to the 1851 census, only 2.5 per cent of the heads of families were born in Ireland and yet 7.2 per cent listed their occupation as 'pigkeeper'. In the 'Potteries', 'pigs were certainly the most visible feature of the local landscape, outnumbering people three to one in 1849.'[12] Not until the early 1870s was it decided in Quarter Sessions that pig-keeping was a sanitary nuisance and the pig-keepers were finally driven from the area.[13] In Ipswich so many pigs were penned in the small washhouses in the backyards of working-class dwellings that the sub-soil became saturated and the wells were contaminated; in Leicester 'the very universal practice of keeping pigs in or near dwellings in the borough' gave rise to 'intolerable stenches'; in West Hartlepool pig-keeping was stoutly defended by the poor, who with some reason argued that they were judiciously putting their money into bacon rather than beer — 'a fat pig is better than a barrel of ale' went the argument, although it was one which carried more weight on Smilesian than sanitary grounds. In Stratford-upon-Avon the residents lived with their pigs in a fashion little different from Shakespeare's time, and the local MOH's reports, like those of so many officials in other communities, were a long chronicle of repeated battle against domestic pig-keeping. In Southampton, when a doctor visited a patient who lived within 7 feet of an open cesspool into which flowed all the wash and blood of a local pig-killing establishment, he reported that the 'smell was so pestiferous that he (not being stink-seasoned) could not remain five minutes without fainting.'[14]

In Scotland things were little different; in Stirling the authorities in 1857 waged an all-out war against the pig-keepers but in 1874 there were still over a hundred pigsties in the town.[15] In Ireland pig-keeping was as much an urban as a rural way of life. In Waterford, a town of some 26,000 residents in 1891, there were 300 'piggeries' within the town's confines, only fifty of which had drainage for the manure; in Killarney in 1891 over a hundred pigsties nestled among the houses and there, as elsewhere, the manure was prized and heaped up alongside the houses.[16]

Adding their own special pungency to the air were the cowsheds. Within the city limits of Edinburgh, for example, there were, in 1865, some 2000 cows, and it was not until the Dairies, Cowsheds and Milk Shop Order of 1885 was finally implemented in the mid-1890s that the dairies (partly to escape more stringent controls on tubercular cattle) moved out.[17] For most of the century the condition of the cowsheds was notorious, but overwhelming all other animal odours was the stench of the abbatoirs. Despite the increasing importation of chilled and frozen meat in the final third of the century, slaughter houses still existed, though in diminishing numbers, in the centre of towns until the end of the century. In Manchester the blood and offal from the centrally located slaughter houses 'drained unchecked into the sewers and thence into the rivers', but when the city tried to close them down and construct a public abbattoir it was baulked by the strong opposition from the local Butchers' Guardian Association.

In 1873 London had 1,500 privately run slaughter houses; by 1897 there were still 500. For much of the century London's streets resembled those of a country town on market days. In 1876 some 349,435 cows and bulls, 1,659,324 sheep, and 14,394 pigs were brought into London to the central Metropolitan cattle market and the foreign cattle market at Deptford. Even though many were brought in by train and not on the hoof, they were, nevertheless, led through the streets from the central train termini to the cattle markets and private slaughter houses. As late as 1892 well over 13,000 cows, calves, sheep, lambs and pigs were slaughtered *each week* in London's abbatoirs. These slaughter houses were supervised by the MOH, but their waste products and blood still all too often found their way onto the streets. The slaughtering of cattle was one of the free spectacles that made town living exciting, but it augmented the filth and stench of the city.[18]

Added to all this was the filth resulting from the horse-drawn traffic. 'So long as horse traction continues', wrote one St Pancras official, streets were bound to be filthy.[19] In the 1830s 3,000,000 tons of droppings were estimated to fall on the streets of English towns, and by 1900 some 10,000,000 tons.[20] The problems of street cleaning were enormous. At the end of the century St Pancras had almost 200 men employed full-time in street cleansing at a cost of over £24,000.[21] As the century progressed increasingly sophisticated machinery was employed. In Glasgow at the end of the century horse-pulled rotary brushes were used; but the city still had to employ over 1000 men in the task.[22] The paving of the streets, which was accomplished in most

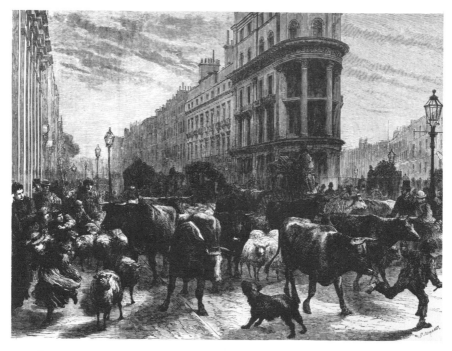

5. The 'Cattle Nuisance' was, as in this London scene, an integral part of Victorian urban life and contributed to the excitement and odour of the city as well as to the traffic congestion.

Source: The Graphic, 27 January 1877

towns by mid-century, and the later introduction of automatic washing machines, contributed to the improvement in the state of the streets, but it was not until the much maligned automobile replaced the horse that the city streets ceased to be a significant contributor to the health hazards of the age – at least until the volume of motor traffic increased to the point where carbon monoxide presented a new threat.

The disposal of all this manure presented as great a problem as its collection. As much as possible was sold to farmers, but the residue had to be carted to great dumps. Here, too, in the late nineteenth century improvements were made, for by the end of the century the largest cities possessed 'dust destructors'. In Leeds the Horsfall Destructor not only saved the Corporation 9d a ton over the old carting method but proved an invaluable means of cheaply and efficiently disposing of stray pets and diseased meat and animals. In one year it disposed of thirteen foxes, 285 dogs, 109 cats, eleven cows, seventeen sheep, twenty-nine pigs, five turkeys, and nine cwt. of pickled tongues, twenty-eight quarters of beef, 218 cwt. of shellfish and a 'sea-serpent'. Oldham's Horsfall destructor was typical. It burned street and household refuse at 2000°F, and the heat generated helped to supply part of Oldham's municipal electricity, while the clinker left as deposits was mixed with lime and used for mortar and street building.[23] Occasionally the towns could recoup some of the cost of the 'destructors' by selling the clinker and mortar.[24]

The furnaces served as symbols of municipal progress and thrift, for by generating enough energy to produce electricity they proved that light could indeed come forth out of darkness. The Shorditch dust destructor, for example, generated cheap electricity for lighting and heating the new municipal baths. The furnace was officially started with a ceremony in which prayers and piety mixed with jubilation and pride. To great cheering it was declared that Prometheus, who had stolen the heavenly fire from the earth, had now been outdone: 'for it had been reserved to the Shoreditch Vestry . . . to use the dust of the earth for light and power for the use of man.'[25]

The efficient cleansing of the streets and removal of refuse added to the pleasantness of city living and, more important, helped cut down the breeding places of flies. But of greater importance to general public health was the removal of human excrement, for of all the factors in the high death rate from preventable diseases none was more significant than faulty or inadequate sewerage. At mid-century Victorian England was in danger of becoming submerged in a huge dung-heap of its own making. Bad sanitary habits, a legacy of more casual, less densely-crowded living, where sanitary defects did not automatically produce ill-health, were encouraged by bad sewerage. According to health authorities perhaps as much as one-third of the nation's deaths were attributable to defective or inadequate sewers and drains, and to the omission, in general, as Simon put it, 'to make due removal of refuse-matters, solid and liquid, from inhabited places'.[26]

Domestic filth was an accepted and unremarkable part of the lives of the majority of Victorians for much of the century. As late as 1889 the South Shields MOH commented on how many of the houses of the poor were still without *any* sanitary conveniences so that 'filth has to be stored up in the living rooms of the family until the idea of living under any other arrangement fades from the minds of the inmates, until all-pervading filth presents itself to their minds as a law of the universe, against which it is hopeless to contend.'[27] As in other aspects of slum living, the environment bred mental depression, the depression gave rise to apathy, and the apathy resulted in a dull acceptance of existing conditions.

If many of the working-class dwellings lacked adequate sanitary arrangements, things were often not much better in the larger houses, deserted by the middle classes in their flight to the healthier suburbs. As medical officers were quick to point out, behind the seemingly respectable facades of former one-family residences, there now lived up to forty families, and the dwellings had not in any way been adapted to the sanitary needs of the new occupants. One toilet for forty families had inevitable results: the poor, wrote L. C. Parkes, 'were in the habit of depositing their excreta in a newspaper, folding it up, and throwing it with its contents out of a back window. This points strongly', he added, in a model of understatement, 'to the desirability of strictly limiting the number of people who may use one closet.'[28] No such legislation was passed, however, and for many of the urban poor what we might call conditions of sanitary overcrowding always prevailed. The General Board of Health's inspector was horrified at the conditions in mid-century Darlington: 'In 1 yard 66 persons are obliged to use 1 privy; in another 65, and in the third 63, in a fourth 54, in a fifth 45, in a sixth 41, in a seventh 35 and so on', and he pointed out that since the closets were up against the walls of the house and were undrained, the filth permeated the walls.[29]

The continued existence of large mounds of human excrement in close proximity to dwellings is all the more surprising in view of the prevailing effluvia or pythogenic theory of disease. According to this theory, which was a dominant one both in medical circles and among the general public down into the 1880s, diseases arose spontaneously from the miasma, or effluvia, or noxious gases emanated by accumulated organic matter. Put simply, bad air from putrefying matter vitiated health and produced disease. Dr Southwood Smith put it most succinctly: 'No fever produced by contamination of the air can be communicated to others in a pure air.'[30] In 1850 a surgeon told the Board of Health, 'I am of the opinion that the accumulation of excrementitious matter in privies in yards near to houses is injurious to health.' The reason he advanced was, of course, pythogenic: 'it vitiates the atmosphere and renders it unsuitable for the purposes of respiration.'[31]

The pythogenic view focused attention on the sanitary state of things, and although the theory of the propagation of disease which it advanced was incorrect, it nevertheless achieved much good. As Professor Michael Flinn has written:

87

miasma might not actually convey germs from a diseased to a healthy body; but in the absence of an exact and accurate knowledge of the means of infection, it was not a bad guide. The eradication of miasma – not entirely achieved even by the mid-twentieth century – was a sound instinct, and could do nothing but good.[32]

That smells and stinks caused disease was not proven, but where excrement lay there also were the breeding grounds for disease-carrying flies and air- and water-borne germs. Although the effluvia theory offered little stimulus for empirical biological research, by its stress on a pure environment it encouraged the public health movement and the sanitary reforms we associate with Edwin Chadwick. 'Sewer atmosphere', 'filth clouds', and 'miasmic gases' were pollutants, obvious to both eye and nose. William Farr at the Registrar-General's Office gave expression to this when he wrote:

> Every population throws off insensibly an atmosphere of organic matter . . . and this atmosphere hangs over cities like a light cloud, slowly spreading – driven about – falling – dispersed by the wind – washed down by the showers . . . The exhalation from sewers, churchyards, vaults, slaughter-houses, cesspools, commingle in this atmosphere, as polluted waters enter the Thames; and notwithstanding the wonderful provisions of nature for the speedy oxidation of organic matter in water and air, accumulates, and the density of the poison (for the transition of decay is a poison) is sufficient to impress its destructive action on the living – to receive and impart the processes of zymotic principles – to connect by a subtle, sickly, deadly medium, the people agglomerated in narrow streets and courts, down which the wind does not blow, and upon which the sun seldom shines.

It was, in Farr's opinion, to this cause that the high mortality rates in towns could be ascribed:

> the people [in towns] live in an atmosphere charged with decomposing matter, of vegetable and animal origin; in the open country it is diluted, scattered by the winds, oxidized in the sun; the vegetable world – the great organizer – incorporates its elements, so that, though it were formed proportionally to the population, in greater quantities than in towns, it would have less effect comparatively.[33]

Some twenty years later Farr was still emotionally writing of effluvia as if it were a murderer at large, a rabid beast prowling the back alleys of the congested cities: 'zymotic poisons, as dangerous as mad dogs, are still allowed to be kept in close rooms, in cesspools, and in sewers, from which they prowl, in the light of day, and in the darkness of night, with impunity, to destroy mankind.' Farr even thought that one could draw up an effluvia map for London, with the darkest clouds hovering over the low-lying, densely-packed, riverside parishes, and the lightest wafting high over Hampstead and other outlying parts.[34] When the germ theory of disease first gained currency in England in the mid-1870s, it merely reinforced the existing horror of filth and stench, for, as Ransome, one of the leading health reformers, put it in 1878, some believed that 'germs of disease . . . arise spontaneously from the filth that surrounds them, and others . . . allow that putrefying animal matter is their foster parent . . .'[35]

Whether, as in Simon's earlier career, one believed that disease was spread by 'sewer atmosphere' or (as Simon came to accept by 1873), by 'molecules of excrement' and 'miscroscopical forms', whether, that is, one held the miasmic or the new germ theory, it was apparent that street scavenging and cleaning, pure food acts, and other reforms would have only a limited success so long as old methods of excrement removal prevailed.[36] Yet these methods did persist well into the second half of the century, and not only lessened the impact of reforms in other areas (especially on infant deaths), but also added immeasurably to the physical discomforts of the close living quarters of the masses.

In the first half of the century cesspools were the most common form of excrement disposal in small and large communities alike. But as urban populations became more densely-packed so these cesspools became choked, adjoining land became saturated, and near-by wells contaminated. To Simon cesspool gases formed 'a climate the most congenial for the multiplication of epidemic disorders. . . .':

> It requires little medical knowledge to understand that animals will scarcely thrive in an atmosphere of their own decomposing excrements, yet such . . . is the air which a very large proportion of the inhabitants of the City are condemned to breathe . . . in a very large number of cases [the cesspool] . . . lies actually within the four walls of the inhabited house; the latter . . . receiving and sucking up incessantly the unspeakable abomination of its volatile contents. . . . where the basement . . . is tenanted, the cesspool lies – perhaps merely boarded over – close beneath the feet of a family . . ., whom it surrounds uninterruptedly, whether they wake or sleep, with its fetid pollution and poison.

'Now here', he concluded, 'is a removable cause of death.'[37] In 1841 London had some 3,000 known cesspools and countless unknown ones, and even within one relatively efficient Metropolitan Commission, that of Holborn and Finsbury, only about one-third of all the houses in the 1840s had communications with main sewers. Parts of the City of London, in Simon's memorable phrase, had a 'cesspool city' beneath them.[38] In Leeds, during the cholera fear of

1832, when an effort was at last made to cleanse some of the town's many cesspits, over seventy-five cartloads of filth were taken from one cesspool alone. Yet not until the second half of the century were cesspools cleaned out on a regular basis in Leeds.[39] In Chichester in the 1860s, even though it had a population of only 9,000, the cesspools were located so close to the wells that the drinking water was contaminated.[40] As late as 1876 in Stockport the railway workers' dwellings were 'surrounded with swamps (not merely pools) of sludge, slops, and other offensive matters, resulting from a want of drainage and privy accommodation.' These pools were so large that 'the women and children were obliged to navigate their way on planks, blocks of wood, and old doors.'[41] In Ipswich the MOH literally and metaphorically uncovered immense cesspools in the centre of town which had not been cleared out and were bursting with the accumulated filth of twenty or thirty years' use. Perhaps this state of affairs was not surprising, for although it had a population of some 45,000 inhabitants, Ipswich employed only four men to remove all of its cesspool filth. Even when these cesspools were cleaned, only the solid matter was removed, leaving the liquid matter to saturate the sub-soil and seep into the water table. The Ipswich MOH, like so many other MOH, considered that the first priority was to cleanse the cesspools and only then to move on to alternative forms of excrement removal. In his first three years he had improved almost 2500 open middens, roofing them over and making them water-tight. Yet in 1893 the Local Government Board could still complain that the Ipswich authorities were lax in their system of excrement removal and that they cleansed the cesspools only at very irregular intervals and then only 'when full'.[42]

It would be wrong to suggest that cesspools were found only in working-class neighbourhoods. Gwydyr House, where the first Board of Health sat in 1848, had nine cesspools, 'all full and overflowing' in its basement. At Bowood, the country seat of Lord Landsdowne, the basement was a virtual sewer, as was Earl Grey's at Hawick. As we have noted, Windsor was notoriously ill-drained. Marlborough House, Spencer House, and the town house of the Marquis of Bristol in London all had leaking and dangerously inadequate sewers, and Cambridge was described in the 1880s as 'an undrained, river-polluted, cesspool city.'[43]

The cleaning of cesspools created such a stench that it is easy to understand why local authorities would hesitate to begin the vile task. Most towns in the early Victorian period left the job to private contractors, and despite the cholera visitations of 1832 and 1848 which drew attention to the cesspools as possible sources of fever, there was no concerted nation-wide movement to clean up the cesspools until well after mid-century. As late as 1890 the sanitary authority for the villages in Pembrokeshire did not offer any free cleansing service, and so the deep cesspools there were overflowing. As elsewhere the Pembrokeshire farmers tapped the liquid manure when they needed it, but that was irregularly, and so the villagers lived on top of semi-liquid pools of excrement.[44] When local authorities tried, as did Derby, to recover the cost of cesspool cleansing from the house owners they were refused permission by the Local Government Board.[45] Since the private contractors would charge up to 3s for removal, few working-class tenants or slum landlords would, or could, pay the price. In any case, the cleansing process was dreaded. 'Night-soil men' were described, not surprisingly, as 'very filthy in their appearance and habits', and their labour filled the air with nauseating smells and was, in the opinion of one Leeds doctor, 'horribly disgusting, a reproach to a civilised community . . . an offence against common humanity.'[46] Given the effluvia theory, the stench every time a cesspool was cleaned out must have encouraged the sentiment that it was better to let sleeping dogs lie.

However harmful to health urban cesspools were, the only readily available alternative at the beginning of Victoria's reign – the dung heap – presented even greater health hazards. Just as subterranean swamps polluted the subsoil beneath the Victorian town, so dungheaps polluted the atmosphere above. Those who picked over these mountains of filth and assorted rubbish for something salvageable or saleable were, in the eyes of the Victorians, the 'residuum', just as the heaps themselves represented another type of residuum. There were few communities, rural or urban, without heaps of accumulated excrement as an all-too apparent feature of their topography. In 1865 the Privy Council turned its attention to Seacroft, whose sanitary condition was similar to that of so many picturesque villages. 'None of the cottages have any drains whatever. It is the practice to throw everything in the shape of sewage, garbage, refuse, and even solid excrement into the highway, onto the Green and the adjacent midden heaps, and into a ditch if such be handy. . . . Almost every cottage has in front of it a midden-heap.'[47] In the northern colliery towns at the same time the Privy Council discovered that

> Middensteads and privies are rarely met with, many long rows of cottages have no convenience of either kind. The whole of the roadway, both before and behind the rows, is generally a succession of dust heaps,

on to which are thrown all slops, garbage, and refuse, and the emptyings of such chamber utensils as are used. The heaps and neighbouring roadway being far oftener used for all purposes of personal easement without the medium of any utensil.

Thus 'throughout the hot summer months [dung-heaps] are allowed to reek in the sun immediately under the windows and close to the pantries or food cupboards of the cottages.'[48] In Greenock, which had almost 50,000 inhabitants when the Privy Council visited it in the mid-1860s, the majority of houses were without any toilet facilities whatsoever. Consequently

> the common method of getting rid of refuse in houses is by depositing the contents of chamber vessels with ashes and other filth in the roadway between the hours of 10.00 pm and 8.00 am. For the fourteen hours of the daytime, such matters have, for want of other means of disposing of them, to be voided and retained inside the close and crowded rooms, no matter whether the inmates be grown men or women of various families, or whether they are in sickness or in health.[49]

The old cry of 'gardez-loo' sung out from the windows of Edinburgh warned of a custom that continued well into the Victorian era. As late as 1892 the MOH for Lanark was complaining about the slops, including faecal matter, which were being thrown out of windows and doors. Convictions for 'emptying chamber utensils in the street' were still 'fairly numerous' in Manchester in 1845.[50]

While the density of houses and people made the lack of toilets and sewers more potentially dangerous in the towns, rural conditions were even more primitive. Simon summarized in 1864 the findings of the Privy Council:

> The most various accumulations of animal filth in closest proximity to dwellings, entire absence of drainage, and drains inoperative and stinking, ponds and ditches equivalent to open cesspools, drinking-water polluted and made poisonous with refuse – such are the evils which . . . local authorities are doing nothing, or nothing adequate, to remove.[51]

In Cambridgeshire it was customary for landlords to provide no privies at all for their rural tenants but 'only a hole dug at his cost, over which the tenant may erect a sort of sedan chair, which he carries away on leaving.'[52] In this, as in other areas of life, the distinction between classes was enormous, for the total absence of privy accommodation, or at best a mere hole in the ground, continued to an age when the more affluent were providing themselves not only with modern dry-closets, but with w.cs. The sanitary habits of the poor, reinforced by want of proper facilities, only served to confirm class prejudices and to heighten the sense that the poor were a race apart, as much removed from the privy pails of respectability as they were beyond the pale. Thus effect was confused with cause, and the filth of the human pigsty could be blamed upon the degraded habits of the pigs.

Old habits of course die hard, and just as in our own century the cry was raised that it was no use whatsoever for local councils to provide the poor with baths since these would inevitably be used for storing coal, so in the nineteenth century it was argued that when conscientious landlords did take the trouble to provide adequate privies the poor only destroyed them or preferred dung heaps which brought in some money or could be exchanged for a potato patch.[53] Well into the century thousands of labourers were not given any alternative to the dungheap, though. Dr Hunter at the Privy Council might condemn 'the constant . . . habit of indoor defecation' among the mining community of Northumberland and hold it 'unnecessary', but in the same breath he could describe how, in one community of six hundred pitmen's families, there was not a single privy: 'The women and children dung', he wrote, using a word generally reserved for animals, 'into pots, which are emptied into . . . bays (or recesses sunk immediately in front of the house), the men dunging away from home, valuing their dung and depositing it in the garden if they have one.' Hunter commented that he suspected that 'they do not really feel the want of privies . . . privies, except as a means of storing valuable dung have hitherto been a failure among them.'[54]

In Dublin the MOH claimed that the poor relieved themselves in 'any utensil handy', and then made 'use of the same vessel for the [drinking and cooking] water', and that while the children went outside to relieve themselves in the garden or on the floors of the outside privy (if one existed), the women preferred to use pots within the house.[55] In Croydon's town centre the poor inhabitants used alleyways for urinals, much to the disgust of one member of the local board who complained that he was obliged to keep his blinds down to shut out the scenes of animalistic conduct.[56] Given the inadequate facilities it is difficult to think what alternative was available, either in Dublin or in Croydon or elsewhere. In Neath, for example, there were almost 500 dwellings which had no toilet facilities whatsoever, not even a common cesspool, and in another 200 or so houses, with a combined occupancy of almost 1000 residents, there were only forty privies, but 'nearly all in such a state as to be unsuitable'. Little wonder that over half the inhabitants were 'compelled to exist in [a] daily state of discomfort and degradation.'[57]

As late as the 1870s Simon was in despair over the lack of toilet facilities and the consequent habits of the poor. In Wakefield, even in the broad daylight, he wrote in 1869, 'people are seen easing their bowels into the beck which afterwards supplied them with drinking water' and he commented that such things existed throughout England, and entailed 'such filthiness of life as can only be stigmatized as bestial: but against which, in the present state and circumstances of the law', it was impossible 'to take systematic and really effective action.' By this time Simon was convinced that much of infant mortality, loosely dismissed by coroners as 'convulsions', was really 'excremental poisoning' and he called, in increasingly urgent and eloquent terms, for a massive assault on the primitive methods of excrement disposal still existing:

> It has long been among the most fixed of certainties which have relation to civilised life that wherever human population resides, the population cannot possibly be healthy, cannot possibly escape recurrent pestilential diseases, unless the inhabited area be made subject to such skilled arrangements as shall keep it habitually free from the excrements of the population.[58]

The following year Simon's team of investigators was drawing the government's attention to 'arrangements for excrement disposal and water supply such that people must drink their own excrement' (this, in Nottinghamshire); or to 'little or no drainage . . . [and] want of privy accommodation' (in Cornwall), or to 'widespread fouling of earth and air with excremental filth' (Lancashire).[59] In 1874, when Simon came to write up his first annual report as MOH to the newly formed Local Government Board he was still harping on the same theme. Based upon an extensive sanitary survey of some of the largest towns and also representative villages throughout Britain, Simon concluded

> There are houses, there are groups of houses, there are whole villages, there are considerable sections of towns, there are even entire and not small towns, where general slovenliness in everything which relates to the removal of refuse-matter, slovenliness which in very many cases amounts to utter bestiality of neglect, is the local habit; where within or just outside each house, or in spaces common to many houses, lies for an indefinite time, undergoing foetid decomposition, more or less of the putrefiable refuse which house-life, and some sort of trade-life produce: excrement of man and brute, and garbage of all sorts, and ponded slop-waters; sometimes lying bare on the common surface; sometimes unintentionally stored out of sight and recollected in drains or sewers which cannot carry them away; sometimes held in receptacles specially

provided to favour accumulation, as privy-pits and other cesspools for excrement and slop-water, and so-called dust-bins receiving kitchen-refuse and other filth.

Both air and water were being polluted, Simon insisted, and he earnestly called upon the nation 'to introduce for the first time, as into savage life, the rudiments of sanitary civilisation', Simon argued that if the existing state of sanitary knowledge were applied uniformly throughout the nation about 125,000 lives a year could be saved: failure to isolate infectious diseases and poor excrement removal were, he held, jointly responsible for most of the unnecessary deaths.[60]

Public health historians, perhaps focusing too narrowly on the splendid creation in the 1860s of a system of main sewers in London, have assumed that significant improvements took place throughout Britain in that decade. Simon's investigations revealed a much slower and uneven pace of reform. Primitive and defective privies and the dry conservancy methods of disposal continued to exist down to the end of the century, and at the end of Queen Victoria's reign w.cs were still unknown to the majority of her subjects.

Nevertheless there were marked improvements and these tended to take place in three stages. The first was the drainage of cesspools, making them smaller, water-tight and air-tight and thus self-contained. The second step was to introduce a system of dry conservancy into the homes of the poor. Only after water was laid on could the w.c, the third stage, be adopted.

Leicester was typical of many towns in the way it tackled the problems of excrement removal. At mid-century it had almost 3,000 uncovered cesspits, covering 1¼ acres. These were emptied more regularly, properly covered and drained and gradually made smaller. Then they were slowly replaced with the pail system, which put an end to seepage into the sub-soil; then followed a period of experiments with different cleansers for the pails – ashes, earth, disinfectants and deodorants; only in the last few years of the century was the final stage, the replacement of the pails by w.cs, begun in earnest. In 1895 Leicester had 6,700 pails, 11,000 ash-pits, 17,000 ash-bins and 13,000 w.cs.[61]

Of the dry conservancy methods, the privy midden was both the most primitive and most common in the first half of the century. At its worst the privy midden was little better than a small, private cesspit, with poor drainage and considerable leakage into the soil around. It was designed to have brick or metal sides and base, but these were often poorly constructed. As late as 1900, for example, the local medical officer wrote that most of the 6,418 privy middens which were still to be found in York were in a dangerously insanitary state. Many of them were either leaking badly from their porous walls and bases or were so full of excrement that they were overflowing. In either case they were saturating the soil around.[62] After Victoria's death the York MOH was still complaining about the state of the town's middens. 'Have you', he asked his colleagues in the pages of *Public Health*, 'watched flies and other insects playing about the middens, and seen them go into the house and into the pantry, depositing filth on food?'[63] York was by no means unusual in its number of privy middens: Manchester in 1869 still had 38,000 privy middens and these outnumbered the w.cs four to one.[64]

The pail or pan system was clearly an improvement over middens. Pans could be supplied to the houses, regularly collected, emptied, scoured, and disinfected, and re-used. They were relatively clean, saved the sub-soil from saturation, and above all did not require offensive and prolonged cleansing operations near dwellings. They also offered an alternative to costly sewers, did not depend upon water supplies and could not be damaged if bulky objects were thrown into them. Their removal was also much easier than the old scavenging of the cesspits in narrow courts and alleyways of towns like Liverpool, where almost one-quarter of the inhabitants lived in the 2,000 unsewered courts of the town.[65]

It would be tedious and repetitious to describe in detail how the pan or pail dry conservancy method was adopted in town after town after mid-century, but it is instructive to take a quick look at some of the larger communities. In Edinburgh over 14,000 houses had been converted to the pail system by 1873. Collection began at 6.00 am, and householders could be fined 40s if they did not have their pails ready on collection day. The tenants, however, appear to have been nervous about their pails being stolen, and so they were known to dump the contents outside the house rather than leave the pails outside. It seems also that in most working-class flats there was no special closet or privy for the pails, and so they were placed in the living or sleeping rooms. The early hour of collection was dictated by the smells which inevitably accompanied the process, but in Hull people could not be persuaded to have their pails ready at 5.00 am, when collection began; similarly night-time collection ran into difficulties.[66] Like many other towns, Edinburgh had at first relied upon private contractors to collect the pails, but then did the job itself, and in so doing had saved £2,800 a year. Nevertheless, although the Corporation in 1873 managed to realize £5,493 from the sale of manure, this did not go very far towards the costs of collection which, with some 200 collectors and sixty-eight horses, amounted to £21,605. By this time Edinburgh was removing some 56,000 tons of excrement a year from its dwellings.[67]

In Leeds, in 1871, there were still 20,000 privies, ashpits, and middens. Ten years later when it was finally decided that these ought to be cleaned out, 28,000 tons were removed during the first year's operations, and another 46,000 the following year. Although Leeds slowly adopted the pan method, the great middens still existed into the 1870s, and according to one contemporary report 'the stench in Leeds from 10.00 pm to 4.00 am' when these were periodically cleaned out, was 'something fearful.'[68] The cost of converting from middens to pails acted as a deterrent: in the mid-Victorian period a hundred pails and lids cost only £23 but it cost a further £2 a privy to convert from midden to ash-pail, and these were considerable costs for a large town. Contrary to expectation, the costs of cleaning and removing (generally on a weekly basis) the pails was often higher than the cost of cleansing cesspits. In Leeds, for example, it cost 7s a ton to remove and clean the pans as against 2s 6d per ton to empty the cesspits. Similarly, when Bolton went over to the pail system costs jumped from 3s 6d per house for cleaning the old cesspools to 53s 6d per house for removing the pails.[69]

Manchester decided in 1845 to undertake the cleansing of its privies and cesspools rather than contract out to private firms; at that time this was a task which involved cleaning about 30,000 privies of roughly 70,000 tons of excrement a year.[70] A by-law of 1845 required a separate privy for each new house, and between 1845 and 1847 Manchester installed privies in almost eight per cent of the existing houses.[71] The city hoped that it could make a profit, or at least break even, from its removal operations, and it set about the task with vigour, employing in 1846 112 men to clear the accumulated filth – a chore which took a quarter of a year, during which the crews averaged 1000 privies a week.[72] In 1874 and 1875 15,000 separate cesspools were cleansed and in 1877 40,000 midden closets were converted to pails.[73] By the 1880s Manchester was collecting over 80,000 tons of 'nightsoil' and almost 50,000 tons of street filth and manure each year in its Holt Town collection depot alone.[74] Over 60,000 privies had been reconditioned or converted to the dry conservancy method by 1881 (the year Manchester obtained legislation requiring w.cs in all new dwellings). As late as 1911 two-thirds of Manchester's working-class population lived in houses which still had the pail system, ash-boxes, or a privy midden. Great improvements had certainly been made, but in the opinion of Manchester's MOH, the failure to introduce a comprehensive sewer system backed up by w.cs accounted for the high incidence of typhoid, scarlet fever, and diarrhoea in the city's working-class neighbourhoods.[75]

In Birmingham there were still almost 20,000 middens in 1871, covering some thirteen acres; many were little better than open cesspools, but there was no local by-law governing their construction or location. The Privy Council commented in 1870 that 'it is common to find huge, wet, foetid middens, uncovered, undrained, some of them as deep and big as the foundations of an ordinary cottage.'[76] Conditions had not improved ten years later. Writing in the mid-1880s the local MOH, Dr Alfred Hill, described the typical cesspit:

> The pit is unnecessarily deep and large, it is open to the rain, it is not watertight, sometimes not drained, or, if drained, the outlet becomes obstructed, a volume of liquid filth, stagnant and horribly offensive from decomposition, accumulates, poisoning the air for a considerable distance, while soakage goes on into the ground, polluting it to an extraordinary degree, and finding its way to the surface wells from which the tenants draw their domestic supply . . . The pollution is not, however, limited to air, soil, and water, but owing to the improper situation of the pit, the interior of houses are invaded by the liquid contents.

Such cesspits were numerous in the city. Dr Hill's programme for Birmingham was similar to that adopted in so many other towns — first, the substitution of small shallow middens for the huge pits, then the substitution of removable pans and pails for the small middens. Birmingham in 1875 had 8,000 w.cs but these put a great strain on its sewer system and as late as the 1870s it was thinking of imposing a special tax on w.cs. In 1875 Birmingham still had 7,000 pail privies and 35,000 privy middens. It took well over a hundred men to cleanse the city of its 'night-soil' and remove it to the 127-acre sewage farm on the outskirts of Birmingham.[77]

The dry conservancy system required a considerable work force. In Dublin, where in the early 1880s there were over 18,000 ash-pits (the only way to clean half of them was to carry the contents through the house), the city had to employ 110 men and engage thirty-nine horse-driven carts to remove the filth. The cost of removing and processing under this dry conservancy method was considerable. About one-fifth of the total amount spent on public health measures in Newcastle between 1865 and 1882 went on ash-pit cleansing.[78] Glasgow, which,

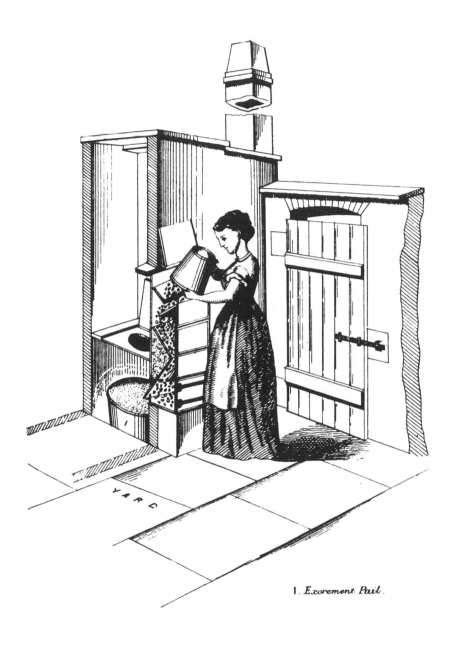

6. Dry-Ash Closet, Manchester. As late as the First World War over half of
  Manchester's working-class population relied on similar methods.

Source: Parliamentary Paper XXXI (1874), 'Supplementary Report to the
  Local Government Board, Appendix 7', plate XIX

with the 1862 Police Act, had given the police the task of refuse removal, was employing 240 men, called 'wheelers' by the mid-1880s, in the removal of 'night-soil'. The town had to use 175 horses and 600 railway wagons to get the 700 tons of refuse it collected daily out of the city. At this time there were 3,000 pails in the houses and another 1,200 in the town's factories. All told it was costing Glasgow well over £20,000 a year in removal.[79] Not until the very end of the century did Glasgow proceed with a system of w.cs to replace these pails; it did not have a modern and comprehensive sewer system until 1893. At the end of the century the predominant form of excrement removal in Nottingham was still *via* pails, and it cost the town £18,000 a year to process the 40,000 pails in the city. It was estimated that if these could be converted to w.cs, the town would save roughly £10,000 p.a. Similarly in Leicester at the close of the century the Borough Surveyor estimated that if the town went over from pails to w.cs it could save at least £600 p.a. At that time it was costing Leicester £3,000 to move the 10,000 tons of excrement which accumulated every year.[80]

The municipalities hoped that there was some truth in the popular saying 'where there's muck there's money' and that they would be able to defray some of the costs of collection by selling the excrement as manure to farmers. The town was thus, in a certain sense, still dependent upon the countryside. But the towns produced far more waste-products, both animal and human, than the country could use, and the market for town-made manure, at best uncertain, was further dislocated by the importation of cheap fertilizers, such as South American guano.[81] An acre of market garden could absorb forty or fifty tons of manure annually, however, and in the 1860s ash-pail excreta could fetch as much as £3 a ton (and this was much cheaper to the farmer than phosphate fertilizers, which could cost over £7 a ton). It was natural, therefore, for municipalities to hope that they could market excreta. Tamworth, as late as 1872, was putting its excrement up at public auction![82] When Manchester took over the operation of excrement removal in 1845 it hoped to make at least £10,000 a year, at the going rate of 3s a cartload, from its sale to the local farmers. It was, for a town of Manchester's commercial nature, a grave miscalculation: by mid-century the cost of excrement removal was *twice* the potential value as manure.[83] Yet at the beginning of the present century Manchester was still driving 'a large and thriving trade' in the sale of its waste-products. True to its commerical traditions it marketed excrement as 'special concentrated manure', fish and animal refuse was made into oil, tallow, soap, and sold 'on a commercial basis', and clinkers from street refuse were turned into mortar and sold 'at a fair profit'. Nevertheless, the city spent over £177,000 on the processing of these products and realized under £43,000 on their sale, and the local market for manure was so depressed that the Corporation had to give its excrement away.[84] Dublin, Glasgow, Nottingham, and other cities suffered similar disappointments.[85]

The recycling of the towns' excrement back into the land was thus, despite the high hopes entertained for it by Edwin Chadwick and optimistic town officials, a failure, or at best a clumsy, smelly, expensive operation. If the dry conservancy method was to be at all hygienic the pails had to be sanitized (often with sulphuric acid), and this reduced its value as agricultural manure. When in 1878 the Local Government Board conducted an extensive survey into town sewage systems it discovered that none of the large towns it inspected had managed to break even on sales to farmers.[86]

Despite the problems involved and the fact that (as the Local Government Board put it), 'it is liable to be a nuisance during the period of its retention, and a cause of nuisance during its removal', the dry conservancy method was the predominant form of excrement removal throughout Britain in the second half of the nineteenth century.[87] Only in the last decade did the third stage of sanitation – water-borne sewage and modern filtration and treatment plants begin to replace the older system in the major cities of Britain.

Certainly one reason why sewer systems were not adopted earlier was their cost. Ratepayers' associations, such as the Land and Houseowners' Association in Liverpool, were generally opposed to a system which called for massive engineering expenses and attendant increases in the local rates.[88] The rates were a major concern, but they were by no means the only argument used against the adoption of w.cs. The effluvia theory, for example, could work as much against the building of sewers as for it, for while it was argued by some that drains were an effective and safe way of getting miasma underground and effluvia flushed out of residential areas, others maintained that defective pipes brought sewer gases, and hence disease, right into the home. To some the sewer was a symbol of sanitary progress; to others it was simply a costly and dangerous fad. While Ruskin rhetorically declared that 'a good sewer' is 'far nobler and a far holier thing . . . than the most admired Madonna ever painted', others drew a somewhat different picture of the family, serenely sitting around the family hearth unwittingly breathing in the noxious vapours from the sewer system.[89] In 1848 the Dublin Sanitary Association bitterly opposed the idea of w.cs, arguing that 'it was erroneous in principle and highly detrimental to the health of towns to permit under any circumstances the discharge of excretory matter into sewers.'[90] In a period when drains were often laid with no sound knowledge of how to trap them to prevent the flow-back of gases, one can well understand why some householders would be reluctant to take advantage of the opportunity to connect to main sewers, and why they would not wish to extend the sewers into working-class districts, where the quality of connecting pipes would be lower. It was only after a design breakthrough in 1862 that the cistern for storing water (for drinking and washing) could be kept separate from the w.c.[91]

One hardly needs to resort to the elaborate Freudian anal speculations which have recently been offered to explain Herbert Spencer's stand against laws which would compel house-owners to link up with the main sewer system.[92] As late as the 1860s outbreaks of fatal typhoid had been traced to defective drains and sewers, and well-informed and well-intentioned men could argue, with conviction, that 'the connection of the dwellings of the inhabitants with the main sewer [was] a fruitful source of disease'. Some towns even imposed fines if houses were connected to main sewers, and, as was the case in Manchester, one of the first tasks of the MOH was often to *disconnect* house drains from storm sewers (which had never been designed to accommodate anything but rain water) and convert the town to the apparently safer and more effective dry conservancy method.[93] To be effective, w.cs had to be kept in good working order, and in an age of cheap and shoddy fixtures and often ignorance or carelessness on the part of the user, sanitary officials were rightly concerned that broken fixtures would make the w.cs far less safe than the reliable and simple pans or pails. In 1885 90 per cent of the houses inspected by the Jewish Sanitary Committee had broken or unflushable w.cs, and in 1890 only *one* per cent of 3000 houses inspected in London was 'free from defects in plumbing and draining'.[94]

Above all else, the abandonment of the dry conservancy system for w.cs was not practical until a system of running water had been laid on. In Liverpool an act of 1854 empowered the Council to insist that a house-owner convert the house to w.cs: yet not until some three years later did Liverpool begin to draw a really satisfactory water supply. After that it could begin the conversion to w.cs. in some earnest, and in 1860 it turned down all new house plans which did not provide for w.cs. In 1863 the process of conversion to w.cs began; by 1866 some 56,000 inhabitants had benefited from the change.[95]

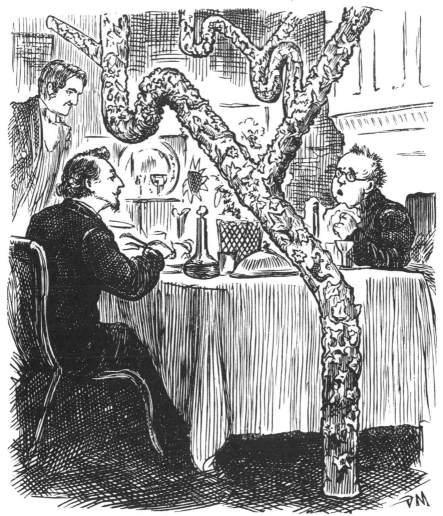

UTILE CUM DULCE.

Inquisitive Gent. " YOU WILL—A—THINK ME VERY INDISCREET—BUT I CAN-NOT. HELP WONDERING WHAT THIS ELABORATELY-CARVED AND CURIOUSLY-RAMIFIED STRUCTURE IS FOR. IS IT FOR ORNAMENT ONLY, OR INTENDED TO HEAT THE HOUSE, OR SOMETHING? "

Fastidious Host. " O, IT'S THE *DRAINS!* I LIKE TO HAVE 'EM WHERE I CAN LOOK AFTER 'EM MYSELF. POOTY DESIGN, AIN'T IT? MAJOLICA, YOU KNOW. . . HAVE SOME CHICKEN? "

7. Domestic sewers. The guest's horror was probably prompted not so much by the indelicacy of the dinner conversation as by the fear, commonly held, of noxious vapours escaping from the sewer pipes.

Source: Punch, 6 January 1872

103

As in so many areas of public health, so in the treatment of sewage the Victorians were pioneers and they had to approach their work cautiously, watching each other's experiments, and learning by trial and error, for example that hastily converted storm sewers were not up to carrying sewage, or that simple sand filtration might work for water but was not as effective as a combination of settlement tanks, lime, sand, and gravel for sewage. The scope for error was enormous and it is little wonder that sanitary authorities moved cautiously on the adoption of sewer systems. In 1874 alone some thirty-two patents were taken out for sewage treatment systems, and how was a local authority to know which was the best? The technical difficulties involved, the scale and cost of sewering, the fear of failure, the uncertainty about their effectiveness (the Local Government Board claimed in 1876 that even *after* treatment the typical town's sewage smelled of cabbage water, except in warm weather when it took on the stench of rotten eggs), all combined to serve as a deterrent to the amateur local governments of the day. To add to their fears was the fact that a system of water-borne sewage (unless the town was fortunately situated on an estuary or on the coast) would pollute the local river and might give rise to law-suits. Birmingham, for example, realized that the wholesale conversion of the town to w.cs would further pollute the Tame and possibly involve it in costly litigation. It even contemplated imposing a tax on w.cs to slow down their adoption, but compromised by continuing as much as possible with the dry conservancy method so as not to overburden its sewers and the river Tame.[96]

When, in 1844, Leeds first contemplated sewering the town it was nervous about the high compensation (and attendant legal) costs, the effects of diverting water from the all-important factories, the possibility of sewer seepage into cellar dwellings, and the costs and problems of processing the sewage at the outfall. Above all, many members of the Corporation wondered whether the whole thing would work. Then there were conflicting opinions to be resolved on the use of the river as an outlet for the drains, and added to all this was the suspicion, which in the event proved correct, that the estimate (of £80,000) which they had been given was too low. With all these fears and doubts gnawing at them, the Corporation voted 32 to 2 for postponement of the plan. The agitation and inspections accompanying the Royal Commission on the Sanitary State of Large Towns and Populous Districts (1843–5) inspired and re-activated interest in the sewering of the town. The Corporation appointed its own engineer to draw up plans, but then prudently decided it ought to call in a second opinion, and approached an outside consulting engineer. The *Leeds Intelligencer* accused the Corporation of being 'guilty of a most criminal delay', but one can certainly sympathize with any municipality which took a good long look before leaping into what must have appeared the financial abyss of sanitary engineering. Even though towns could learn much from watching one another, they each had their own peculiar problems associated with terrain, soil composition, and property rights and thus they were, in a sense, on their own.[97]

The trials and false starts of Leeds were by no means confined to the larger towns, for, if we are to judge by the experience of Farnham, a Surrey town of some 5,000 inhabitants in 1881, similar problems beset any community ambitious enough to undertake a sweeping change in its sanitary arrangements. Throughout the 1850s the sanitary condition of Farnham had been a cause of dispute between the local Board of Guardians and the vestry, and when in 1866 Farnham finally established a local board of health the town's excrement removal was still an unwholesome mixture of open sewers and cesspits. The new Board decided that the proper sewering of the district was its most important and immediate responsibility, and it placed advertisements in *The Times*, the *Engineering Journal*, and the *County Chronicle* for plans to be submitted by qualified engineers. Prizes of £100 and £50 for the two best plans were offered. This was, no doubt, as good a way as any of going about the task, but when the replies, in a bewildering variety, started to come in, the local Board found itself faced with the daunting task, for which it was unqualified, of judging the entries. It soon realized that it had ventured into something well beyond its competence, and hired a civil engineer, at forty guineas, to evaluate the plans. Unfortunately his report was, like the plans, too technical for the Board to act upon with any confidence, and so they turned to a local farmer who had some practical knowledge of drainage and who, presumably, could communicate in terms comprehensible to laymen. Had they turned instead to the Privy Council they would have received excellent free advice, for Simon's team was building up considerable expertise in sewage disposal and was only too happy to travel to local communities to help. Perhaps Farnham thought that it was too small, or, more probably, it simply wished to handle its own problems without government interference. In any case, faced with conflicting advice and a variety of possible schemes, the local Board dithered, then lost interest. In 1877, some two years after Farnham appointed its first medical officer, there was another show of interest, and again a civil engineer was hired, this time for ten guineas; but, again, no action was taken. Then in 1879 an influential landowner, a Mr Potter, through whose land the polluted river Wey flowed, threatened under the recently passed Rivers Pollution Act (1876) to restrain the Board from using the river for its untreated sewage. Alarmed by the spectre of litigation, the Board was thrown into confusion, and then at last acted, travelling to Taunton and Chiswick to examine their sewage systems, and it showed its good faith by taking the plunge and writing to the Local Government Board for advice. Presented with the alternative of precipitation or irrigation and filtration methods, the Board was again indecisive, and nothing was done until another local landowner, a Mr Bateman, brought suit against the Board under the Rivers Pollution Act. Although the Board argued in its defence that it now had under serious considera-tion some fifteen drainage schemes, the judgment in Bateman *versus* Farnham (1883) went against it, and it was at last compelled to act. Again an engineer was appointed to draw up plans and at last work began, only to be accompanied almost immediately by numerous problems – construction difficulties, disputes over the site of the sewage farm, haggling over the cost of the land and over the injury which the sewage site (against which, understandably, there was much prejudice) might cause local farmers, squabbles with house-owners who fought to preserve the integrity of their gardens against the upheaval of sewers and connecting drains. In all, some nine months elapsed between the initial drafting of the engineer's plans and their approval by the Local Government Board and accompanying sanc-tions of a loan of £14,000 payable over thirty years. Once the plans were put out to bid they attracted thirty-six engineering firms, mostly located in the Midlands, for the boilers and pumping engines, ranging from a low of £1,119 to a high of £2,270, and for the laying of sewers a further twenty bids, from £9,342 to £14,888. In both cases the lowest bids were accepted. The problems of Farnham must, however, have struck the local Board as just beginning, for the contractor for the sewer went bankrupt, local inhabitants somehow managed to fall into unfinished sewers, and compensation costs for damage done to prop-erty by the laying of sewers and legal costs of arbitration began to soar.

Finally in 1887 the sewer lines were completed and in the summer of 1888, when the total costs were all in, the Board discovered that the scheme had cost £18,000 and it was forced to go to the Public Works Loan Commissioners for an additional loan. Unfortunately, its difficulties did not end there, for several leaks appeared in the sewers, the sewage farm smelled, and the wash from the local breweries caused the sewege to ferment. The Board discovered also that in several cases where householders had made connections into the main sewers they had failed to install flushing toilets. Although the Board could compel the connection, it had no power to force landlords to install w.cs, and since hand flushing rarely had the force to cleanse the pipes fully, the whole new system did not work quite as efficiently as the Farnham authorities hoped. At the beginning of this century there were still many houses in Farnham which were connected to the main sewers but were without w.cs.[98]

Until many more local studies are done we cannot say how typical the many trials and set-backs at Farnham were. Many Victorian towns had similar experiences, and when London, which other towns were watching closely, embarked upon its great sewer system (begun in 1858 and finished in 1865, by which time there were over eighty miles of sewers), it ran into innumerable difficulties, not least of which were the bankruptcies of various contractors.[99]

Indeed, with all the problems, known and unknown, facing them, the major municipalities of Britain were remarkably active, and rather than criticize the slow adoption of large-scale sewer systems we should perhaps wonder at the adoption of so many in the mid- and late-Victorian years. *Punch* might have fun at the expense of London's Metropolitian Board of Works and write in 1858 that its progress on the great work of sewerage was 'slow but sewer', (and that what was needed was a 'Stinking Fund'), but we are in a position today to see that it was anything *but* slow.[100] The progress of Bazalgette's great scheme for two intercepting sewers running south and north of the Thames, carried on by some 6,000 men, was reported in the daily and periodical press and served to publicize the 'sanitary idea' to the entire nation. Not entirely inappropriately, the opening ceremonies at the southern outfall down the Thames were attended by the Prince of Wales, Prince Edward of Saxe-Weimar, the Lord Mayor, the Archbishop of Canterbury, the Archbishop of York, and 500 guests, who dined on salmon, while the city's excreta gushed forth into the Thames beneath them.[101]

A year after London had completed the majority of its sewering, the Privy Council reported that significant advances had taken place in many towns over the past few years. In Bristol it reported (1866) there was now a thorough system of sewerage by large sewers, and w.cs were beginning to augment the old cesspools. Similarly in Cardiff, Croydon, Carlisle, Penrith, Newport, Dover, Warwick, Penzance, Salisbury, Ely, Rugby, and elsewhere there were the beginnings of a sound sewer system and the introduction of w.cs. In most of these communities the changes had occurred in the late 1850s and early 1860s.[102] Although the Privy Council was careful to stress that these improvements marked a beginning only, its 1866 Report was in marked contrast to its earlier report in 1860 of a survey which disclosed conditions of filth and archaic sanitary methods, and which concluded that over the past decades there had been too much energy devoted to the 'removal of local uncleanliness' (that is, the emptying of cesspools) and not enough to 'the promotion of local cleanliness', in other words to the construction of new systems.[103] One indication of the rate of progress is that by 1880 the Doulton company alone was manufacturing approximately 3,000 miles of sewer and drain pipe annually.[104]

In the Welsh towns of Llanelli, Neath, and Swansea, the improvement was slower, but here, too, there was evidence of progress, mainly in the 1870s.[105] Progress was generally slower in the north of England also, and when in 1886 the Local Government Board conducted a survey of northern towns it found the principal improvement in the draining of cesspools and their reduction in size rather than the conversion to w.cs. Throughout the Black Country, for example, pail closets continued to outnumber w.cs well into the Edwardian period.[106] And although the Royal Sanitary Commission noted in 1871 that towns everywhere had built or were in the process of building sewers, this did not necessarily mean that they were replacing the dry conservancy method with w.cs. The Privy Council's observation about Leicester: 'in the poorer neighbourhoods there are far more privy middens than water closets', could apply equally to most towns, however well-sewered they may have been.[107]

An analysis of the introduction of the w.c (which had been patented by Bramah as early as 1778) indicates how much progress was being made in the mid- and late-Victorian years and yet how much still remained to be done. In Liverpool 115 miles of main sewers and fifty-six miles of pipes in courtyards were constructed and some 2,639 privies were converted to w.cs, all in the decade from the mid-1850s to the mid-1860s. By 1871 about 15,000 privies had been converted to flushing toilets, and the city government had spent £40,000 in subsidies to the house-owners. Yet in that year there were still over 30,000 houses in Liverpool without w.cs.[108] In Manchester in 1871 only 10,000 of the 70,000 houses had w.cs, and almost four times that number still used midden closets. Most of the w.cs were in the better houses and as late as 1911 less than half of Manchester's houses had w.cs. In the working-class districts two-thirds of the population were still making do with pails, ash-boxes or even midden privies. Although at the end of the century w.cs were replacing pail closets at the rate of 5,000 a year, there was still much to be done.[109] In Crewe pail closets outnumbered w.cs and there were still 264 cesspools and almost 2,000 privy middens at the turn of the century; not until 1920 were newly-constructed houses required to have w.cs in Crewe.[110] Edinburgh began its process of conversion from dry conservancy to w.cs in the very late 1860s and by 1873 almost 28,000 houses had them – yet at that time well under half the houses below an annual rental of £5 had water laid on and only one-fifth of them had w.cs.[111]

In Glasgow over 40 per cent of the population in 1870 lived in houses without w.cs, but this was much better than Rochdale, where there were only 300 w.cs in the town's 9,000 houses.[112] Birmingham in 1875 had 8,000 w.cs compared to its 35,000 old midden privies and 7,000 privy pails, but by the end of the century it had over 50,000 w.cs.[113] In York over 20 per cent of the houses, irrespective of class, were still without w.cs at the end of the century and in the working-class neighbourhoods there were still innumerable midden closets. Until 1901 the York council made a charge of 1s each time an ashpit or midden was cleaned out, 'thus giving the householder a strong inducement to allow refuse to accumulate for as long a time as possible.' Things would not have been so bad if the privies had been in good order, but as the local MOH complained, many were 'more or less foul or leaking, with uncemented walls and floors . . . a large number of them are found inches deep in liquid filth, or so full of refuse as to reach above the cemented portions of the walls.'[114]

Somewhat surprisingly, perhaps, the Irish towns appear to have made more extensive progress at the end of the century. Dublin in 1880 had only 743 w.cs in the entire town, but it then started an energetic programme of conversion and two years later it had 15,000 w.cs, and these outnumbered the privies. By the end of the century w.cs outnumbered the older privies by two to one in Ireland's major towns.[115]

In rural areas throughout the British Isles hand-flushed privies and dry earth or ash privies were still common. One of the author's earliest recollections as a young boy was the incredulity of the old lady who found herself hostess to a family of evacuees from the Blitz, on being told that in London a pull of the chain flushed the toilet and that men did not come around to clean out the toilet. Whether she later checked with my mother to confirm her suspicions that I was a child with a large imagination I don't know. That something taken for granted by one person was in the realm of the improbable to another represented the meeting, so to speak, of two sanitary standards which emerged in the nineteenth century.

By the 1880s the major cities had built new sewage treatment plants to process the outpourings of their sewer systems. Leyton in north-east London, which was one of the fastest-growing communities in the land, was said to have had the most modern. There the sewage was mixed with sulphurous powder and water and agitated, then permitted to flow into precipitation tanks and mingled with milk of lime. The lime helped to contract the solid particles in suspension and precipitate them to the bottom of the tank in the form of sludge. When the sludge had settled the water was drawn off into the river Lea, and according to tests the deposits flowing into the river were purer than the water initially drawn from the river for the purification plant. After further treatment the sludge was pressed into 'cakes' and spread over the adjoining fields, but this method was found to be too smelly and so Leyton began to burn its sludge in a 'Destructor'.[116] In Nottingham the 900-acre sewage farm was so impressive that it attracted foreign visitors. Livestock was fed on the grass grown there and some 60 horses, 400 cows, 320 sheep and 70 pigs grazed on it. Birmingham's sewage farm presented a less bucolic scene, for the site was poorly drained and consequently the sludge built up to a depth of four feet in the 1860s. During the next decade the town was forced to build larger filtration tanks.[117] After much experimentation most authorities settled on Italian rye grass as the best crop to grow on sewage farms. The farm, with its land treatment system, was an effective way of dealing with the sludge left over from the precipitation tanks; it constituted a secondary treatment system with a natural bacterial treatment of sewage, and though the fields had to be rested to get a good crop growth, it did constitute perhaps the most effective use of human excrement and represented a highly scientific culmination of an idea advanced in rudimentary form by Chadwick earlier in the century.[118] Manchester's Carrington Moss sewage farm, a peat bog of over 1,000 acres, cost the Corporation almost £94,000 to develop in the 1880s. The Corporation kept 400 acres for itself, and rented out the remaining 700 acres in small holdings to local farmers. By the 1890s Carrington Moss was receiving 70,000 tons of excrement a year.

In 1844 the engineer in charge of drawing up plans for Leeds's sewer system rightly stressed that its efficiency was dependent upon a regular and adequate flow of water: 'the supply of water in a town, and the discharge of the refuse, are two branches of the same subject', he wrote, 'and unless the water be abundant enough, and distributed enough to cleanse the drains, these last would often be more offensive than useful.'[120] While progress was made, especially during and after the 1860s, the amount of water available in most towns rarely met the sanitary experts' standards for a sufficient flow. Private water companies could often act most arbitrarily or at odds with the best interests of the town. Thus in Leeds the local waterworks company refused to give the Council favourable rates and so the main sewers were flushed only once a month, and the Leeds Water Works Company refused to supply water for w.cs unless a domestic water supply were also laid on. The Corporation had no power to coerce them. The municipal ownership of waterworks goes back at least to the fifteenth century, when Southampton, Hull, Bath, and Plymouth were all operating their own water supply. In the seventeenth century Rye and Oxford owned theirs. Nevertheless, at the beginning of the nineteenth century, most waterworks were in private hands, and of the forty towns inspected by the Select Committee on the Health of Towns, thirty-one were considered to have deficient water supplies, and only six were held to be good. Chadwick in his 1842 survey concluded that 62 per cent of the towns had inadequate or impure water and he rated only 12 per cent of the towns as good.[121]

The 1848 Public Health Act permitted local authorities to take over water companies, but only if the companies agreed. The expense of the private bills necessary acted as a deterrent and it was not until the Public Health (Water) Act of 1878 that a really easy legislative path was provided for the municipal purchase of private waterworks.[122] In 1840 only five municipalities in England and Wales had their water supply in their own hands, but by 1871 about one-third of all the urban sanitary authorities owned or were developing their own water supply. With the Public Health Act of 1872, 'for the first time a definite obligation to provide a proper water supply was placed on the shoulders of local authorities', and by the end of the decade slightly under 44 per cent of the 944 urban sanitary authorities in the country were running their own waterworks. By the end of the century about two-thirds were doing so. The purchase of private companies by local authorities naturally provoked some opposition (generally based on concern for local taxes), but there does not seem to have been any great philosophical debate over what was, after all, an important step towards municipal socialism. Perhaps that is because the municipally-owned waterworks was not a new or untried concept and because stock-holders were generously compensated when a local authority bought a waterworks company. But even the advocates of *laissez-faire* private enterprise appear to have accepted the merits of municipal ownership of a resource as precious and vital as water. The argument of Samuel Holme in 1844 for the muncipalization of Liverpool's water companies was a difficult one to answer: 'water is as essential to the health and comfort of mankind', he wrote, 'as the air we breathe, and when mankind congregate in masses counted only by tens of thousands, it is essential to the public health that it should be most abundant, not doled out to yield 30 per cent interest, but supplied from the public rates and at net cost.'[123]

The costs involved in the municipalization of water were enormous. By 1884 Leeds had spent well over £1,500,000 and when London finally purchased, at the beginning of this century, the several water companies in its area, it had to spend £47,000,000.[124] Preston spent £135,000 to purchase a company which was supplying only half the houses in the town.[125] Liverpool spent over £500,000 on the purchase of the city's two private waterworks companies: Manchester's Longendale Scheme involved the borrowing of £650,000 against the rates and the Rivington Pike water project, which was begun with an original estimate of £200,000, cost £1,345,969 by the time it was finished.[126] By 1900 annual municipal expenditure on waterworks had doubled from the 1884 figure and stood at £1,500,000. Municipal loans from the government for water supply stood at £53,000,000 at the end of the century.[127] The substitution of municipal ownership for private did not necessarily produce an immediate improvement in the quantity or quality of water supplied. Manchester gained control of the Manchester and Salford Waterworks Co. in 1851 and yet as late as 1904 only one house in fourteen had water laid on.[128] But by and large by the 1880s the large towns were receiving enough water for their sewer systems to function efficiently and for the conversion to w.cs to be feasible and desirable, and the water was of much improved quality – 'increasingly homogeneous and delivered in a sufficiently safe condition to ensure that large-scale water-transmitted outbreaks of the disease [typhoid] had now become rare.'[129]

John Simon rightly regarded the public works loans contracted by local authorities as a barometer of their activities and of general sanitary progress, and basing his views on this criterion, he allowed himself a rather cautious optimism in 1874 when he noted that the loans under general sanitary acts had risen from an average of £330,000 p.a. (1858–1864) to double that (£692,000 p.a.) between 1864 and 1870. In the years 1870 to 1872 the loans had averaged £884,000 each year, and in 1873 nearly £1,000,000 were borrowed by local authorities for sanitary purposes.[130] Just as impressive, the amount of loans sanctioned under the Local Government Act (1858) for sanitary purposes rose from £260,905 in the first year to £1,212, 890 in 1870; during that period over £7,000,000 was loaned under the Act and well over £10,000,000 in all.[131] Thus the period from mid-century to the 1870s saw the beginnings of a strong commitment, involving heavy expenditure, on the part of local authorities. When in 1874 the Local Government Board conducted a survey of the estimated cost of sanitary work in England and Wales it found that local authorities had contracted for over £3,500,000 of work, of which almost £2,500,000 was for sewerage and water supply.[132]

The significance of government loans goes beyond the fiscal, for before the Local Government Board would recommend a loan to the Public Works Loan Commissioners, it conducted a local investigation by its own sanitary engineers. This was an invaluable way not only of discovering defects and inadequacies, but of pressuring or encouraging local improvements. The Public Works Loans Act of 1875 (38 and 39 Vict.c.89) imposed on the Local Government Board the obligation to ensure that the work for which the loan was requested was actually carried out, and this required both inspection beforehand and overseeing afterwards. The Local Loans Act of the same year (38 and 39 Vict.c.38) enabled local authorities to issue debentures and annuities certificates for the purpose of raising loans, and here again the Local Government Board was the sanctioning body. Thus the Board was in a strong position to advise, direct, and gently control, and it used these methods, rather than bullying or litigation, to encourage sanitary work at the local level. Under the 1866 Sanitary Act the Privy Council was empowered to force local authorities to carry out sewage work and supply water and the Local Government Board inherited this right, but enforcement through legal processes was difficult and expensive, and rarely contemplated or used.[133] Generally it preferred to exert pressure in its preliminary inspection and to use its technical expertise to persuade. By the late 1870s it had built up considerable experience in all matters relating to sanitary engineering, and bewildered local bodies turned to it for advice on sewage removal, the construction of sewers, outfall works, and processing plants. This expertise, together with the power of the purse, enabled it to exert considerable influence as the central sanitary authority for England and Wales.[134]

By 1875 the Local Government Board was beginning to express considerable satisfaction with the rate of sanitary progress. This progress was maintained over the next two decades. Between 1871 and 1891 over £50,000,000 was borrowed by local authorities from the Public Works Loan Commissioners (roughly £2,500,000 was for housing purposes and the rest for sanitary work). Urban authorities accounted for roughly £43,000,000 of the total.[135]

These large sums represent a remarkable level of local sanitary activity. Between 1880 and 1891 urban sanitary authorities borrowed £3,225,500 for waterworks and £7,738,522 for sewage and sewage disposal; the figures for rural authorities were £576,502 and £1,145,278 respectively.[136] The scale of urban sanitary problems was much greater than in rural areas, but to offset the costs was the growth in rateable value as the towns developed. In 1872 urban sanitary districts, excluding London, could raise over £3,000,000 in local rates, while all the local rural districts could raise only £23,540. The borrowing capabilities of rural districts were proportionally less than the towns, therefore, although not all towns automatically qualified for government loans. Dublin, for example, was denied a much-needed loan in 1875 for its proposed main drainage system because the Treasury did not consider its financial state healthy enough to guarantee repayment. Not until the 1878 Public Health Act was Dublin able to obtain from the government the money it so desperately required to put its house in order.[137] Despite the financial difficulties of many of Ireland's towns, the Local Government Board for Ireland sanctioned loans of well over £1,000,000 in the decade between 1875 and 1884; the majority of the money went for waterworks. These loans often threw a considerable burden on the rates – to take one example of many, Wrexford's loan for sanitary purposes amounted to *twice* its total rateable value. In the last quarter of the century the Irish Local Government Board sanctioned over £4,000,000 for sanitary improvements in Ireland – about twice the amount Scotland borrowed in the same period from the central government.[138] The enormous difference between the loans granted by the Public Works Loan Commissioners to urban areas on the one hand and to rural on the other is somewhat misleading, for many rural areas preferred to raise money commercially than to involve the central government in its local affairs, and they also resorted to local acts which did not involve the Government's money.[139] Of the almost £11,000,000 which was spent on public health throughout England and Wales in just the one year, 1872–3, for example, rural communities spent roughly one-half the amount spent by the urban authorities, certainly no inconsiderable sum.[140]

The greater expenditure involved in sewerage and water systems presented a challenge to ratepayers' associations and all those who were fearful of central government interference and growth. On the one hand the government loans carried with them a certain loss of local autonomy and for insanitary areas the embarrassment of public exposure; on the other they were generally too tempting to turn down. Caught between spiralling costs and the complexities of modern sanitary engineering and urged on by the momentum of the public health movement, there was really very little else urban communities could do but turn to the government for loans, and so assist, however unwillingly, in the growth of government interference in local affairs. In Exeter the sewage treatment system begun in 1896 cost £88,000, a gigantic and unprecedented sum for a city which had spent just a little over £10,000 on excrement removal over the past several decades. It was all very well for the *Flying Post* in Exeter to write, 'We live in a sanitary age and whether we like it or not, municipalities are called upon to spend money freely. Sewage works, water supply and gas supply are the three leading questions before every municipal constituency in the Kingdom', but it was understandable that local authorities would hesitate to spend freely, when to do so meant placing a strain on the rates and calling in the government in a capacity which, through advice and the sanctioning of loans, could lead to active intervention and possibly dictation. It is equally understandable that well-intentioned men could advocate no change at all, on the grounds that the past was infinitely worse, for it took vision and an understanding of the potential of modern sanitary science to embark on costly and difficult schemes.[141]

In his classic *Report on the Sanitary Condition of the Labouring Population* Chadwick earnestly pleaded that 'the primary and most important measures, and at the same time the most practicable, and within the recognized province of public administration, are drainage, the removal of all refuse from the habitations, streets, and roads, and the improvement of the supplies of water.'[142] Within twenty years of his report, major improvements had been made in all these areas and within forty years the sanitary standards of all the major cities had undergone radical improvement. As the medical officer for Glasgow, Dr Chalmers, put it, in giving evidence before a government committee in 1904: 'One talks of insanitary areas at the present moment, but although it is the same phrase, it means something different from what it did thirty years ago.'[143] The sanitary revolution which had occurred revealed the effectiveness of preventive medicine, for by 1881 the general death rate, which in the two decades of the 1860s and 1870s had been 22.5 and 21.5 respectively, had fallen to 18.9. Even more encouraging was the fall in the death rate from the principal zymotic diseases (smallpox, measles, scarlet fever, diphtheria, whooping cough, and 'fever' – which included typhus, typhoid, and simple continued fever): it was cut almost in half between 1860 and 1880. As the County MOH for Yorkshire wrote, the zymotic death rate 'is generally looked upon as an index of the sanitary state of a district because all these diseases are preventable'; by 1881 the usually cautious Local Government Board allowed itself a rare moment of optimism:

> We cannot but regard this progressive diminution in the mortality from zymotic diseases and especially from fever, which is probably the most amenable of all to sanitary control, as a special matter for congratulation.[144]

There was, of course, much still to be done – the high level of infant deaths and the 30,000 deaths which occurred in 1901 from gastrointestinal diseases sadly testify to continued insanitary conditions – but it was indisputable that at the end of Victoria's reign England was an infinitely more sanitary and healthy place to live in than at the beginning, or in the middle, of her reign.[145]

5
Fever! Fever!

'The Cholera is the best of all sanitary reformers, it overlooks no
mistake and pardons no oversight.'
The Times, 5 September 1848

Cancer, heart attacks, and traffic accidents are part and parcel of our
modern society and we tend not to brood on them unless they strike
close to home. The fear and threat of untimely death lies submerged in
our consciousness. Similarly in the nineteenth century, more time and
thought were devoted to the immediacy of the enjoyment or struggle
of living than to the possibility of early death. The Victorians ritual-
ized death to help innoculate themselves against its shock: the rich
turned funerals into ornate pageants calling for a special kind of
etiquette and even decorative arts, the poor turned them into occa-
sions, partly for the same psychological imperatives, to be with family
and neighbours, to apply the comforting balm of tradition, to drink,
eat, gossip, pray and commiserate. Wakes enabled homage to be paid
to the dead and mitigated the feelings of loss and despair experienced
by the survivors. The possibility of sudden and often painful death
from one or other of the many epidemic diseases of the day simply was
one of the inescapable facts of nineteenth-century life.

But to say this is not to suggest that the shock of death to the
survivors was slight. When 'fever' struck it might leave its mark on
entire neighbourhoods and the sight of parents, siblings, or young
children slowly succumbing or suddenly dying could not help but
affect surviving family members. The sadness and grief could be
softened only partially by the fatalism of the age. Social and medical
historians tend to dwell on the cold figures of mortality, but such
statistics give little indication of the debilitating weakness of those
who survived or of the misery, both pecuniary and psychological,
which illness or death brought. To the poor disease could mean
dropping into the ranks of pauperism and the stigma of poor relief. To
society at large it could mean the disruption of normal life and a sense
of stress and urgency which approached that of a community under
siege.[1]

117

During the eighteenth century a series of good harvests and thus improved food supplies had resulted in a decline in major epidemics, a falling death rate and a sustained growth of the population. Even the rapid urbanization of the early stages of the industrial revolution had not altered the pattern of general progress. But all this changed sharply just before Victoria ascended the throne. The alarming return to an age of epidemics was well publicized and placed in a statistical context by the figures released from the annual census data, the newly-formed office of the Registrar-General, and the investigations of the Statistical Society of London. The resulting awareness of high mortality did much to make urban development under the late Georgians, with its relatively high-density, inner-city living, suddenly suspect and encouraged the exodus of the wealthier classes to the suburbs. The rise, once again, of widespread infectious and contagious diseases, and especially of cholera, a disease new to the English experience and the first national epidemic since the seventeenth-century plague, served to remind the Victorians that their society, however progressive, was not immune to the scourges of the past.

The major epidemic diseases, though conveyed in a variety of ways (by contaminated water, foodstuffs, clothes and utensils, by body lice, flies, or droplets from the mouth) and thus calling for a variety of remedies and preventive measures, were all influenced by cleanliness, diet, personal hygiene, public sewerage, or domestic living arrangements. These diseases called for more than the doctor's healing art or the research chemist's endeavours. They called for the state to inspect and ultimately control the excesses of unregulated urban growth and rural neglect: in short, they projected the state into public health and placed it, in the position of guardian, over the environment.[2]

Of the fatal diseases of the period, cholera had an impact out of all proportion to its statistical importance. Following an inexorable progress from Asia across Europe, it first struck in England in 1831–2, again in 1848–9, and, with diminished virulence, in 1853–4 and 1866–7.[3] Roughly 32,000 people died from cholera in 1831–2, 62,000 in the epidemic of 1848–9, another 20,000 in 1853–4 and about 14,000 in 1866–7.[4] But as important as the number dying was the high percentage of fatalities among those contracting the disease – between 40 and 60 per cent – and the speed with which cholera could strike.[5] The victim could be dead within a few hours of the first apparent symptoms. But more generally he died after several days of suffering from violent stomach pains, vomiting, diarrhoea, and total prostration, during which the body turned cold, the pulse became imperceptible, and the skin wizened.[6] During the final stages the afflicted might well be taken for dead, and gruesome stories circulated of premature burial and the poor victim's anguished attempts to claw free of the coffin. The sudden death of apparently healthy people added still further to the fear. As the *Methodist Magazine* wrote in considerable alarm in 1832:

> To see a number of our fellow creatures, in a good state of health, in the full possession of their wonted strength, and in the midst of their years, suddenly seized with the most violent spasms, and in a few hours cast into the tomb, is calculated to shake the firmest nerves, and to inspire dread in the stoutest heart.

Cholera was thus a 'shock disease'.[7]

Reports from the Continent of attacks on the authorities or doctors and hyperbolic accounts such as those in the *Lancet* ('No rank escapes its attack . . . whole families are exterminated – civilised nations changed to savage hordes . . . all grades and bonds of social organisation disappear.') added to the general unrest. *The Times* was certainly exaggerating in 1831 when it wrote of 'great panic' and 'complete panic', but the following year thirty riots associated with cholera occurred in London, Liverpool, Manchester, Exeter, Birmingham, Bristol, Leeds, Sheffield, Glasgow, Edinburgh, Greenwick, Cathcart, Paisley, and Dumfries.[8] By contrast, the outbreak of cholera in Hull, Selby and Leeds in the spring of 1832 did not prevent the inhabitants of nearby York attending the mass rallies on the 1832 Reform Bill, nor did it put a damper on Race Week.[9] The majority of the riots were inspired by fears that medical students and doctors were taking advantage of the cholera to obtain bodies for their anatomy classes, and it was rumoured that they were murdering cholera victims. 'Choleraphobia', which could strike miles from the centre of the epidemic – when cholera first appeared in Sunderland in the north, panic almost immediately erupted in Caernarvon, Gloucester, Norwich, and Plymouth – was almost always linked with fears of body-snatching ('Burking'), premature burial, or burial in unconsecrated ground.[10] The wake required that a decent amount of time should pass between death and burial and the authorities' insistence upon expeditious burial of cholera victims cut into the custom of a good 'send off'.[11] The very numbers dying prevented burials being accorded the dignity and ritual which custom demanded. Clergymen said hasty prayers from a safe distance outside the graveyeard and funerals were not well attended, for, as Charlotte Yonge commented, 'the living had

to be regarded more than the dying'. The Irish especially were outraged by the improper and hasty burials and they sometimes managed
to hold off the authorities when they came to bury the body. In the
notorious London slum, Seven Dials, the police refused to go near the
body of a cholera victim which the relatives were protecting from a
hasty burial. The local magistrate called for special constables to go in
and get the body but was told by the beadle 'the parish couldn't git a
special constable no how; none of the householders wouldn't serve'.
Eventually some watermen volunteered to carry off the body for a
payment of 5s each, the large sum (equivalent to some two or three
days' work) representing the 'wages of fear'.[12]

With the whole neighbourhood in a frenzy of whitewashing, with
the pungent smell of burning pitch, used for fumigation, hanging over
them, and with the constant, mournful rumbling of hearses, the
impact of cholera was highly visible. Dumfries, where several
thousand inhabitants fled the town at the first signs of cholera, took on
the character of a ghost town: 'Scarcely an individual was met with in
the street', observed Dr Alison, 'the medical men's gigs and the hearse
only were heard. . . .'[13] In Bilston, near Wolverhampton, the vicar
wrote that 'all kind of business is at a stand; nothing reigns here but
want and disease, death and desolation', while in Wolverhampton
itself a local doctor described how:

> In all quarters there were the sick, the dying, and the dead. . . . The
> general silence of the city, save when broken by the tolling of the funeral
> bell . . . was most remarkable; the streets were deserted, the hurried
> steps of the medical men and their assistants, or of those running to seek
> their aid, alone were heard, while the one-horse hearse, occasionally
> passing on its duty, was almost the only carriage to be seen in the usually
> busy streets.[14]

It is remarkable that there was in fact so little panic. Indeed the first
two cholera epidemics, occurring as they did in time of political and
social unrest, reveal the inherent stability of English society.[15]

This is all the more remarkable in view of the complete inability of
the authorities to contain, let alone prevent or cure the dreadful
disease. Cholera was contracted by swallowing water or food which
had been infected by the cholera vibrio, a minute bacillus. The vibrio
could last up to five days in meat, milk, or cheese, less in green
vegetables, and up to sixteen days in apples, and it could dwell up to a
fortnight in water. It was most often spread by water contaminated by
the excreta of cholera victims, or by flies which hatched in or fed upon
the diseased excrement.[16] When the sanitary conditions described in

the previous chapter are recalled it is clear why cholera spread so rapidly.

Medical opinion was hopelessly divided on the causes of cholera. The fact that between 1845 and 1856 over 700 works on cholera were published in London suggests not only that it was a 'shock' disease but that its causes and prevention were subject to a wide variety of interpretations.[17] The contagionist theory met with great opposition, partly because it implied the need to establish internal quarantine and quarantine meant loss of trade. A *cordon sanitaire*, it was argued, would result only in greater poverty and unemployment for the masses, thereby increasing the risk of spreading cholera. In any case, there was hardly the bureaucracy available for satisfactory inland quarantine; the army raised the spectre of repression and martial law and the local constabulary was woefully ill-prepared for such measures. When in Stratford-upon-Avon the authorities decided to cordon off the town they had to rely upon a posse of old men, a rag-tail element not entirely inappropriate for that Shakespearian town.[18] But, more important, cholera affected some members of a family but not others and so contagionist theory was damaged. The alternative theory, that cholera was spread from miasmas of filth – as Chadwick put it, from 'epidemic atmosphere' or 'deleteriously impregnated air' – at least moved in the right direction of focusing attention upon filthy conditions, especially inadequate sewerage and accumulations of excrement.[19]

Adequate excrement removal was, however, a long-term proposition and the epidemics called for immediate action. A variety of remedies was offered, and most of them suggest that in combating epidemic disease the Victorians were closer to the Middle Ages than to our own time. The *Lancet* in a flurry of optimism, reported in 1831 that a community of East European Jews in Wiesniz had escaped the cholera raging all around them by rubbing themselves with a liniment composed of wine, wine vinegar, camphor powder, mustard, ground pepper, garlic and cantarides (made from crushed dried bodies of beetles, and better known as the aphrodisiac, 'Spanish Fly').[20] Purveyors of patent medicines had a field day: among the concoctions offered as remedies for cholera were Daffey's Elixir, Moxon's Effervescent Magnesium Aperient, and Morrison the Hygienist's Genuine Vegetable Universal Mixture. Many, no doubt, turned to the more inviting and readily available 'remedy' of twenty drops of laudanum in a wine glass of brandy![21]

Hardly more effective, but at least offering some spiritual solace, were the prayers and fast-days suggested by churchmen of several denominations. Cholera, it was thundered from a thousand pulpits, was God's punishment for moral and spiritual laxity, drunkenness, failure to observe the sabbath, and other sins, including advocacy of enfranchisement for the Jews and marriage with the deceased wife's sister! The evangelicals especially asked the poor to place their trust in prayer, and the Congregationalists offered 'Moral Preservatives against cholera' – temperance, cleanliness, industry, fortitude, and gospel reading.[22] The Unitarians took a more rational approach: the obvious sin, they argued, was the general 'condition of the lower classes' which was 'an invitation to disease'; prayer 'may heal the wounded spirit but not the maimed body. It may purify the heart but not the atmosphere. . .'[23]

Much the same attitude was taken by Lord Palmerston when, during the visitation of 1853, he was asked by church groups to declare a national day of fasting. 'The Maker of the Universe', the Home Secretary replied, 'established certain laws of nature for the planet in which we live; and the weal or woe of mankind depends upon the observance or neglect of those laws.' Palmerston suggested it would be far more efficacious to set about the 'purification and improvement' of the working-class districts of all towns in order to destroy the

> sources of contagion which, if allowed to remain, will infallibly breed pestilence, and be fruitful in death, in spite of all the prayers and fastings of a united but inactive nation. When man has done his utmost for his own safety, then it is time to invoke the blessing of Heaven to give effect to his exertions.[24]

Sir John Simon, looking back on events at the end of his long career, took Palmerston's stand to be symbolic and 'characteristic of a new era'.[25] That era, marked by the determination of the central government to guide and direct local communities, had its beginnings in the cholera epidemic of 1832 and the demands it made upon the government to act. While the central government had done nothing about the 'fevers' which were endemic in all large towns and which were, in the long run, responsible for far more deaths than cholera, it was now compelled to take action. A temporary Board of Health was quickly established after hurried consultation between the Privy Council and the Royal College of Physicians. It was composed of the President and four Fellows of the Royal College of Physicians, the Superintendent-General of Quarantine, the Director-General of the Army Medical Department, the Medical Commissioner of the Victualling Office and two non-medical civil servants.

In 1831 and 1832 this temporary Board of Health issued a series of recommendations in the form of Sanitary Regulations. These called upon local governments to establish boards of health and it was suggested that their personnel include one or more magistrates, a clergyman, a certain number of 'substantial householders', and (a recommendation which distinguished these boards from earlier local bodies) one or more medical men. The local boards, it was recommended, should appoint district inspectors – the first such to be suggested on a national scale by the central government – to report on 'the food, clothing and bedding of the poor, the ventilation of their dwellings, space, means of cleanliness, their habits of temperance'. Houses were to be whitewashed and limed, and linens cleaned, and cholera hospitals were to be established; quarantine of the stricken was called for, although in a very half-hearted fashion, and food and flannel clothing were to be distributed to the poor. These recommendations suggest that under the extreme pressure of the cholera crisis the government did realize that domestic cleanliness and adequate clothing and good nutrition were necessary to increase resistance to disease. Over the next two decades, however, the emphasis moved, under Chadwick's influence, to the more public areas of water supply and main drainage.

Most of the Board's recommendations were sensible, but the authorities were in the dark about the causes of cholera, and so together with sound advice about personal and domestic cleanliness it offered a veritable stew of dietary advice:

> take for dinner a moderate quantity of roast beef in preference to boiled, with stale bread and good potatoes, two glasses of wine with water, or an equivalent of good spirits and water, or of sound porter or ale. Eat garden-stuff and fruit sparingly, and avoid fat, luscious meats. In short, whilst under apprehension of cholera, use a dry nutritive diet, sparing rather than abundant, observe great caution as to eating suppers, for cholera most frequently attacks about midnight, or very early in the morning.

The same circular acknowledged frankly that 'no specific preventive against cholera is known to exist' and its recommendations conjure up visions of rather desperate quackery: moderate bleeding (10–12 oz) by leeches, warm baths followed by flannel rubs, a mixture of castor oil and laudanum, and plasters of mustard, peppermint, and hot turpentine. Interestingly the *Lancet* found little to criticize in these remedies, but commented that the Board had not put sufficient emphasis upon the role of doctors.[26]

Across the country local communities were sufficiently frightened to set up temporary boards of health and to wage somewhat haphazard war on filth along the lines suggested by the General Board. Unprecedented amounts were spent on cleansing operations: Edinburgh for example spent £19,000 to combat the epidemic of 1832.[27] But the local boards were temporary and, as devastating as cholera was, once it disappeared it tended to be forgotten, and reforms hastily improvised to meet the challenge were not made the basis for a comprehensive approach to public health problems in general. Looking back on the year, the *Annual Register* for 1832 declared that there had been too much fear: 'everywhere it [cholera] was much less fatal than preconceived notions had anticipated', it wrote, and 'the alarm was infinitely greater than the danger. When the disease gradually disappeared . . . almost everyone was surprised that so much apprehension had been entertained'.[28] When cholera appeared again a decade and a half later it ruthlessly exposed how little the local authorities had done.[29] Even the 1848 epidemic failed to produce local boards of health across the country and far too many centres of population muddled along with their archaic, hopelessly inefficient, and ignorant commissions of police or of sewers, lighting, or paving.[30]

In 1885 when Dr Ballard undertook a special survey of cholera for the Local Government Board he concluded that 'we can now look forward with less dread than perhaps the population of any other European country to the introduction of epidemic cholera.'[31] It was certainly a rough barometer of the general sanitary improvements (which we noted in the previous chapter) that although cholera appeared in sixty-four communities in 1893 it was confined to just a single attack in forty-two of them. As the MOH of the Local Government Board wrote in relief and jubilation, 'such a result, altogether unique in the history of cholera, was, I believe, largely due to the improved sanitary circumstances of England.'[32] By 1896 the government could dismiss cholera as one of the 'exotic diseases'.[33] While the mean annual death rate (per million living) from cholera was 231 in the period 1848–72, it had dropped to an insignificant 0.006 between 1901–10.[34]

Between the first and second cholera epidemics both the contagionist theory of disease and the belief that it was simply a punishment from God were far less widely voiced, but the miasmic theory continued to exert its hold on medical opinion right up to the pathbreaking experiments by Dr William Budd and Dr John Snow in 1849. Budd, who had done extensive research into the causes of typhus and typhoid concluded in 1849 that cholera was 'a living organism of a distinct species, which was taken by the act of swallowing it, which multiplied in the intestine by self-propagation', and Snow gave this new theory wide currency in his *On the Mode of Communication of Cholera* (1849). In 1854 Snow was given the opportunity to prove his theories when he dramatically and conclusively traced cholera deaths to houses supplied by the suspect water of the Southwark and Vauxhall water company. When he managed to persuade the local authorities to lock the handle of a pump in Broad Street in Soho (a compact area where over fifty people a day were dying of cholera) the deaths there came to a sudden halt, and although it was not until 1883 that Koch succeeded in isolating the cholera bacillus, Snow's work marked a triumph for the young science of epidemiology.[35]

Although cholera had a dramatic impact unequalled by any other diseases it was 'fever' which throughout the nineteenth century stimulated the most action from both central and local authorities. Cholera came and went, but, as the Privy Council noted in 1864, 'typhus fever appears never to be wholly absent. . . .'[36] Frequently rising to epidemic proportions, the various fevers were always endemic, always lurking as a threat to the nation's health. Fever drew attention to filth and to poverty and so forced authorities to come to terms with *public* health, that is, with social and environmental conditions, with living standards broadly construed.

Typhus, known also as Irish fever, goal fever, ship fever, putrid fever, and camp fever, was a rickettsial disease, spread mainly by the faeces of the body louse; conditions of overcrowding greatly encouraged the spread of the disease. The mortality rate was high – even quite late in the century about one-third of all notified cases ended in death.[37] The decline of typhus in the 1870s was widespread throughout England. In 1869, when typhus was first differentiated from typhoid, there were 4,281 typhus deaths in England and Wales. During the 1870s typhus deaths averaged almost 1,400 a year. Over the next decade the average was further reduced to under 400.[38] Together with typhoid and continued fever this reduction accounted for almost one-quarter of the total decline in deaths between 1851–60 and 1891–1900.[39] In Liverpool, a port city of poor immigrants, casual labour, and overcrowding, and hence a good indicator of the hold of a filth disease, the annual average death rate for typhus declined from 748 (1856–65) and 652 (1866–75) to 238 (1876–85) and just twenty-five (1896–1905). Between 1906 and 1913 fatalities from the disease dwindled to an insignificant number, under six a year.[40]

Significantly, though typhus continued to exist it had obviously been controlled – its presence in a Liverpool court no longer carried the threat of an uncontrollable epidemic.

How are we to account for this remarkable decline? It has recently been argued that 'the dramatic decline of typhus in the 1870s was probably more powerfully determined by the natural history of the disease itself than by any consciously planned modification of the physical environment' – an argument based in part on the chronology of the decline, which, it is claimed, occurred *before* the effects of better sewerage and water supply could have made themselves felt over a wide population.[41] In support of this argument it is suggested that the areas suffering most from epidemic typhus were often the last to receive proper water supplies and it was not until the 1870s, for example, when the disease was already in decline, that running water was laid on in working-class districts of London where typhus had been endemic. This interpretation, with its stress upon 'an exogenous change in the virulence of the infective micro-organism itself' and its de-emphasis of 'consciously planned programmes of urban reform', does not dismiss the latter entirely but only seeks to rearrange 'the hierarchy of causal factors'.[42]

Certainly there is much to support this revisionist thesis, for the decline in typhus deaths was, though far from uniform, widespread from 1870 onwards, while improved sanitation in the 1860s and 1870s was not. Typhus became less virulent and fatal even in those areas untouched by sanitary improvements. And yet one may question whether typhus could have declined as dramatically as it did where it was most prevalent – in the densely-packed courts and alleys of the great cities – if improved excrement removal had not accompanied the weakening of the micro-organism itself. Typhus declined at a slower rate in those towns (Belfast, Dublin, Sunderland, Liverpool) which were slow in the mid-Victorian period to effect improvements in sanitation and water supply, or where widespread poverty and filth co-existed. If a micro-organism is in decline it needs only the slightest additional factors (dietary improvements, for example) to weaken its impact further, and while it is true that typhus weakened its terrible hold before the introduction of comprehensive sewerage and water schemes throughout Britain, even the smallest improvements made in the 1860s – especially the attack on polluted heaps of exposed excrement and polluted wells and leaking cesspits, the introduction of much more sanitary dry conservancy pans and pails, taken together with increased use of cotton (more easily washed than woollen) under-clothing and bedding – probably hastened its decline. If nature itself was a major factor in the decline of typhus as a killer, it was nature assisted and encouraged by the efforts of the municipalities.

Throughout the first half of the nineteenth century typhus and typhoid were confused with one another.[43] Whereas typhus was a rickettsial disease spread by the body louse, typhoid was bacterial, and was spread, like cholera, by ingesting contaminated food and drink. The carrier from person to person could often be immune to the disease and this added to the mystery of typhoid. The typhoid patient displayed all the tell-tale signs of 'fever' – he became listless, lost his appetite, developed a high, continuous fever, often accompanied by a rash, and profuse diarrhoea (which never accompanied typhus).[44] It could be water-borne, and unlike typhus, it not only continued as a major disease throughout the nineteenth century, but it also affected all classes. Prince Albert died of it and Edward, Prince of Wales, contracted a severe case in 1871 after staying at the country home of the Countess of Londesborough, near Scarborough. Both his groom and the Earl of Chesterfield, who had also stayed in the house, died of the disease. That the Heir Apparent so narrowly escaped death served as a timely warning to the more comfortable classes to look to their own house drainage. Two years later an outbreak of typhoid hit Caius College, Cambridge, and drew attention to the primitive sanitary conditions of the colleges from which England drew her leaders.[45] Although it could be conveyed in a number of ways, typhoid must also be termed, like other diarrhoeal diseases, a filth disease. Probably the greatest number of typhoid deaths throughout the nineteenth century were caused by water that had become contaminated by diseased human faeces. In Stockport, for example, the incidence of typhoid in houses rated under £5 which were equipped with inefficient privy pits was almost four times higher than in the same class of house equipped with w.cs, and eightfold higher than in houses rated between £5 and £8.[46] When in 1870 the Privy Council sent Dr Buchanan to investigate what it thought to be an outbreak of typhus (it was in fact typhoid), he found conditions that made diarrhoeal disease inevitable: 'arrangements for excrement disposal and water supply such that people must drink their own excrement.'[47]

The provision of sewers, which no doubt helped to reduce the number of fatalities from typhus, may, ironically, have increased the number of typhoid deaths, for all too often the sewers poured contaminated filth into the rivers which were a major source of drinking water (see Chapter 9).[48] Whatever the reasons, typhoid continued to be endemic down to the end of the century.[49] Local authorities and the Local Government Board were puzzled by the disease and as soon as they turned to one possible source of transmission another would become suspect – water supplies, milk, foodstuffs like watercress and shellfish, were all at one time or another held responsible for outbreaks of typhoid.[50] The counties of Northumberland, Durham, and Yorkshire struggled against recurring epidemics of typhoid, and Darlington, Stockton, and Middlesborough were among the towns that continued to have epidemic typhoid down to the end of the century – all three towns drew their water from the Tees, a river into which some twenty villages sent their untreated sewage. In general, deaths from typhoid were twice as numerous in towns as in the countryside.[51]

Thus typhoid continued to serve as a barometer of inadequate water supplies and sewerage down to the end of the century. When, in communities like Maidstone, epidemic typhoid appeared, the Local Government Board or the local MOH would seize the occasion to conduct what amounted to a trial of the local water authority. Even where other sources of infection were suspect (such as milk, or the general contamination of the soil by excreta) typhoid was often a prelude to pressure on the local water company to improve the quality of its supply.[52]

Despite all the uncertainty and ignorance surrounding the origins and transmission of typhoid, improvements in water supply and sewerage did succeed in reducing its virulence. The death rate from typhoid in the decade 1891–1900 was almost half that of 1871–80 and by 1904 the death rate was well under one-third the rate that had prevailed throughout the 1870s.[53]

So far we have considered epidemic diseases which are intestinal, but among the major diseases of the nineteenth century there were several which were respiratory or pulmonary. Influenza, for example, was endemic throughout the century and pandemics occurred in 1830–1, 1836–7, 1843, 1847–8, 1855, 1870, and again in 1889–92. In the outbreak of 1847–8 there were 50,000 deaths in London alone from influenza, a figure some five times greater than that for cholera deaths in 1849. Influenza was greatly encouraged by the diet of the poor which lowered their resistance, and by their general social condition, particularly the necessity to walk to and from work, their damp houses, and the high cost of fuel. For most of the century influenza was accepted with resignation; it did not begin to arouse the concern of public health officials until the present century.[54]

Several other diseases became epidemic as a result of the generally low standard of nutrition and therefore lowered resistance, none more so than scarlet fever. Scarlet fever was viewed with dread, for the chances of a child (95 per cent of all cases were of children under ten years of age) who contracted it dying of the disease were very high. As late as the 1880s in Edinburgh about one child died for every fourteen catching the disease, while in the great epidemic of 1880 it carried off almost one child in five who contracted it.[55] Although contaminated milk was suspected, the exact cause of the disease was unknown, and it remained a major killer throughout the century. In 1863, 34,000 died of it and in 1874 over 26,000. In London alone it caused over 1,000 deaths as late as 1891.[56] John Simon, frustrated by the failure of sanitary measures to contain it, called in 1869 for a quarantine system as strict as that applied to diseased animals and for the establishment of quarantine hospitals. Quarantine was obviously impossible to enforce in the crowded dwellings of the poor, and although the need was pressing, local authorities, partly out of ignorance about the transmission of the disease, partly out of parsimony, were very slow to provide isolation wards, either in children's hospitals or in general hospitals. Some thirty years after Simon first made his plea, local authorities were still failing, against the wishes of the local MOH, to isolate scarlet fever cases.[57] Children thus moved freely from homes where scarlet fever (and measles, another highly contagious child-hood disease) had struck to school and back again.[58] Where isolation facilities, backed up by immediate notification and stricter control of milk supplies were introduced, the results could be dramatic.[59] In general, between 1861 and 1891 scarlet fever deaths declined by 81 per cent. This was partly due to the decline in the potency of the scarlet fever streptococcus or to the heightened immunity of urban popula-tions.[60] The various factors combined to make scarlet fever's decline responsible for some 19 per cent of the total decline in death rates over the second half of the nineteenth century.[61]

Also dreaded and fatal was diphtheria, called 'croup', 'inflamma-tion of the throat', 'putrid sore throat', 'malignant sore throat', 'dis-ease in the throat' or 'throat fever', names which suggest by their vagueness the ignorance which surrounded the disease.[62] From a sore throat diphtheria could quickly develop into blood poisoning, heart failure, or the growth of a membrane across the tonsils, which required a tracheotomy, often performed, when time was vital, by a pen-knife or hat-pin.[63] Diphtheria was listed with scarlet fever by the Registrar-General until 1860 and it was not until the second half of the century that it began to receive serious scientific attention. In 1883

Edwin Krebs succeeded in isolating the bacterium and in 1894 an anti-toxin was introduced into general use. Just like scarlet fever, the percentage of those contracting diphtheria who died was very high – some 20–25 per cent, and, again like scarlet fever, its cause and transmission continued to puzzle public health officials, who tended (with cause) to blame insanitary milk supplies.[64] The rapid increase in deaths of children under fifteen from diphtheria in the last two decades of the century was particularly frustrating to MOH and, as with measles and scarlet fever, a controversy raged over the impact of the Education Act of 1880 upon the increased morbidity. The 1880 Act put teeth into the 1870 Education Act by compelling local authorities to mark school attendance, and it was argued that it was the increased contact of children with one another which was causing the rise in death rates.[65]

Of all the killers, respiratory or intestinal, tuberculosis was the greatest, perhaps accounting for one-third of all deaths from disease in the Victorian period. It thus remained the 'White Plague', the 'Captain of the Men of Death' so feared by John Bunyan in the seventeenth century.[66] Although it had been long associated with artists and poets, and although it affected all classes, it was intimately connected with nutritional standards, and it hit hardest in those urban working-class districts which were ill-ventilated and overcrowded. It spread most rapidly and was most virulent where there was repeated exposure to a diseased person in confined quarters. The prevalence of consumption among tailors had caught the attention of Dr Guy early in the century, and its incidence among others working in crowded conditions – potters, miners, hosiers – attracted the attention of the Privy Council. It is difficult to chart the course of t.b. with any confidence, for it was often confused with other diseases, including cancer, and it was not a fully notifiable disease until 1912.[67] Nevertheless, it seems that between 1851–60 and 1901–10 t.b. mortality was roughly halved.[68] Encouraging though this decline was, the fact remains that t.b. grew in *relative* importance until at the end of the century it lay second only to heart disease as a major cause of death. It was claimed in 1894 that every single year it accounted for three times as many fatalities as were recorded in total, from action and disease, in the Crimean War.[69] Nevertheless, its decline was significant: it accounted for about half of the *total* decline in the death rate over the second half of the century.[70]

Even more than the other diseases so far mentioned, tuberculosis provides a 'sensitive index of living conditions in a community'.[71] In order to be controlled it required long-term improvements in housing conditions, dietary standards, and the quality of milk. As we have seen there were improvements in these last two areas, and if the general stock of housing did not improve significantly and if over-crowding remained a grave problem, at least the very worst slums and back-to-backs (where deaths from t.b. ran some 50 per cent higher than in other types of housing in the same area) were less typical of working-class housing conditions after mid-century (see Chapter 11).

The efforts of voluntary associations and MOH to improve standards of personal hygiene probably helped in the decline of t.b. Local authorities at the end of the century tried to control the 'promiscuous expectoration which transmitted t.b.' In Oldham the authorities issued and circulated a handbill to every house which stressed that t.b. was highly infectious and could be conveyed by matter spat up by the consumptive person: the handbill forbade spitting in public rooms, railway carriages, and other public places, advised that handkerchiefs and rags used by consumptives should be destroyed immediately after use, and informed the public that the local authority would disinfect houses occupied by t.b. sufferers. Similarly, the Brighton public health authorities issued 'Precautions for Consumptive Persons', in which they urged people not to spit 'except into receptacles the contents of which can be destroyed before they become dry'. The local MOH hoped that England would follow the example of the U.S.A and prohibit spitting in all public places.[72] Some aspects of preventive medicine cannot be quantified: the admonition to use handkerchiefs and not to spit no doubt played some small part in the decline of air-borne infections. Perhaps health authorities were slow to enforce codes against spitting and to insist upon strict controls on milk because they were so slow to adopt the germ theory of disease. Some seventeen years after the discovery of the tubercle bacillus in 1882 the President of the State Medicine section of the British Medical Association could declare:

> I say that we can fight phthisis on the old lines, by improving heritage when that is possible, by improving the homes and conditions of life and labour which are always possible and always call loudly for interference. But this insane hunt after the tubercle bacillus, as if it could be bottled up in a twopenny-halfpenny spittoon and got rid of, is the insanest crusade ever instituted on illogical lines.[73]

Correct in his view of what lowered resistance to t.b., he displayed an all-too common unwillingness to accept the basic cause. Meanwhile the fear of t.b. remained and the poor resorted to folk remedies, such as eating live snails and maggots or breathing the air emitted by pigs, cows, or horses, and to quack medicines.[74] To do so was doubtless more comforting that to wait for long-term improvements in living standards.

Of all the major epidemic diseases of the nineteenth century only smallpox was contained and turned back by means of a medical discovery. The decline of smallpox deaths accounted for 5 per cent of the total reduction in mortality from disease in Victoria's reign, and it was accomplished through means – compulsory vaccination – which brought the state into public health in the most direct and, in the opinion of some contemporary critics, most dictatorial fashion.[75] Vaccination, following the process first used by Jenner in 1798, came into general use by the time Victoria ascended the throne. Indeed, state medicine had its first early rumblings when in 1808 a Resolution was passed in Parliament to the effect that 'public benefit would be derived from the establishment of a Central Institute in London for the purposes of rendering Vaccinia Innoculation generally beneficial to his Majesty's subjects.'[76] In 1832 the National Vaccine Establishment (under the direction of the Royal College of Physicans until taken over by the Privy Council in 1860), issued over 100,000 charges of Jenner's lymph, and between 1837 and 1839 another 800,000.[77]

More than anything else it was probably the smallpox vaccination centres which introduced the Victorians to the notion of government intervention in matters of health. *The Graphic* wrote in 1871 that a 'whole nation solemnly baring its left arm and waiting to be scratched – it is a ludicrous image. The very earnestness with which people go about it tends to make it laughable.' But although the *Graphic* found a vehicle for its humour in the 'calm satisfaction' of those vaccinated, the 'gloomy resignation' of those preparing for it, and the 'shrinking terror' of those 'actually under the lancet', the scene, whatever elements it might hold of the human comedy, had some highly significant aspects.[78] It represented and revealed, after all, a willingness on the part of the general public to put its faith sufficiently in medical science to allow itself to be injected with elements of a dreaded disease, and in fact the entire process represented a remarkable breach in the general concept of *laissez-faire* and freedom from government intervention. Not unexpectedly a powerful anti-vaccination movement sprang up to preserve the sanctity of the human body and the integrity of the body politic. On both religious and political grounds it was argued that the rights of the individual had to be defended against this new menace of a doctoring state. Rather like today's opposition to the compulsory wearing of crash helmets for motorcyclists, it was maintained that the individual must be allowed to take his chance on death rather than be coerced into submissive conformity by a busybody, police state. Women like Ann Supple, who received twenty-five summonses for refusing 'to be party to the poisoning of her baby' as she put it, and who faced gaol rather than submit to vaccination, became martyrs to the cause.[79]

The Victorian state did not impose compulsory vaccination on the nation without first going through a trial period of voluntary vaccination. The smallpox epidemic of 1837–40, in which almost 42,000 people died, represented a challenge which had to be met: the response was a *permissive* vaccination act (1840) which enabled anyone to be vaccinated at public expense and which placed upon the already busy poor law authorities the burden of carrying out the vaccinations.[80] It was not until 1853, following a study by the Epidemiological Society of London, that a *compulsory* vaccination act was passed. This made it obligatory for parents to have their infants vaccinated within three months of birth. Although it made the process of vaccination much more common throughout the nation it was still administered in a haphazard fashion and a further smallpox epidemic occurred between 1870 and 1873 (in which some 44,000 people died, almost a quarter of these in London alone).[81] The appearance of this epidemic had coincided with a select committee on smallpox from which another Smallpox Act (1871) had resulted, designed to tighten up the compulsory nature of vaccination by making it obligatory for local boards to appoint vaccination officers, by imposing fines of up to 25s on those who refused to have their children vaccinated, and with imprisonment for non-payment of the fine.

One would have thought that the epidemic of 1870–3 would have been sufficiently frightening to persuade the nation to adopt vaccination on a comprehensive and thorough scale, but in fact the reverse happened, and the anti-vaccination movement gathered momentum and strength in the final quarter of the century, with the result that the percentage of infants receiving vaccination declined from 85 per cent of all births in 1873 to slightly over 70 per cent in 1897.[82] The efficacy of smallpox vaccination was hardly in question: in the epidemic of 1871 the mortality rate in London among those contracting the disease who were vaccinated was only 10.7 per cent: the mortality rate among the non-vaccinated was 45.9 per cent.[83] Obviously the opposition was based on other considerations.

The anti-vaccination movement began in earnest following the appointment, under the 1871 Act, of vaccination officers throughout the country, and the growing practice of the Privy Council of sending out inspectors to check up on local vaccination stations. This 'interference' by the central government, coupled with the obligation now put on local authorities to appoint vaccination officers, and the impossibility of opting for alternative methods, such as the Leicester method of notification and isolation, all smacked of a violation of local liberties. The underlying fear, for so long evident in the country at large, that government interest in public health might lead to dictatorial decrees, had, in the opinion of many, finally been realized. The government, hitherto an agent of information and persuasion, had now emerged in its true colours, as a monster of control. To these arguments were added cries about the dignity of the human body and the 'unnaturalness' of vaccination (to which the *Lancet* responded that it was 'unnatural' to wear clothes or to ride in a train!). Opposition to compulsory vaccination was also based on religious principles, namely that it was sinful to inject impurities into the blood – an argument that eventually won recognition under the 'conscience clause' of the 1898 Smallpox Act, despite the counter-argument that such beliefs amounted to 'omissional infanticide'.[84]

The leading force behind the anti-vaccination movement was Leicester. Despite its generally poor sanitary condition, Leicester, a town of relatively full employment and little overcrowding, had had a good record against smallpox, achieved by the 'Leicester method' of compulsory isolation of smallpox victims, the quarantining of all those who had had any contact with the patient, and a vigorous programme of cleansing, disinfecting, and, where necessary, burning of infected bedding and clothing, and the disinfecting of houses. In 1869 the Leicester Anti-Vaccination League was formed, and together with the London Society for the Abolition of Compulsory Vaccination it carried on an energetic and dedicated campaign against the central government's policies. Between 1869 and 1884 sixty-one imprisonments occurred in Leicester for non-compliance with the smallpox acts, and the movement culminated in a great demonstration in 1885, which drew together anti-vaccination forces from over fifty towns.[85] Although the decline in smallpox was due far more to vaccination than to any sanitary improvements, the Vaccination Act of 1898 introduced the 'conscience clause' which enabled parents to avoid compulsory vaccination of their children. By the end of 1898 the number of certificates granted to conscientious objectors under the Act was 203,143, with Lancashire accounting for over a quarter; Leicester requested 28,524 certificates.[86] Even though it was often difficult to get life insurance, rent a dwelling, or get a job without proof of vaccination (it was required for all London County Council and London council housing), there were thousands of unvaccinated babies at the end of the century. From a low of only 3.8 per cent of all registered births in England and Wales in 1875 and 5.7 per cent in London in 1881, the percentage of unvaccinated babies rose steadily to 22.3 per cent and 26.6 per cent respectively in 1898.[87] The reduction in the number of vaccinations suggests not only the decrease in its urgency with the decline of the disease (and the number of carriers) itself, but the degree of apathy, or ignorance toward preventive medicine which still prevailed and the strength of feeling about being bullied by a paternalistic state into good health. The struggle over vaccination suggests that improved national health depended on more than vigorous government commitment or even scientific discoveries. Also needed were the co-operation of local government and health officers, the support of the medical profession as a whole, and the willingness of the public at large to accept the judgment and policies of state medicine.

It is clear that different diseases required different government action.[88] Typhus, typhoid, cholera and other diseases spread by micro-organisms in water, milk or food, and affecting the bowels, or spread by fingers and flies, were capable of being contained by a vigorous purification of water supplies, better excrement disposal, and improved personal hygiene. But other infectious diseases were spread by viruses in air-borne droplets of saliva, and if, as one medical authority has recently written, 'probably with every breath we take in a room where there are more than one or two people, some of these flakes from other people's saliva pass into our noses', a process which is greatly accelerated by coughing and sneezing, it is clear that measures other than sanitary engineering were necessary. Several diseases – t.b., measles, smallpox, scarlet fever – could be rendered less dangerous by a system of early notification and isolation. These preventive measures, no less than the attack on filth, required close co-operation between central and local health authorities and between health officers and the general public.[89]

Aggravating the problem of air-borne disease was the enormous amount of overcrowding which prevailed in almost all the major centres of population, the lack of adequate isolation facilities, and the extensive population movements of the nineteenth century, which on the one hand injected new waves of healthier and younger country men and women into the towns, thus raising general health standards, but, on the other, placed in close proximity to one another immigrants who had built up little resistance or immunity to a variety of diseases which flourished in the densely-packed industrial towns. There was perhaps little the government could do about internal migration movements (in any case their impact upon the etiology of disease is certainly most complex); the solution to the problem of overcrowding lay, as we shall see in a later chapter, in a variety of long-term solutions arrived at painfully through a process of much trial and error; notification and isolation were, however, something that the government could advocate and enforce. Unfortunately they were slow in coming.

As early as the 1860s Simon was calling for an effective system of notification and isolation to combat infectious disease, but his call went unheeded, and in 1874, from his central perspective at the Local Government Board, he attributed the persistently high death rates to two main factors – the omission 'to make due removal of refuse-matters, solid and liquid, from inhabited places', and the license permitted 'to cases of infectious diseases to scatter abroad the seeds of their infection.'[90] Despite Simon's constant urging, the provision of isolation hospitals or isolation wards in already existing hospitals, was a matter of too little too late. In 1883 only thirty-four towns, with an aggregate population of only 2,500,000, had introduced a system of compulsory notification of infectious diseases.[91] The system of notification had been left a matter for local option and had clearly been found wanting. Huddersfield had adopted notification as early as 1879, and a system of notification was in force in Bolton, Burton, Nottingham, Jarrow, Llandudno, Derby, Leicester, Oldham, Preston, Edinburgh, Warrington, Blackburn, Norwich, Rotherham, and Blackpool from 1879, but it was not until the passage of the Infectious Disease (Notification) Act of 1889, almost twenty years after the Association of MOH first began their agitation for it, that the system was adopted throughout England.[92] Interestingly, t.b. was not included in the list of notifiable diseases, partly, it seems, because it was felt that it would impose an economic hardship (through enforced isolation) upon the large number of sufferers.[93] One of the reasons for the slow adoption, on a voluntary basis, of a system of notification was that the medical profession was divided on the issue, for while both the groups saw the necessity for notification, the local MOH wanted the responsibility for notification to fall on the general practitioners and the GPs wanted it to rest squarely on the shoulders of the house-owners.[94] In a rare example of working-class interest and intiative in public health affairs, the Trade Unions Congress of 1883 passed a resolution in favour of compulsory notification, containing the demand, well ahead of its time, that any resulting loss of wages should be compensated for out of the local rates.[95]

The Infectious Disease (Notification) Act of 1889 made notification by doctors to the local authority compulsory in London and optional throughout the rest of the country. It was immediately adopted by seventy-five local authorities and, by 1891, by 555 urban and 372 rural sanitary districts. In that year the Local Government Board estimated that the acts had been adopted (but not necessarily enforced), in areas populated by some 20,000,000 of the 26,000,000 people living in England and Wales.[96] Of the 141 provincial towns with populations of over 25,000, all but thirteen had adopted the Act and by 1893 some 25,000,000 people were, theoretically, living under its protection.[97]

This broad adoption of a permissive act marks a commitment by local authorities to preventive medicine that obviously went well beyond the improvement of drains and sewers, water supplies, and paving, all of which, loosely speaking, could come under the heading of 'town improvements', or 'civic beautification'. In part it represented the growing acceptance at the local level of the germ theory of disease and it may well have been inspired by an awareness, after the compulsory Education Act of 1870, that without notification and isolation infectious diseases caught and conveyed by children might become more widespread. With more children going to school – between 1870 and 1889 the percentage of children between five and fifteen attending school increased from 22.7 to 55 per cent – and mingling with one another in crowded classrooms, diseases such as scarlet fever and measles became more widespread. With both the promotion of teachers and with government grants dependent upon full attendance, there was very little incentive for teachers to report cases of infection.[98]

The adoption of a permissive act was one thing, but the provision of isolation facilities to make it effective was quite another, for that involved the local authority in additional expense and left it wide open to the charge of extravagance from the ever-vigilant rate-payers. There was, in any case, considerable anxiety, often amounting to fear, concerning isolation hospitals, for it was by no means certain that hospital authorities could guarantee that the diseases supposedly bottled up inside would not escape to pollute and threaten the surrounding neighbourhood. Thus in Edinburgh local rate-payers argued that the sewage from the infectious disease ward of the Lauriston Place

Infirmary might flow into the main sewers and so infect the whole town. When the Metropolitan Asylums Board first embarked upon the provision of isolation hospitals in 1870 local inhabitants raised a fierce enough opposition to close some and delay the opening of others, and at the end of the century Windsor had to erect its temporary, corrugated-iron smallpox hospital alongside the sewage farm, far away from the residential areas. One manual for healthy living, written in 1885, included 'infectious hospitals' in its lists of 'cemeteries, sewage works, dust yards, and bank holiday neighbourhoods' as things to avoid when considering the site for a new house![99]

Thus the actual provision of special isolation wards and hospitals was very slow in coming. As late as 1879 only 296, or about one-fifth, of the 1,510 provincial sanitary authorities possessed some means of isolating infectious diseases and even as late as 1891 the total had advanced to only 400 or so.[100] Once again, as in so many other areas of public health, the problem was predominantly one of money, for although government loans were available, the ultimate burden was still on the local rates. In Derbyshire, for example, there were two local health authorities with rateable values of only £4,000 p.a. each, and four or five other districts with rateable values of between £4000 and £8000. 'Such districts', wrote the County MOH for Derbyshire, 'could not possibly afford to put up proper hospitals, nor to maintain them if put up.' There was, consequently, only one authority in Derbyshire, a county with a population of over 426,000, which had erected a permanent isolation hospital by 1895. The Isolation Hospitals Act, 1893, enabled county councils to establish isolation hospitals, but here again the costs involved dampened the enthusiasm of all but the most ardent advocates of preventive medicine.[101] In 1882 the Local Government Board estimated that it cost between £200 and £300 a bed to build a hospital, and this was well beyond the means of most small rural districts as well as many towns. When Liverpool belatedly provided some 300 beds it had to spend over £80,000.[102]

In the 1890s the Local Government Board thus discovered that in most areas of the country facilities for isolation of epidemic infectious diseases were woefully inadequate. In Bishop Auckland, in Durham (population of 10,000 approximately), there was an isolation hospital, but it was a converted dog kennel, with only five beds and no disinfecting apparatus. Carlisle had just thirty-two beds and no disinfecting equipment for a population of some 40,000. Burslem and Burton-on-Trent, both pottery towns with high incidences of infectious lung diseases, had just eighteen and thirty beds apiece for populations, respectively, of 32,000 and 46,000. Llanelli, a town with a population of 24,000 had no isolation hospital at all. Wigan was better served, with sixty beds for a population of 50,000.[103] The bigger towns were not much better provided for. Leeds (population over 367,000) had one 'house of recovery' with sixty-four beds, a smallpox hospital with thirty-six beds, and a small convalescent shelter for children suffering from scarlet fever. Bolton (115,000) had been the first town in England to obtain powers for the compulsory notification of infectious diseases (in 1877), and it imposed a dual obligation on both doctors and householders to report infectious diseases, but it had no effective isolation wards until the Borough Fever Hospital was built in 1882. In 1895 it had thirty-two beds and a few cots.[104] Liverpool, like so many other towns, had relied on the local workhouses to provide accommodation for patients suffering from infectious diseases. In 1885 the Local Government Board sharply rapped the Liverpool Corporation over the knuckles for its failure to provide isolation facilities and suggested that some 750 beds were required.[105] Eventually the town was stirred into action, and by 1892 had provided three isolation hospitals with a total accommodation for 298 patients, out of a total population of almost 518,000. Manchester (505,000) did not provide any municipal hospital, but relied upon subsidies to the Manchester Royal Infirmary, which had 372 beds in isolation wards. Birmingham (478,000) had provided some 400 beds. Preston, a notoriously insanitary town with a population of over 107,000, had provided no isolation facilities whatsoever.[106]

However inadequate these facilities were, they were superior to rural areas, where there was no alternative to the parish workhouse. In London things were much better, for the 1867 Metropolitan Poor Act provided the town with a network of infectious diseases hospitals, organized by the Metropolitan Asylums Board. The Board's first fever hospital, for smallpox and scarlet fever patients, and for paupers only, was erected in 1870, and the Board's work was extended gradually until a range of infectious diseases was provided for, and admission to the Board's hospitals was no longer restricted to paupers only – the removal of the stigma of pauperism had been strenuously urged by the Metropolitan MOH.[107] By 1893 the Metropolitan Asylums Board actually possessed, or was in the process of building, over 5,000 beds in 'fever' hospitals. Whereas in 1873 only about two per cent of all scarlet fever deaths occurred in hospitals in London, and only 11 per cent in 1883, by 1894 that figure had risen to 74 per cent; similarly, for diphtheria, the percentage rose from about four per cent in 1888 to 38 per cent in 1894 – an indication not so much of the ineffectiveness of the hospital treatment or the insanitary state of hospitals as of the greater numbers of sufferers from these infectious diseases, many in the advanced stages, being admitted to the municipally-run hospitals. The compulsory Notification of Infectious Disease Act prompted the Metropolitan Asylums Board to step up its work and more people were placed in its hospitals in the year 1893 than during the entire decade, 1881–90.[108]

The compulsory Notification Act of 1889 was passed right after the Local Government Act of 1888 which, among other things, established County MOH. These county officers could sometimes bring pressure to bear on local authorities. Thus the County MOH for the West Riding of Yorkshire concentrated in his early years on infectious diseases and urged local authorities to put the Notification Act into immediate effect and to build adequate isolation facilities. Under his constant urging, the number of local authorities in the West Riding adopting the Act rose from seventeen (at the end of 1889) to ninety-six by 1891, and between 1895 and 1901 the percentage of notified cases of smallpox, diphtheria, scarlet fever and typhoid which were admitted to hospital rose from 14 per cent to 30.4 per cent.[109]

The provision of hospital accommodation for patients suffering from infectious diseases was never a top priority for local authorities, and it was only after considerable prodding from the Local Government Board and the introduction of comprehensive legislation that isolation hospitals were built. One cannot say that local authorities responded with quite the same vigour to the germ theory of disease as they had, some thirty years earlier, to the pythogenic. Sanitary engineering, however costly, could at least appeal to the Victorian's sense of energy, and his civic pride, to say nothing of his sense of smell. Notification and isolation hardly had the same dramatic appeal; indeed they had connotations of quarantine and incarceration.

Yet if halting and erratic, the Victorian response to the major epidemics was quite remarkable. With the exception of smallpox these diseases had to be contained without the benefits of anti-toxins, yet they *were* contained. In an age of rapid urban and population growth this must surely be seen as a triumph for preventive medicine. It is a testimony also to the resourcefulness and earnestness of the Victorians. Of course they did not bow gracefully to the necessity of following central government directives, nor did they swallow willingly the bitter pill of compulsory legislation. Indeed relations between the central government and local authorities were often strained and bitter

– a struggle between two growing bodies, one using the vocabulary of national health and strength, efficiency and progress, the other using the vocabulary of low rates, local option, independence, and freedom. It is to these two growing instruments of public health, the central government and the local authorities, that the next two chapters turn.

6

State Medicine

'Sanitary Science [is] the product of the English Mind.'
Dr Ballard, MOH, Local Government Board, 1885

The bureaucratic and legislative development of state medicine has been recounted several times.[1] It is a story of the incoherent and fitful growth of central government powers and of reforms generally pushed through in the face of both political and general indifference or open hostility. Most public health measures did not form a central plank in any ministry's platform. General elections and the fortunes of ministries hardly hinged upon issues of public health and neither party developed a comprehensive ethic, or philosophy, of public health.[2] Yet the central government's involvement with public health grew, in response to the widely exposed needs of the day, to such an extent that it was not until the advent of compulsory education late in the century that the daily lives of Victorians were as widely affected by any government action as by state medicine.

While the development of the medical departments of the Privy Council and the Local Government Board under the direction of John Simon has been thoroughly examined, the interaction between these central agencies and the local authorities has not.[3] This chapter deals with that interaction and the guidance and leadership offered by the central government and its general legislative enactments to local authorities. It was (as Chapter 7 also indicates) a relationship which was marked more by suspicion and distrust than by mutual affection or respect.

The presence of fever in the working-class districts of London stimulated Chadwick to use (or, in the opinion of his critics, abuse) his powers at the Poor Law Board to investigate the connection between epidemic disease and environmental factors – investigations which he followed up in 1842 in his remarkable survey of the sanitary condition of England. He was assisted in his task by the panic which the first cholera epidemic initially caused and the precedent which it set for government intervention. Chadwick's arrogance and high-handed

142

methods provoked much opposition and his impatience with medical science and use of phrases like 'sanatory police regulations', coming fast on the heels of the formation of the suspect metropolitan police force, were hardly diplomatic, but it would be hard to exaggerate his influence. He was the guiding force behind the early Victorian sanitary reform movement. Some historians, perhaps stressing too much the *ad hoc*, essentially pragmatic character of much British reform, have questioned the influence of Benthamite philosophy on the course of social reform. But that influence is certainly apparent in the public health movement – and it *was* a movement, with a sense of organization and *esprit de corps* among a small group of like-minded men, sharing an underlying ideology and a sense of mission. Chadwick had served as Bentham's secretary and from him had adopted the philosophy that the right ordering of society aided individual happiness and that certain matters (in this case health) required communal, rather than individual or family action. Chadwick and his Benthamite circle used a variety of methods over the years to capture and direct the public health movement – influencing politicians like Althorp ('irridation'), manipulating opinion through parliamentary investigating committees ('suscitation'), such as the Royal Commission of the Sanitary State of Large Towns (1843–5) and through organizations like the Health of Towns Association, and finally 'permeation' of government agencies, like the Poor Law Board and the General Board of Health (Chadwick was Secretary of both). It was throughout a calculated and finely engineered effort to give purpose and direction, a coherent philosophy, to the role of the state in the life of the nation.[4]

Chadwick was aided in these efforts by the statistical work of William Farr at the Office of the Registrar-General and by the strong reformist tendencies of the early group of statisticians in the Statistical Society of London. The Registrar-General's Office was established in 1837 and Farr was virtually in charge of it from 1839. Though Farr had a keener appreciation than Chadwick of the influence of poverty upon disease – 'Diseases', he wrote, 'are the iron index of misery' – and he advocated a variety of remedial measures, like Chadwick he stressed environmental engineering as a way of bringing down death rates from infectious diseases and, like Chadwick, he used his official position to urge comprehensive sanitary measures. In the First Report of the Registrar-General he wrote:

> It may be affirmed without great risk of exaggeration that it is possible
> to reduce the annual deaths in England and Wales by 30,000 and to

increase the vigour (may I add the industry and wealth?) of the population in an equal proportion.

A quarter of a century later Farr was still stressing the same theme – if the death rate of the thirty large towns which he selected for his comparative statistics could be reduced (as he believed it could) to the same level as that for his 'Healthy Districts' then almost a third of a million lives could have been saved between 1851 and 1860.[5] It was a message which Farr tirelessly presented, year after year, in both rhetorical and statistical form. Like Chadwick, Farr believed that the skilful use of statistics, especially *comparative* statistics, had persuasive force. Statistics, he argued, were 'an arsenal for sanitary reformers to use', and in the eyes of a leading MOH his medical statistics 'reoriented the whole business of State Medicine'.[6] In his appendices, in the form of a letter, to the annual reports of the Registrar-General, Farr injected a strong moral tone which conveyed a sense of both urgency and commitment that was to be taken up by Simon and his co-workers at the Privy Council and Local Government Board. In 1843, for example, Farr wrote:

> Over the supply of water – the sewerage – the burial places – the width of streets – the removal of public nuisances – the poor can have no command . . . and it is precisely upon these points that the Government can interfere with most advantage. The Legislature would enact the removal of known sources of disease, and, if necessary, trench upon the liberty of the subject and the privilege of property, upon the same principle that it arrests and removes murderers, who, if left unmolested, would probably only destroy lives by hundreds, while the physical causes which have been averted to in this paper, destroy thousands – hundreds of thousands of lives.[7]

His analogy was carefully chosen for he was arguing for a system of medical policing to protect the only valuable property the poor possessed, their lives.

This opening phase of sanitary reform was thus infused with the enthusiasm and moral fervour of a small group of men, well-known to one another, and approaching the work ahead of them with optimism and proselytizing zeal. Typical was the Metropolitan Health of Towns Associations which was formed in 1844. Inspired by Dr Southwood Smith, a Benthamite and close associate of Chadwick's, it brought together political leaders and aspiring politicians – the Duke of Norfolk, Marquis of Normandy, the Duke of Cambridge, Earl Grey, Earl Granville, Viscount Morpeth, Ashley (Shaftesbury), and the idealistic Young England members, Bulwer Lytton and Disraeli – and doctors of the prominence of Gavin, Guy, Liddle, Simon and Southwood Smith. The purpose of the Association was principally propaganda: 'To diffuse among the people the valuable information elicited by recent inquiries, and the advancement of science, as to the physical and moral evils that result from the present defective sewerage, drainage, supply of water, air, and light, and construction of dwelling-houses.' Within a couple of years the Association had branches in Edinburgh, Liverpool, Manchester, York, Halifax, Derby, Bath, Marlborough, Walsall, Plymouth, Worcester, and Rugby.[8]

The early reform movement was thus an amalgam of forces. At its centre was Chadwick and the statisticians he used in such a calculating fashion, statisticians who 'time and again . . . embarked upon surveys the major conclusions of which were anticipated and preconceived'.[9] Statistics were, they argued, irrefutable facts, which could not be ignored or denied. They presented a convincing picture of 'intolerability' that demanded remedy. Between 1853 and 1862 fully one-quarter of all the papers read at the Statistical Society of London were on public health and vital statistics, and when the moralizing of the early statisticians in the Society gave way to more objective presentation, the combination of statistical evidence and moral pleas was taken up in good measure by the Social Science Association.[10] This projection, through statistics backed up by moral outrage, of 'intolerability', found a response in the evangelical passions of the age. With its stern attitudes towards sabbath observance and its strict attitudes towards morality, accompanied as these often were by a patronizing and unsympathetic attitude towards the poor and their plight, evangelicalism has been criticized by both contemporaries like Dickens, who accused the evangelicals of 'taking possession of the people' and placing them in 'religious custody', and by later historians. But as George Eliot saw, evangelicalism also stimulated a sense of social responsibility and duty (the 'principle of subordination, of self-mastery'), and a belief, grounded in Scripture, that 'there was divine work to be done in life'.[11]

As early as 1772 John Heysham of Carlisle had noted that disease was 'the off-spring of filth, nastiness and confined air, in rooms crowded with many inhabitants', and Dr Currie of Liverpool had drawn attention to the way typhus seemed to thrive on 'want of cleanliness and ventilation'.[12] But it was not until the first year of Victoria's reign that the government explored the apparent connection between filth, poverty and disease. In the typhus epidemic in London (1837–8), when the numbers applying for poor relief dramatically increased, the poor law guardians of East London had spent public funds to remove accumulations of filth and to prosecute negligent landlords. The auditors had disallowed the expenditure and the matter had been referred to the Poor Law Commission. There Chadwick, the Secretary, had argued that the prevention of diseases resulting in pauperism came within the competence of the Commission and he persuaded his superiors to go beyond the strict definition of their duties to authorize a detailed study of fever conditions in London. Once he had obtained his authorization Chadwick moved carefully and set the stage for self-generating reform, for his investigating team was chosen for its predisposition to reach conclusions agreeable to Chadwick and conducive to reform based upon sanitary engineering. All three doctors chosen by Chadwick had already distinguished themselves as sanitarians. Neil Arnott (the inventor of the water-bed and one of the Queen's physicians) had worked for the East India Company, James Kay (later Kay-Shuttleworth) was the author of *The Moral and Physical Condition of the Working Classes*, and Thomas Southwood Smith had served for over a decade as Physician at the London Fever Hospital. Arnott and Kay's investigations in Wapping, Ratcliff and Stepney, and Southwood Smith's in Bethnal Green and Whitechapel, with their conclusions that there was an indisputable connection between filth, disease, and pauperism, set the stage for Chadwickian solutions.[13] Underlying the reports was the reiterated argument that, however expensive sanitary reform might prove to be, unless something was done to prevent illness and its resultant unemployment, the cost of pauperism would always be higher. Thus in his report of 1838 'On some of the Physical Causes of Sickness and Mortality to which the Poor are particularly exposed, and which are capable of removal by Sanatory Regulations', Southwood Smith wrote:

> It becomes, then, a question whether, setting aside all higher considerations, it is not expedient, even on the ground of economy, to appropriate a part of the money expended on the poor in protecting them from fever, by removing from the immediate proximity of their dwellings the main cause that produces it, rather than relieving a few individuals after they become affected with the diseases.

A year later he was even more explicit:

> It is plain this disease [fever] is one of the main causes of the pressure on the poor rates. This pressure must continue and the same large amount of money spent year after year for the support of families afflicted with fever, as long as the dreadful *sources* of fever which encompass the habitations of the poor are allowed to remain.

and he set the tone for the arguments used throughout the century by Simon and other sanitary reformers when he concluded that 'the prevention of evil, rather than the mitigation of the consequences of it, is not only the most beneficent, but the most economical course.' It was a persuasive argument and one that Chadwick never tired of using.[14] In its annual report for 1838 the Poor Law Commission officially endorsed Chadwick's team's plea to alleviate the pressures of pauperism by preventive medicine.[15] Throughout the century the advocates of public health reform used the fiscal argument as one of the key weapons in their arsenal against the counter-arguments of the ratepayers' associations and 'economy' parties. They even claimed they could calculate the cost of ill-health to the community down to the last pound. Thus in 1894 the MOH for Renfrew reminded his local authority that the outbreak of typhoid the previous year had cost the district £21,496 in lost wages, hospital costs, lost production and burial costs – a far higher sum, he stressed, than its prevention would have required.[16]

Chadwick's commissioners' reports, followed by the first report of the Registrar-General in 1839 and Slaney's Health of Towns Committee in 1840, established a statistical and analytical basis for the public health movement. This basis was broadened considerably and public opinion was first widely awakened to the need for remedial measures in 1842 when Chadwick published his remarkable, one is tempted to say epic, *Report on the Sanitary Condition of the Labouring Population of Great Britain*. Drawing upon the evidence gathered by approximately 1,000 Poor Law MOH, Chadwick skilfully wove the most lurid details and evocative descriptions, damning statistics and damaging examples into a masterpiece of protest literature. The *Report*, which covered 372 pages of text and another 85 of appendices, powerfully portrayed the inadequacy of existing systems of sewerage, water supply, and drainage, and stressed the connection between these and overcrowding on one hand, and epidemic diseases on the other. Chadwick argued 'that the various forms of epidemic, endemic, and other diseases caused, or aggravated, or propagated chiefly amongst the labouring classes by atmospheric impurities produced by decomposing animal and vegetable substances, by damp and filth, and close and overcrowded dwelling prevail amongst the population in every part of the Kingdom . . .', and he dramatically claimed that 'the annual loss of life from filth and bad ventilation is greater than the loss from death or wounds in any wars in which the country has been engaged in modern times.' Through the shrewd use of carefully-chosen comparative death rates and life-expectancy tables (contrasting town and country, and working-, middle-, and upper-classes), he vividly evoked the vast amount of unnecessary and preventable loss of life in the country. But he went beyond an analysis of mortality and struck a note he knew would have an effect upon his fellow-countrymen when he emphasized:

> That the population so exposed [to disease] is less susceptible of moral influences, and the effects of education are more transient than with a healthy population: That these adverse circumstances tend to produce an adult population short-lived, improvident, reckless, and intemperate, and with habitual avidity for sensual gratifications: That these habits tend to the abandonment of all the conveniences and decencies of life, and especially lead to the overcrowding of their homes, which is destructive to the morality as well as to the health of large classes of both sexes.

Playing down the broader, underlying issue of poverty as a root cause of much ill-health, Chadwick stressed the environmental, miasmic causes of disease and resultant pauperism and maintained that these causes could be removed:

> That the primary and most important measures, and at the same time the most practicable, and within the recognised province of public administration, are drainage, the removal of all refuse of habitations, streets, and roads, and the improvement of the supplies of water.[17]

In short, the *Report*, which Chadwick made sure was widely circulated (it sold over 100,000 copies) presented a compelling indictment of the sanitary condition of England and offered a coherent programme for reform.

In 1844 the Duke of Buccleuch's Royal Commission on the Sanitary State of Large Towns and Populous Districts confirmed the findings of Chadwick's *Report* and in particular exposed the totally inadequate sewerage provisions in the fast-growing towns throughout the country. It recommended that the central government should be given powers to inspect and supervise local sanitary work and that local sanitary districts, with authority over drainage, paving, cleansing, dwellings, and water supply, should be formed with powers of local rating for water and other schemes. Underlying the report was a cry for extensive remodelling of the role and functions of both central and local administration. It marked, close to the mid-century, a realistic and Chadwickian appraisal of the sanitary state of the nation and the measures required to tackle the problem.[18]

This early sanitary movement bore legislative fruit in 1846 in the first of a series of Nuisances Removal Acts, which gave justices in petty sessions summary jurisdiction to prosecute those responsible for 'nuisances' (defined broadly as unwholesome houses, accumulations of filth, and the existence of foul drains or cesspools), and established the Poor Law authorities for rural areas.[19] In the same session the Public Baths and Washhouses Act enabled local authorities to provide these amenities. In 1847 the Towns Improvement Clauses Act and the Towns Police Clauses Act consolidated and defined the rights of towns to lay water supplies and main drainage schemes and to control nuisances. Along similar lines to these acts, which helped to expedite private acts by offering a standard legislative format were the Water Works Clauses Act, the Commissioners Clauses Act and the Cemeteries Clauses Act, all of 1847.

This first stage in the public health movement culminated in the Public Health Act of 1848 which established a General Board of Health and empowered local authorities to establish local boards of health, to manage sewers and drains, wells and water supplies, gas works, refuse and sewerage systems, and slaughter houses, and to regulate offensive trades, remove 'nuisances', control cellar dwellings and houses unfit for human habitation, and provide burial grounds, recreation areas and parks, and public baths – powers which were backed up with the right to levy local rates and purchase land.[20] London, ever jealous of its ancient liberties, operated independently under an act of 1848 establishing the Metropolitan Commissioners of Sewers: the City was given the further privilege of operating under its own special City Sewers Act.

The fact that, among the members of the General Board of Health were Chadwick and Southwood Smith (the great evangelical, Shaftesbury was also a member), indicated that a new era of preventive medicine and sanitary engineering was about to dawn. To many contemporaries it suggested a period of intolerable state interference. Even Simon, who certainly understood Chadwick's impatience with local government, thought his plans represented 'papal forms of civil government'.[21] In fact the Board could dictate to local authorities only in exceptional circumstances. The clauses providing for local boards of health were not obligatory and before the Act could be adopted a preliminary enquiry had to be carried out and before that could take place at least ten per cent of those rated for poor relief had to petition to have it. And under the Act each ratepayer, according to the value of his property, had from one to six votes on the issue of whether or not to petition. Only where the death rate in a district exceeded 23 per thousand living did the General Board of Health have the right to force local authorities to establish local boards, and this was a *general* or overall death rate and thus might not include those towns which had a high death rate in their crowded central districts, but which had considerably less morbidity and mortality in the suburbs and environs. In Simon's view, the power enjoyed by the central Board to force districts with high death rates to establish local boards was a distinct handicap, since this 'coercive, not to say penal' clause 'tended to bring on the Board whatever odium attaches to coercive central interference with local government.' Simon was certainly correct to add that the clause achieved little in practice, for there was little the Board could do to force those local authorities which had resisted the formation of a local board to take action in the field of public health.[22]

In 168 communities, where the death rate was under 23, local boards were established in response to petitions from at least ten per cent of the inhabitants rated for poor relief.[23] Between 1848 and the end of 1853 the General Board of Health had received applications from only 284 places for permission to establish local boards of health.[24] In Lancashire, only twenty-six towns took advantage of the Act, and in 1858 only 400,000 of the approximately 2,500,000 people living in Lancashire were under some public health board, and some of the most insanitary industrialized parishes were without any public health authority whatsoever.[25] In 1848, of the 187 incorporated towns in England and Wales only twenty-nine placed the powers of draining and cleansing and paving in one central body; in thirty towns the corporation had absolutely no power over these functions (they were in the hands of independent commissioners) and in another sixty-two towns there was absolutely no public health authority whatsoever. In some communities the corporation cleansed the streets, but only the commissioners of paving or sewers could water them; in others, health committees might be able to inspect or repair drains but not sewers, and to clean roads but not pave them.[26]

Where local boards were established that was not in itself any guarantee that the town would now steer a new course in public health, although the Act empowered the local boards to undertake a variety of actions – arrange for ordnance surveys, maintain streets, construct sewers, license slaughter-houses, and lodging-houses, control cellar dwelling and 'nuisances' and appoint surveyors, inspectors of nuisances, and MOH.[27] Generally, upon adoption of the Act, the existing town corporation simply became the local board of health, and so the same interests which governed the one governed the other.

In part, the unwillingness of the local boards to employ the 1848 Act with any determination and vigour can be accounted for by their composition which will be discussed in the next chapter. In part they moved slowly and cautiously because that had been the traditional tempo of local government. The various investigations carried out by Chadwick's special fever commissioners, by Chadwick himself, and by the Select and Royal Commissions had amply demonstrated that where local improvement Acts prior to 1848 had been applied for they had generally been implemented in the most tentative and hesitant fashion. Sometimes this was due to the nature of the private improvement Acts, for they did not permit the local authority to construct house drains at the owners' expense or force connections to main sewers, or to recover the costs of cleansing from house-owners, but generally it was a case of parsimony compounded by ignorance and fear of engineering innovations. The example of Darlington, which was subjected to a General Board of Health investigation in 1850 may be taken as typical. The inspector, William Ranger, found that only thirteen of the fifty-four streets in the town were fully sewered and that

> In the sewers already laid there appears to have been no regard paid to any general system, inclination, depth, capacity, form, or construction; some are four, five, and even ten feet deep, whilst others are level with the surface of streets, and in form are square with stone sides and tops, but *without bottoms*. Drains 9 or 12 inches square, placed to receive the discharge of circular and other sewers are of much greater value.

That Darlington was still employing square-shaped sewers rather than the more easily and efficiently scoured and flushed egg-shaped ones which he had for so long advocated must have smacked of heresy to Chadwick: that they were using sewers without bottoms must have struck all sanitary officials as madness. One can only imagine what the sub-soil was like. In only one street were the sewers capable of draining the cellar dwellings which were so numerous in the town. Ranger went on to give details of up to sixty-six people sharing one privy and of lean-to privies saturating the wall they shared in common with dwellings – all this in a town that had almost trebled its population during the first half of the century.[28]

Clearly there was considerable need for a central body like the General Board of Health to serve in an advisory capacity on engineering matters and to pressure local authorities to adopt the 1848 Act. Conscious of the fears of centralization which it aroused, the General Board of Health was reluctant to force unwilling communities to adopt the Act, perhaps because it knew that local boards set up under

duress would remain inactive or be no more effective than the anti-
quated bodies they replaced. Thus when the General Board went
down to Tamworth in 1853 (in response to its high death rate and
reports of miserable sanitary conditions, including mounds of uncol-
lected pig manure), it discovered that though the town council had
adopted a local improvement Act in 1833 it had done little to implement it, and that half the roads remained unpaved and the water
supply was still dependent upon wells, many of which were contaminated from leakage from adjoining cesspools. Despite these appalling
conditions and the resultant death rates, the General Board of Health
still felt unable to impose a local board on the town in the teeth of
concerted opposition.[29]

In other communities the 1848 Act was welcomed locally as an
opportunity to galvanize the town into action, and local reformers
were only too happy to conduct the General Board's inspectors on a
tour of the worst spots. If Stratford-upon-Avon is at all typical, the
General Board's inspectors carried the Chadwickian message with
them, for among the arguments they used there on behalf of the 1848
Act was one based on financial grounds – that as a result of the sanitary
conditions, outdoor poor relief had doubled between 1845 and 1848
and yet it would take only £10,538, or a shilling in the pound on the
rates, to set things aright. This argument and the organized efforts of
the reform party secured the adoption of the Act and the establishment
of a local board against the wishes of those who insisted it 'would
entail a vast expense on the ratepayers'. Interestingly, and by no means
untypically, the wealthier ratepayers were for adoption, the smaller
ratepayers against. It was only after Stratford set up its local board
that it discovered that the Board's original estimate was much too
low![30] In other towns, such as Hanley in the Potteries, the visit of
Robert Rawlinson, one of the Board's inspectors, was enough to stir
the town to sanitary improvements, even though the local opposition,
headed by the existing Commissioners of Sewers, was strong enough
to stop the creation of a local board of health.[31]

The contribution of the General Board of Health to the public
health movement cannot be measured so much by the number of local
boards of health that were established by its prodding as by the
generally improved *attitude* towards sanitary reform which often
followed in the wake of one of its inspections. Men like Rawlinson had
the experience in engineering which local communities for the most
part lacked and their advice on water supplies, glazed brick sewers,
and earthenware pipes helped to extend the Chadwickian revolution

throughout the country. The Board's main influence undoubtedly lay in the advice it offered on sanitary engineering and on such practical matters as how to put water and sewer projects out to bid and in its inspections which could scare or shame communities into activity.[32]

But the Board tried to do too much too quickly. Simon later reflected that it was rightly criticized for its 'tendency to build overmuch on foundations of small experience, a liability to one-sidedness on questions of science and administration, a failure to listen duly to dissentient voices, a deceptive trust in central dictation as the short and ready road to success, and a too despotic tone in the affairs of local and personal interest.' These, Simon sympathetically argues, were only 'faults of over-eagerness'. Certainly in view of the foot-dragging attitudes of the majority of local administrations the impatience and imperious attitudes of the Board are understandable.[33] But in its tone and approach it was clearly out of joint with the times. Opposition to the Board never weakened, and in 1858 it was dismantled.

The successful attack on the General Board of Health and the absorption of its functions by the Privy Council have been interpreted as a blow to the concept of central direction in local affairs and a decline in the vigour of centrally-administered preventive medicine.[34] It is true that the decade of the 1850s and 1860s witnessed a series of *ad hoc* pieces of legislation and the powers conferred by this legislation were often confusing in conception and application. And at the local level there was, without doubt, a general lack of any overall plan for public health improvements. But at the centre the Privy Council was far more active and influential than has generally been allowed.

The Nuisances Removal Acts of 1855, 1860 and 1863 were designed to tackle the problems of accumulations of excrement and street refuse, industrial waste and smoke, polluted rivers, slaughterhouses, and filth, and to guard against a sweeping range of other 'threats', to use Chadwick's phrase, to 'the health, personal safety, or the conveniences of the subject'.[35] These Acts gave the local authorities a wide range of powers – the definition of nuisances was widened, local governments could enter and inspect both business and private premises, and seize unwholesome fish and meat. In the same period the Sewage Utilization Act of 1865 gave town councils and other health authorities power to dispose of sewage for agricultural purposes and the Sewage Utilization Act of 1867 enabled authorities to dispose of sewage outside their boundaries, purchase land for the purpose and band together with other authorities where common interests were involved. Coupled with the right (granted in the Local Government Act of 1858) to take land under compulsory purchase for sanitary purposes, the local governments between 1858 and 1866 enjoyed considerable sanitary powers, but these were contained in widely-scattered, general, and permissive legislation. It is clear that many of the local authorities needed encouragement and prodding from the central government (see Chapter 7). How effective in this role was the Privy Council which took over from the late, but hardly lamented General Board of Works?

In the decade between the passage of the 1848 Public Health Act and the end of the General Board of Health only 103 towns had elected (or been compelled) to establish local boards of health. Over the next ten years a further 568 did so.[36] In part this impressive improvement represents a pragmatic turning, on the part of local authorities, to more efficient and concentrated administration after the futility or ineffectiveness of operating under the partial powers granted in local improvement acts administered by paving and sewer commissions. But if on the one hand the growth of local boards of health indicates the acceptance by an increasing number of local authorities of the need for more powerful local public health bodies, on the other it suggests that these local communities no longer harboured quite the same hostility either to the concept of uniformity in public health administration or to the direction and possible interference from the central government which it entailed. This generalization needs considerable qualification (see chapter 7), but the bitter hostility towards the Chadwickian General Board of Health, so apparent in the attitude of the local communities, was not directed towards the Privy Council, and slowly the concept of submitting to central inspections and advice caught on. The Privy Council had, after all, already played a role in public health during the cholera crisis of 1831; it was the recognized odd-job man of the Government, a catch-all for domestic policies, and its medical department did not carry quite the same bureaucratic stigma of the General Board of Health.[37] Moreover, the Privy Council enjoyed one important power which gave it considerable leverage over the local communities. Under the 1858 Local Government Act, the Local Government Act Office's sanction had to be sought for all mortgages raised by local authorities to execute public works, and the Privy Council's medical department became the inspecting body for these sanctions. In other words, if local authorities contemplated broad sanitary reforms they might have to enter into correspondence with (and perhaps submit to inspection from) the central government.

It put a new cast on the administration of public health and on relations between central and local government.

Asa Briggs has called the period from the 1830s to the mid-1850s 'the most exciting period in the history of public health', but as exciting as the beginnings of the public health movement undoubtedly were, the *development* and growing intensity and commitment of that movement in the 1860s under the benign guidance of Simon and his team at the Privy Council surely has a special kind of excitement of its own.[38] For it was in that decade that the sanitary idea, hitherto embraced only by a small circle of Benthamites and sanitary reformers, slowly filtered down to an increasing number of communities in the country at large. Judged in terms of new attitudes and advances and measured in terms of real improvements enjoyed by a growing number of Victorians, it was 'the heroic age' of state medicine.[39]

Of course there was still much suspicion and hostility directed towards the central government. In Exeter, for example, the Council, after the sobering experience of the 1866 cholera visitation, formally applied for permission to create a local board of health. This provoked strong opposition from the existing improvement commissioners, who fought under the battle-cry of local autonomy. Their chairman raised the spectre of central control and developed the interesting, if somewhat specious argument that, whereas the existing improvement commissioners were 'uninfluenced by any motive beyond their fitness for office', the election of Council members to the proposed local board of health would be governed by political and party considerations. And, as was generally the case, at the root of the opposition was the question of economy, for the inspector employed by the existing improvement commission cost the community only £12 a year. Despite these considerations, Exeter's Council did declare itself a local board of health and in 1867 took matters of public health into its own hands.[40]

The legislation of the 1850s and 1860s, adding piecemeal to the legislative books as experience with 'nuisances' was gained, was extended in the 1866 Sanitary Act (29 & 30 Vict.c.90), the first public health Act in which compulsory clauses were dominant. The Home Secretary was empowered, in Part II of the Act, to take proceedings for the removal of nuisances where local authorities had failed to act, and in Part III the Home Secretary could do the work of improvement and charge the local authority for the work. The Act marked an important stage in the development of the state in preventive medicine. No longer did it merely direct and advise local authorities. It could now compel action, and in that sense take charge of the direction and tempo of reform throughout England. Simon regarded various parts of the Act as of the utmost importance, especially the duty which now fell on the authorities to provide for sanitary inspections and to suppress nuisances, the greater powers granted the authorities to provide water, and the extension of the term 'nuisance' to include overcrowding. But it was the inclusion of the compulsory clauses that led Simon to write that the Act 'represented such a stride of advance as virtually to begin a new era', and in a telling phrase he emphasized that, 'under the Act, the grammar of common sanitary legislation acquired the novel virtue of an imperative mood.'[41] Simon was jubilant, and wrote from his position at the Privy Council 'that influences which have hitherto been causing about a quarter of our total mortality are now for the most part brought within control of the law.'[42] The tempo and pace of the reform – eighteen years had passed since the first major health Act – and the way it was accomplished, not by any coherent, far-sighted scheme or system, but after a period of piecemeal legislation and trial and error, indicated the essentially pragmatic, halting nature, not only of public health reform, but of Victorian social reform in general.

The 1866 Sanitary Act might mark a significant step forward in the drafting of legislation, but to be a breakthrough, in any real terms, it had to be implemented, and the Privy Council showed great reluctance to enter the field of public health directly under the Act. Simon, at that time, was perhaps more interested in waging his campaign against smallpox and conducting general investigative surveys than in immediately testing local reaction by enforcing the Act in one or two test areas. Simon was in no hurry to give the Sanitary Act a thorough testing. Perhaps the Act was more important as a symbol than as an immediately enforceable piece of legislation, for as a symbol of the new power of the central government to intervene in the affairs of local authorities it stirred them to greater efforts on their own initiative. And probably Simon was quite content to have the Act function in that manner, for he saw the role of his office as one of *stimulating*, not *imposing* action at the local level and if that could be achieved not just by advice and technical assistance but by the trump card, held in reserve, of ultimate power, so much the better. Simon knew full well that the 1858 Public Health Act establishing the medical department of the Privy Council had originally confirmed his authority for a temporary period of one year only and the parliamentary debate in 1859 which extended the life of the department had been considerably heated. His department, he considered, could be most effective and provoke the least resistance if it moved slowly but surely, performing the primary functions of 'inquiry and report', and, through epidemiological research develop 'a scientific basis for the progress of sanitary law and administration.' Simon thus set himself the task at the Privy Council of establishing a '*via media*', between 'officiousness' and 'neglect'.[43] It called for a delicate balancing act but he pulled it off.

Quite apart from what we have already said about its mere presence, armed with the imperative powers of the 1866 Act, as a kind of whip, hovering over local authorities and goading them into action, the Privy Council's contribution to the nation's health was quite considerable. It played a leading role in the investigation of industrial diseases and occupational hazards (see Chapter 10). It generated a steady, proselytizing climate favourable to the passage of further sanitary legislation. Its suggestion, which was acted upon, that the Office of the Registrar-General issue quarterly returns of vital statistics (beginning in 1870) created a much firmer, factual basis for reform. It offered support and the weight of its authority to local reform groups, and scattered throughout its reports and papers are petitions from local ratepayers urging it to start investigations into local conditions or complaining that the local authority was not fulfilling its public health functions.[44] In 1867, for example, Simon corresponded with 113 local authorities to determine what actions had been taken under the Nuisances Removal and other sanitary Acts. In 1870, with relapsing fever raging, Simon engaged in some 200 communications with local governments, sixty-six of them by direct investigation, the others by correspondence. Its inspections often served to shame or stimulate a local authority to much needed action. Thus Leeds switched to the river Washburn for its water supply after Dr Hunter had condemned the existing source, the Wharfe, in a report to the Privy Council, and in response to Hunter's unfavourable comparison between Leeds and Newcastle, Sunderland, and Sheffield, and to his general criticisms, the Leeds Council applied to Parliament for a new improvement act and appointed a MOH.[45] From 1869 on the Privy Council had two permanent inspectors (Drs George Buchanan and John Radcliffe) for general sanitary investigations in addition to a team for scientific laboratory investigations, which, as Simon said, were 'not necessarily connected with our practical business of the moment, but tending to be of powerful indirect influence on our practical business as a whole . . .' Rather than apply constant pressure by continuous interference, Simon preferred to meet challenges and emergencies as they arose, and devote his energies to empirical research on a variety of contagious diseases.[46] In his *A History of English Public Health* W. M. Frazer, summarizing the work of the Privy Council, argues that in 'the calm and non-political atmosphere of the Privy Council . . . Simon performed what is regarded as his best work.' His fourteen annual reports 'lay down the abiding principles of Public Health administration, point the way to farther much needed reforms and, year after year, make urgent demands for the more extensive prosecution of medical research.'[47]

By his Eleventh Annual Report in 1868 Simon declared that the state was now playing a vital role in preventive medicine:

> It has interfered between parent and child, not only in imposing limitation on industrial uses of children, but also to the extent of requiring that children should not be left unvaccinated. It has interfered between employer and employed, to the extent of insisting, in the interest of the latter, that certain sanitary claims shall be fulfilled in all places of industrial occupation. It has interfered between vendor and purchaser; has put restrictions on the sale and purchase of poisons, has prohibited in certain cases certain commercial supplies of water, and has made it a public offence to sell adulterated food or drink or medicine, or to offer for sale any meat unfit for human food. Its care for the treatment of disease has not been unconditionally limited to treating at the public expense such sickness as may accompany destitution: it has provided that in any sort of epidemic emergency organized medical assistance, not peculiarly for paupers, may be required of local authorities; and in the same spirit it requires that vaccination at the public cost shall be given gratuitously to every claimant.

He concluded that 'the principles affirmed in our statute-book are such as, *if carried into full effect*, would soon reduce to quite insignificant amount our present very large proportions of preventable disease.'[48] The phrase 'if carried into full effect' was a crucial one, for the Privy Council built up a massive dossier which revealed a huge gulf between the laws and their application and it revealed conclusively that permissive legislation remained unapplied and that, in general, the sanitary laws needed to be codified and simplified to induce the local authorities to use them.

The widespread recognition among sanitary reformers that what was needed was not more legislation so much as codification of existing laws led to a reform movement for a simplified health act that would integrate all the *ad hoc* legislation over the past two decades in a clear, practicable code of laws. In this reform movement doctors using the Social Science Association as their forum played a leading part and it produced three outstanding works in the canon of public health literature – A. P. Stewart's *On The Results of Permissive Legislation*, E. Jenkins, *Legal Aspects of Sanitary Reform*, and H. W. Rumsey, *On State Medicine in Great Britain and Ireland*.[49] Following a petition to the government by the Joint Committee of the British Medical Association and the Social Science Association, a Sanitary Commission was appointed in 1869. After examining almost a hundred witnesses it reported in 1871 that there was undoubtedly a pressing need for the unification and simplification of existing public health legislation. That it would reach this conclusion was perhaps inevitable, for among the twenty-one commissioners were nine members of the Social Science Association, including both Rumsey and Stewart. It insisted that 'it is desirable to make law concerning public health as simple and uniform as possible', and it called for a special minister to take charge of both the poor law and public health aspects of the nation's health, for a central health authority with a chief MOH and adequate medical staff, and for every local authority to have at least one MOH. At the same time it cautioned that 'The Central Authority . . . must nevertheless avoid taking to itself the actual work of local government: we would leave *direction* only to the Central power.' In what could serve as a summary of prevailing opinion on the proper sphere of government it recommended that the function of the central authority was to:

> direct inquiries, medical or otherwise, to give advice and new plans when required, to sanction some of the larger proceedings of the local authorities, to issue provisional orders subject to parliamentary confirmation, to receive complaints and appeals, to issue medical regulations on emergencies, and to collect medical reports.

Above all the Commission warned that any new central authority 'must steer clear of the rock on which the General Board of Health was wrecked; so completely is self-government the habit and quality of Englishmen that the country would resent any Central Authority undertaking the duties of the local executive.'[50]

Although the Local Government Act of 1871 did not establish a separate ministry of health, as the Sanitary Commission had hoped, it did create a unified public health administration, combining in one body at the Local Government Board the staffs of the old Poor Law Board (with its medical officers), the Local Government Act Office, the Registrar-General, and Simon's Privy Council staff. Simon had from 1868 on urged the unification of all central health authorities, but he now discovered that under the President of the Local Government Board, James Stansfield, he and his medical staff were in a subordinate position to the Poor Law administration. Although one historian dates the beginnings of the modern development of public health administration from the creation of the Local Government Board under a minister responsible to Parliament and from the great unifying Public Health Act of 1875 which, as Simon and the Sanitary Commission had urged, finally consolidated most of the existing sanitary legislation (in a codification that ran to 343 sections and five schedules!), Simon found his new position an increasingly frustrating, 'depressing and bewildering' one.[51]

Even more confining than the attitude of Stansfield or the antagonisms and rivalries between Simon and his staff and the staff of the Poor Law section were 'the demoralizing effects of Treasury control'. The Local Government Board's medical department was responsible for the general overseeing of approximately 1,500 local health authorities and yet they were expected somehow to operate with a staff of ten or so. The Treasury refused to consider increased salaries for the hard-pressed inspectors or funds for a larger staff, and whenever the medical department undertook special sanitary or fever investigations it had to pull its inspectors off their important routine smallpox vaccination work. The tight budget did not even permit Simon or his successors to issue their annual reports free to all the local authorities.[52] Perhaps it is not to be wondered at that in frustration Simon and the other chief MOH to the Local Government Board turned away from the impossible task of trying with an inadequate staff to conduct investigations throughout England and Wales, and turned, instead, to empirical epidemiological research. But here, as well, they ran up against Treasury parsimony. In 1887, for example, the Treasury rejected a request for just £100 to cover 'urgent experimental studies on infection, water purity, and scarlatina'.[53] Quite incredibly, it was argued that the Government simply could not encourage 'speculative inquiries . . . which may or may not prove that disease is in some way connected with sanitary administration.'[54] It took the most determined urging from the Local Government Board to prevent the Treasury cutting back the medical department's important laboratory experiments. Down to the end of the century the central agency responsible for preventive medicine had to operate in an unfriendly atmosphere fraught with the dangers of imminent budget cuts.

In the circumstances it is remarkable that the medical department of the Local Government Board was able to conduct as many investigations as it did. Buchanan was forced to carry out his vital cholera surveys (1884–5), which were, in effect, national sanitary investigations, without special assistants. Similarly, Dr Barry's important investigation into the causes of smallpox in Sheffield was limited by the Treasury's tight rein on the budget, and for want of adequate staff even the vaccination work faltered.[55] Simon complained that his medical department was 'without systematic inspectorial relation to the local workings of the common sanitary law' and had thus 'been unable to make occasional inspections in nearly sufficient number to compensate for the want of system.' Only three per cent of all sanitary districts were visited each year over the first ten years of the medical department's work (about forty-eight per year on an average), although, taking the period 1871 down to the end of the century, the Local Government Board's inspectors visited about half of the sanitary districts in England and Wales, excluding the extensive surveys made as part of the cholera investigation of 1885–6 and the inland survey of 1893–5.[56] The cholera surveys covered about one-third of all the sanitary districts in England. 'The late nineties', Roy MacLeod has concluded, 'found the Medical Department philosophically frustrated and physically exhausted.'[57] At last, in 1898, the Treasury appointed a Department Committee of Inquiry into the medical department of the Local Government Board. It found that between 1872 and 1898 the department had conducted only 1,326 routine sanitary inspections. This average of less than one inspection for each district over a twenty-eight year period was, it concluded, not an indication of negligence or lack of energy but, rather, of overwork and lack of adequate staff. As a result of the inquiry the medical department did finally get a few additions to its woefully insufficient staff, but still by no means enough, and the chief MOH, Thorne-Thorne, still received only £1,500 year, £500 less than Simon had received and less than some local MOH.[58]

It would be most misleading to suggest that we should judge the impact and influence of the Local Government Board's medical department simply by the number of inspections it was able to carry out. Like the Privy Council before it, it could use the *threat* of these investigations to prod local authorities into action. Significantly, not a single town about which it had received complaints failed to make improvements following its inspections between 1871 and 1880, and according to G. Sclater-Booth, President of the Local Government Board, an inspection, or the threat of an inspection, was generally sufficient to galvanize most local authorities into the required action, and thus make a compulsory order unnecessary.[59] Very occasionally a show of force had to be made, as in the case of Lincoln, where a writ of *mandamus* was issued against the Mayor and Corporation for not complying with the Local Government Board's demand to provide an adequate sewage system, but this was a clumsy weapon, and generally a combination of advice, admonition, and threat of public inquiry was effective.[60]

The Local Government Board had a far more effective weapon in its arsenal: all local authorities wishing to qualify for low-cost government loans for sanitary purposes had to submit their plans and schemes to the Board (see Chapter 4) and this gave the medical department some control over local affairs, although Simon would have liked the medical department exclusively, and not the Board as a whole, to have been the sanctioning body. Nevertheless many schemes submitted in application for a government loan called for the Board's inspection and this tied the central and local sanitary authorities more closely together than any compulsory health legislation or powers of legal action.

Between 1848 and 1872 over £11,000,000 had been loaned to local authorities for sanitary purposes, but over the next eight years the Local Government Board sanctioned over twice that amount.[61] The importance of the work of the Local Government Board as an investigative and supervisory body for the sanction of government loans to local sanitary authorities, and its influence upon the steadily improving sanitary state of the nation, can be grasped by the picture presented by the following table:

Loans sanctioned by the Local Government Board for public health purposes: 1871–97

£

1871	267,562	1884	2,460,246
1872	602,271	1885	2,836,109
1873	980,153	1886	2,318,594
1874	1,457,496	1887	2,103,026
1875	1,973,105	1888	2,289,897
1876	2,757,323	1889	2,820,267
1877	4,380,369	1890	2,827,296
1878	3,097,857	1891	3,281,037
1879	3,308,032	1892	4,340,577
1880	2,932,899	1893	7,266,516
1881	2,526,190	1894	5,322,331
1882	2,458,288	1895	6,129,017
1883	2,338,573	1896	5,545,403
		1897	5,886,562

[62]

These loans represented local government expenditure on an unprecedented level – in all, over £84,000,000 was borrowed, of which over £65,000,000 was by urban authorities.[63] From another perspective the loans represented central government influence and assistance on an equally unprecedented scale. Not all these loans were based upon inspections by the medical department – although in 1875 alone it conducted over 400 inspections for loan purposes – but plans were scrutinized, changes made, recommendations suggested, local conditions analyzed. Thus the Board's expertise was brought to bear not only on the local governments but on the central government as well, for, as Ralph Lingen, the Permanent Secretary to the Treasury once confessed in another context, 'I do not know who is to check the assertions of experts when the Government has once undertaken a class of duties which none but such persons understand.'[64] Thus while the loan sanctioning powers of the Board did not enable the medical department to do much about the most backward of lazy authorities they did permit them to influence the improvements made elsewhere.

Perhaps in the long run the Board's greatest contribution was simply that of setting an example, offering general advice, and serving as a clearing-house for accumulated engineering and sanitary information. By 1900 it was receiving nearly 2,000 annual reports from local MOH and another 4,000 from Poor Law MOH, in addition to 1,300 from MOH for educational authorities and another 2,000 from factory surgeons.[65] These reports, though varying enormously in quality, gave the central government an overall, comparative picture of the sanitary conditions prevailing throughout the nation and added enormously to its stock of information. When its inspectors offered advice they could do so on the basis of considerable acquired knowledge. The Local Government Board also had extensive powers to confirm or reject local by-laws and this gave them some supervisory say over the way local authorities handled problems of sanitation and water supply. By 1889 it had confirmed some 370 sets of local by-laws and had the satisfaction of seeing by-laws adopted throughout England and Wales based upon its own detailed model by-laws.[66]

Although it lies somewhat outside the subject of this book, belonging more to epidemiological history, the Board's scientific work should be mentioned. Simon never regarded his epidemiological work to be totally separate from those administrative duties involving inspection or authorization of loans and by-laws, for he maintained that it was up to him and his teams at the Privy Council and Local Government Board to 'develop a scientific basis for the progress of sanitary law and administration, and aim at stamping on public hygiene a character of greater exactitude than it had hitherto had.'[67] Under the guidance of Simon and his successors a series of investigations was undertaken into diet and nutrition, industrial diseases, effects of overcrowding, ague (march fever), tuberculosis, cholera, diphtheria, diarrhoea, bronchitis, infant mortality, hospital hygiene, and a host of other influences upon the public's health. These investigations helped to advance the acceptance of the germ theory and generally served to underline the connection that existed between cleanliness (efficient water supplies and sewerage systems) and good ventilation in the home and factory on the one hand and good health on the other.[68]

Viewed as a whole, the work of the medical departments of the Privy Council and Local Government Board must be seen as an influence both on the central and local level for gradual change rather than for radical innovations or departures. It is the story of routine investigations interrupted by investigations into sudden outbreaks of infectious disease, continuing epidemiological research, occasional pressure on tardy or indolent local authorities, constant encouragement in the form of technical advice and the sanction of loans, and suggestions for by-laws. If the central bodies found it difficult to initiate reforms in the local sanitary districts they could certainly expedite and assist them once they were under way. Theirs was thus the function of an accelerator. They also performed valuable work of publicity, for their printed reports could shame local administrations or suggest where further legislation or sanitary work was most required. Acting as a vast clearing-house for information, the medical departments served also as spring-boards for further reform. Above all the patient, evolutionary pace of the work of Simon and his successors did much to prevent the re-emergence of the fears and antagonisms that had been directed against Chadwick and his General Board of Work. Thus the medical departments of the Privy Council and the Local Government Board must take much credit for the gradual acceptance, between 1860 and 1880, of the role of the central government as a supervisory power in public health. They set the necessary footings for State preventive medicine and assisted in the development of that vital Victorian compromise between State aid and what might be called self-help on the local level. Given the nature both of the composition of the local sanitary administrations in these years and of the political and economic philosophies they espoused, direct control or aggressive use of compulsory legislative powers would have been disastrous.

What was needed was a deft touch – a mixture of the carrot (low-cost loans and free technical advice) and the stick (threatened use of the mandatory clauses in the 1866 Public Health Act): without a doubt Simon and his successors had that touch. Of course they assumed that a new spirit of sanitary reform – the 'sanitary idea' – had wafted, if not exactly swept, over the nation and that gentle advice and encouragement would bear fruit at the local level. How correct they were in that assumption the next chapter attempts to demonstrate.

7

Local Affairs

'I do not believe that the very smallest fraction of those constituting the [local] Boards do so for the sake of the sanitary matters, it is more to get their names before the public, and have the handling of public affairs.'

T. H. Harrison, *Transactions of the Sanitary Institute of Great Britain* (1886–7), p. 208

'. . . of all questions in modern State-Medicine, perhaps none is more deeply important than that of the system on which Members of the Medical Profession should be made serviceable in the administration of the Health-laws. . . .'

J. Simon, *English Sanitary Institutions* (1897), p. 335

However much direction the central government might give from above, ultimately the health of the nation depended on sanitary measures at the local level. Unfortunately, for much of the century the love of local autonomy and its close identification with low rates were nowhere more apparent than in public health. As sanitary needs became increasingly apparent, however, and as the benefits of sanitary measures became clearer, so local attitudes slowly underwent change. In the gradual widening of the sphere of action of local government, its growing professionalism, and responsiveness to society's needs, public health played an important, indeed crucial role.

There were over 1,000 sanitary districts in England and Wales in the second half of the century and only a handful have been examined by historians. The variety of these districts – their size, wealth, location, social composition, growth rates, topography, population densities, access to cheap or open land – make it difficult to offer generalizations. In the following pages I have concentrated mainly upon large towns, where sanitary needs were most urgent, and attempt to present a broad picture of changing attitudes and responses, at the local level, to the challenge of public health.

Neither the 1835 Municipal Corporations Act nor the 1848 Public Health Act made a radical difference in the composition of local bodies responsible for health matters. Generally the existing paving or improvement commissioners remained. Candidates for election to borough councils had to possess real or personal property worth £1,000 or occupy property rated at £30. In smaller boroughs, too small to be divided into wards, the figures were respectively £500 and £15. These qualifications were abolished in 1882, but for much of the century they, and the fact that meetings were generally held during working hours, and services were unpaid, effectively excluded working men.[1] In view of the interest manifested by women in sanitary matters and the role which they played in health-visiting and hygiene, it is worth noting that women were not enfranchised until 1869, but the right of *married* women to sit on borough councils was not established until 1907, and not until 1918 were they given the right to the municipal vote.[2] The municipal franchise was based upon a complex system of rateable values, a system which resulted in a narrow electorate. In 1861 only three percent of the population of Birmingham could vote for the town council which was responsible, among other things, for their health: the figures for Maidstone, Ipswich, and Leeds were, respectively, nine, ten, and thirteen per cent.[3]

The franchise and the property qualifications required to sit on town councils led in some places to 'tight little oligarchies' and in most places to local boards or councils in which property interests (with income derived from rents) predominated.[4] In 1886 the results of a survey of roughly one-fifth of the urban sanitary districts in England and Wales were presented to the Sanitary Institute of Great Britain. The survey indicated that 'the classes who administer the Public Health Acts' represented six main interests. Shopkeepers (30.8 per cent of local sanitary officials) were by far the most dominant single group, followed by manufacturers (17.5 per cent), gentlemen (11.8 per cent), merchants (8.6 per cent), farmers (7.7 per cent) and builders (7.6 per cent). Only 3.2 per cent were lawyers, and 2.2 estate agents. Of the shopkeepers, only 11 per cent could be clearly identified as owners of a small class of property, but shopkeepers stood to gain from low rates, and their competence to decide on sanitary matters was suspect. As one MOH from a district where sixteen of the twenty-four board members were shopkeepers put it:

> I do not believe that the very smallest fraction of those constituting the Board do so for the sake of sanitary matters, it is more to get their names before the public, and have the handling of public affairs. The Medical Officer's Report is read, and no discussion is ever made upon it. The subject of their meetings is generally some wrangle about the Town Hall clock, or other equally absurd subject.[5]

167

Of course there were many exceptions, but as a class shopkeepers seem to have regarded local government service as a way of advancing their business. In all too many communities this meant being known as a staunch defender of the *status quo* and especially of low taxation. The paving and widening of roads, street drainage or the provision of cheap gas lighting might serve their interests, but not so larger, more expensive projects. In Manchester, for example, the ' "economy" party [was] led by and largely composed of shopkeepers'. The 'Small shop element was what he disliked', wrote the MOH for Plymouth in 1900; 'Down with everything was their motto.' To sanitary reformers the shopkeepers and small tradesmen were men of narrow vision who, quite apart from their interest in keeping the rates low, had no appreciation of the scale of work which was necessary to raise the standard of municipal public health. As a writer to the *Salford Weekly News* put it in 1864, it was as unreasonable to expect 'the small trader who deals in units of tens and seldom reaches three figures to comprehend such sums involving some hundreds of thousands' as it was to expect someone who was 'ignorant of geometry and mathematics to calculate the distance and density of Saturn.'[6] In view of their predominance on local sanitary boards, Napoleon's dictum about England being a nation of shopkeepers takes on a special significance.

The second category in the survey, 'manufacturers', is a very large and ill-defined one. Certainly as in Birmingham, Leeds, Darlington, and elsewhere, large or middling manufacturers might have the time, the professional skills, the interest, and indeed the civic-mindedness to work energetically for the improvement of their communities and to be less concerned with rate-increases.[7] But among the manufacturers on local sanitary committees were chemical manufacturers, soap boilers, gas makers, tanners, bone boilers, fellmongers, glue makers, manure processers and 'others too numerous to mention, the nature of whose operations are such as to pollute our water, and load the air of our populous places with noxious gases and smoke.'[8] Even allowing for the reformist slant of the survey one must question why so many manufacturers whose operations were coming increasingly under the public health code (see next chapter) chose to be administrators of that code.

Of the 'gentlemen' making up some 11.8 per cent of local board members, doctors accounted for only 3.3 per cent.[9] The MOH who was having a hard time relaying the actual or potential environmental and health hazards of the community to the local authority could not expect to receive help from a large bloc of medical men on the sanitary committee. Life-insurance men, who stood to gain so much from sanitary improvements, were noticeably absent from public administration. On the other hand the presence of builders should be noted, for, while not a very large group, they did represent an interest which was opposed to the proliferation of local by-laws and the implementation of national health and building codes which would drive up the cost of building or renting houses, especially working-class dwellings.[10]

As for the presence of farmers, the Local Government Board thought that this was by and large detrimental to good health, since farmers, it argued, did not appreciate frequent meetings, and were opposed to change when they did attend.[11]

It would be simplistic to prejudge the attitude of local bodies to public health merely on the basis of the occupations of the elected officials or to categorize or stereotype any single occupational group. Yet the commercial and personal backgrounds of the 'fit and proper' men who contributed so much to the improvement of health in Birmingham and later on in Leeds were not unfortunately representative of the rank-and-file members of most local authorities in Victorian Britain. The corruption, lethargy, innate conservatism, and especially parsimony of local government officials became almost a *cliché* of Victorian public health reformers. But it would be wrong to stigmatize all those who were less than committed to sweeping public health measures as simply members of the 'dirty' party, men without vision who were content to live in communities where the poorer inhabitants were condemned to live amid dirt and disease, men who simply placed a higher value on healthy bank accounts than on healthy citizens. As we have already seen, the engineering and fiscal problems involved in sewerage schemes, the bewildering technological difficulties and the fears associated with committing the budget to relatively untried and unproven experiments could act as a legitimate deterrent. And we might well sympathize with those who found the constant talk of the benefits of water-borne sewage, or this or that method of sewage treatment, either faddism, or, quite simply, boring. The Local Government Board commented that few local boards had competence or interest in sanitary matters and that there would be a general rush for the doors as soon as items concerning public health came up on the agenda![12] The critics of sweeping and costly improvements could also often get support and comfort from comparative vital statistics, for while reformers might claim that conditions were bad, their opponents could always point to some town or other where conditions were worse or could argue that death rates were higher in the past. Thus complacency, as in mid-century Birmingham, could lead to inactivity, and to a kind of psychological myopia, an inability to visualize how things could be improved when they were already better than conditions elsewhere.[13]

Opposition to sanitary reforms might be the product of a number of factors, but it is safe to generalize that 'economy' – the determination to keep the local taxes low – was the greatest obstacle facing reformers at the local level. In his reform tract, *Homes of the Working Classes*, (1866), the Leeds radical, James Hole, justifiably characterized local sanitary bodies in the following manner:

> They and those who elect them, are the lower middle class, the owners, generally speaking, of the very property which requires improvement. To ask them to close the cellar dwellings is to ask them to forfeit a portion of their incomes. Every pound they vote for drainage, or other sanitary improvement, is something taken out of their own pocket . . . to the ratepayers themselves a little claptrap about centralisation, and still more an appeal to their pockets . . . is sufficient to cause the rejection of the most useful measures. . . . When contemplating an ugly, ill-built town, where every little freeholder asserts his independent right as a Briton to do what he likes with his own; to inflict his own selfishness, ignorance, and obstinacy upon his neighbours, and on posterity for generations to come; and where local self-government means merely mis-government – we are apt to wish for a little wholesome despotism to curb such vagaries.[14]

Unless an epidemic or some other emergency created an atmosphere favourable to reform, most public health measures were generally viewed with suspicion, or open hostility, by the ratepayers and the officials who were returned to power on the cry of low rates and economy. Concern for improved health was always modified by concern for light taxation, and, when the spectre of central interference was raised, the cry for 'economy' was linked with the old and compelling cry for preservation of local independence: together they added up to what most local voters and their elected representatives meant by 'liberty'. Indeed, a study of the bitter opposition to sanitary reform might well leave one wondering if it was not local autonomy and low taxation, rather than self-preservation, which was the basic instinct of Victorians.

It would be wrong to assume that only die-hard conservatives or reactionaries put low rates before local improvements, for in Leeds the Chartists, led by the publisher of *The Northern Star* (the Chartist paper) bitterly opposed, on the grounds of economy, the Leeds Improvement Act of 1842, which, together with the Liverpool Improvement Act (also 1842) was 'one of the pioneering measures in the history of public health in England'.[15] The Chartists also initially opposed the sewering of Leeds, and were an obstacle to reform also in Hanley and Macclesfield, where they opposed sanitary measures advocated by the wealthier inhabitants.[16] 'Clean' versus 'Dirty' parties had little to do with the major party divisions or with left-wing and right-wing factions.[17]

But one generalization which appears reasonably safe is that small businessmen and those who derived a substantial part of their total income from rents were advocates of 'economy'. Both groups were active in municipal affairs, and one is tempted to argue that the efficiency of local public health administration was in inverse ratio to their influence on local boards.[18] Local rates were assessed on the rental value of property and thus a man whose sole income was derived from rents paid much higher rates in proportion to his total income than others. E. P. Hennock has persuasively argued that the effect of this was to push middle-class landlords into local government to protect their interests by ensuring that rates were kept as low as possible. Given the fact that they organized themselves into powerful ratepayers' associations, Hennock has concluded that the local rating system 'could not but act as a check to any imaginative approach to the problems of urban life'.[19]

In contrast to the often poorly organized party politics of local government, the ratepayers' associations represented coherent interest groups with clearly defined and focused aims. They constituted an electioneering body which could exert considerable influence and which, consequently, advocates of local reform had to overcome, win over, or somehow accommodate. Occasionally the 'economists' could be menacing, as in Lincoln, where the Corporation, which was thinking of establishing a local board of health in 1866, received threatening letters – one member was told that his coffin had been ordered, and another resigned after receiving a murder threat.[20] More generally the 'economists' were simply hostile to any schemes which placed additional burdens on the rates and viewed with considerable suspicion anything which smacked to them of specialization. Thus, as we shall see, they were generally opposed to, or at least unenthusiastic about the appointment of MOH, inspectors of nuisances, and surveyors: occasionally, as in Oldbury, where the Ratepayers' Protection Society was powerful, they were strong enough to oust the MOH from office;

171

more generally they undermined his position by keeping the salary so low that the MOH had to devote more time to his private practice than to public affairs.[21] In Birmingham the Ratepayers' Protection Society's nominees on the Council prevented the municipal purchase of the Birmingham Waterworks Company in 1854 and a year later the Society, now under the name of the Independent Association of Ratepayers, though defeated in the Council, managed to exert enough pressure in the town to defeat a new improvement bill which would have raised the rates.[22] In Leeds the Leeds Municipal Reform Association had been founded 'principally with a view of lessening expenditure and securing greater municipal purity'. It was so successful at the polls that the rates fell and by 1871 were lower than at any time since 1859. No wonder the *Leeds Mercury* complained that the Council's hands were tied by 'the public . . . crying out "economy, economy" and upbraiding the Council for spending money . . . the great difficulty with which they had to contend was the constant cry of economy.' In Liverpool the powerful Houseowners' Association acted as a barrier to reform throughout the 1860s and 1870s.[23]

Fear of higher taxes thus served to retard the rate of improvement in many communities. In Manchester for example, the incorporation of the city under the 1835 Municipal Corporations Act was fought on the issue of local taxation, for it was feared that the incorporation would result in the higher taxing powers which the Act granted to all borough councils.[24] But, as we have suggested, it was not low taxation alone which motivated the various 'economy' parties. Often, as was the case in Sheerness, there was a willingness to engage in drainage schemes, but the tradition of amateurism and resistance to the new Chadwickian fad of professionalism made the local authority determined to attempt it without the aid of an engineer. Fortunately the Privy Council investigated in time to prevent the adoption of a scheme which would have resulted in the flooding of low-lying cellars.[25] In many towns there was a genuine concern that municipal expenditure was threatening to outpace local economic development. It was on those grounds that a leading 'economist', Thomas Avery (of the scale-making firm), although by no means opposed to necessary public health measures, argued that all municipal works should 'either be suspended altogether or proceeded with more slowly and deliberately'. The first thing Avery attempted when he was elected to the Birmingham Town Council in 1862 was to restrict the borrowing power of the Corporation.[26] The 'economists' also persuasively argued that high taxation would only serve to drive out industry to other towns which were not so concerned with public health and thus result in local unemployment and a lower tax base.[27] In their defence it should be mentioned that public health was just one of many demands on public expenditure, and that as the century progressed so other costly municipal activities increased, among them the provision of libraries, art galleries and museums, new town halls, street building, lighting, the purchase of gas works, the purchase or provision of transport systems, and educational facilities. It was a common cry of reformers like Kingsley and Dickens, Chadwick and Farr that public health measures were the essential foundation for other reforms, but local politicians saw public health as just one of many demands on the rates and it is certainly understandable that in an age of growing complexity of urban life, and accompanying municipal commitments and obligations, they would think that someone had to act as watchdog over the budget. Throughout Britain towns closely watched one another and while the energetic Nonconformist hosiery manufacturers of Leicester, who embarked upon the cleaning up of the town in the mid-Victorian years, may have inspired others to emulate them, the fact that their reforms necessitated a considerable rise in the local rates (from 8d in the £ in 1845 to almost 7s in the £ between 1871–75) provided a clear warning of the costs involved. Large manufacturers could bear the cost (and they often stood to gain from improvements such as pure water: this was true of the Leicester hosiers and the brewing and cloth industries), but the small property ratepayer often could not or would not.[28]

Given all that we have said so far, it is perhaps remarkable, as we have already had occasion to note, that so much was done at the local level. Although each town had its own tempo and rhythm of change there is no doubt that by the late 1860s there was a discernibly new municipal spirit in Britain, and that the opposition to sanitary reforms, so manifest earlier in the century, was less well-organized, less vocal, and less powerful. There are many reasons for this change and for the growth of a civic spirit which was willing to embrace, among other things, the 'sanitary idea'.

Sanitary improvements were often made, not so much willingly and enthusiastically, as sporadically, in response to emergency conditions, especially to epidemics which drew attention to scandalous neglect and which made further delay impossible. It is in this sense that cholera has been called the reformers' best friend: this 'shock disease' demanded action on the part of local authorities. Similarly, outbreaks of typhoid and typhus drew attention to polluted water and dung heaps or cesspits. When, for example, a typhoid epidemic broke out in the comfortable, supposedly healthy Leeds suburb of Headingly in 1889, the fear and alarm led to a committee of inquiry and an attack both upon the negligent medical officer of health and the state of public health in Leeds as a whole.[29] Even when epidemics were not in themselves enough to spur otherwise torpid authorities into a flurry of activity, the fear that unless something were done they might stimulate a Privy Council or Local Government Board inquiry forced local authorities into action.[30] Occasionally a well-publicized government commission, such as the Royal Sanitary Commission of 1869–71, or the Royal Commission on the Housing of the Working Classes of 1884–5 could create a local climate of opinion favourable to reform.[31] Sometimes local governments proceeded with reforms only when threatened by law suits. This was especially the case where local authorities were guilty of river pollution.[32]

These factors helped to bring local governments into the field of public health. Of great importance were two other developments, one the result of central government action, the other of local economic growth – low rates of interest government loans and a higher local tax base respectively. Towns wedded to local autonomy might reject the notion of government loans – Hanley for example preferred to borrow money from the Economic Life Insurance Society at a higher rate of interest rather than submit its sanitary scheme to the central government scrutiny necessary to qualify for a loan from the Public Works Loan Commissioners – but generally the opportunity to borrow money at a lower-than-market rate of interest over a long repayment period proved too tempting to resist, and did much to stimulate local activity and to silence the objections of the 'economists'.[33] Thus the Public Works (Manufacturing Districts) Act of 1863, which enabled large towns to turn to the Public Works Loan Commission for loans for sanitary purposes stimulated considerable action. In the case of Manchester, the government loans offered 'an indirect relief to the local rates, and may have induced the City Council to expedite schemes which would otherwise have been postponed . . .'[34] As we saw in the previous chapter the enormous amounts of money flowing from the Public Works Loan Commission to the local sanitary authorities serve as an indication of the local commitment to sanitary improvement: they mark both a fruitful co-operation between local and central government, and, at the local level, the gradual erosion of the dominant position of the 'economists' ' argument. Similarly, as the income of the thriving towns increased so the opposition to costly reforms became weaker. In Manchester, for example, industrial and commercial growth, accompanied as it was by a population increase, added to the problems of public health, but at the same time resulted in a remarkable increase in rateable value – from under £670,000 in 1839 to over £2,301,000 in 1881, and well over £4,500,000 by the First World War, and did much to weaken the hold of the 'economists' on the civic mentality of the city.[35] In Birmingham and other towns the profits of one municipal venture (in the case of Birmingham, the gas works) were used to help defray the cost of sanitary improvements and other public health measures.[36]

The adoption and implementation of health codes and the filtering down of the 'sanitary idea' to the local level were partly the products of necessity, the need for the town to survive the health hazards associated with rapid urban development and human congestion. But they also indicate a new civic ethos, a desire for municipal improvement, a competitive spirit with other towns, a growing shame at high death rates or insanitary conditions, an increasing embarrassment at exposures and (literally) muck-raking revelations, and, lastly, a growing sense of pride and accomplishment when improvements were effected. Peter Hennock has analyzed, in great depth, the emergence of this urban ethos in Birmingham in the 1860s under the guidance and enthusiasm of Joseph Chamberlain, and, much later, in Leeds, in his brilliant *Fit and Proper Persons: Ideal and Reality in Nineteenth-Century Urban Government*. Many different interests were represented in the new commitment to urban affairs, but binding these interests together and infusing the whole was an evangelical enthusiasm which emphasized the spirit of *community* and of *communal* interest.

We have already noted the evangelical spirit in national politics: perhaps even more important was its engagement in local affairs. Evangelical justification by conduct, as well as by faith, took on a pragmatism that 'emphasized effectiveness in contrast to good intentions'.[37] The preoccupation with effective conduct and the idealistic desire to recapture some of the spirit of the medieval cooperative guild, or the Renaissance city, found its expression in the improvement of the local community. Thus the minister, George Dawson, who had such a profound influence on mid-Victorian Birmingham, stressed throughout the 1860s 'that a town is a solemn organism through which should flow, and in which should be shaped, all the highest, loftiest and truest ends of man's moral nature.'[38] This idealism, with its accompanying pragmatic cutting edge, was powerful enough to lead to a revolution in urban affairs. When, for example, the Birmingham Improvement Act of 1861, was being hotly debated, a group of men in Dawson's Church of the Saviour, founded the satirical paper, *The Town Crier*. They felt:

> that there were certain things, and perhaps certain people [the 'economists'], who could be best assailed and suppressed by ridicule . . . It only dealt with public affairs and with men in their public capacity. Indeed . . . all the men connected with *The Town Crier* . . . were interested in the good government and progress of the town and they used the influence of the paper for the purpose of removing stumbling-blocks and putting incompetent and pretentious persons out of the way.[39]

In Birmingham, the role of evangelical dissent was crucial in the development of a sense of civic mission which encompassed among other reforms, an improved environment – in a sense it was the town corporation as the Sunday school writ large or as the Christian social conscience in action.[40] Already an effective instrument for reform in Birmingham in the 1860s, the evangelical ethos helped to create the necessary civic-mindedness for Chamberlain's reform mayoralty and for the great Improvement Scheme which transformed the inner city in the 1870s.[41]

In London and the great provincial cities the impact of the evangelical conscience on municipal affairs occurred somewhat later. The Christian Socialists and slum missionaries had from the 1840s stressed the importance of a clean environment for the salvation of souls, but it was not until the great agitation of the 1880s, prompted by the Congregationalist pamphlet, *The Bitter Cry of Outcast London*, that the churches began to play a prominent part in sanitary reform.[42] *The Bitter Cry* and the Christian Socialist revival which accompanied it created a religious atmosphere in which dirt and disease and slum housing were regarded as contrary to the basic teachings of Christ. Slums were now condemned from pulpits and at church conferences as products of sin and selfishness, and the town became, in the words of one outraged Methodist (addressing one of the many conferences on the spiritual and physical condition of the urban masses) 'the prize, the citadel, for which the powers of light and darkness must contend'.[43] At Oxford this Christian concern and the development of neo-Hegelian idealism combined to create an intellectual and moral atmosphere which prompted undergraduates to find an outlet for their shame and sense of duty in the settlement house movement and dons to play a role, for the first time, in Oxford municipal affairs.[44]

One direct result of what Beatrice Webb noted as a 'new consciousness of sin among men of intellect and men of property . . . a collective or class consciousness' was the call for a new concept of municipal government, which found expression in Fabian Socialism.[45] Another effect was for men to apply scriptural injunctions to local politics. This was, perhaps, most vigorously expressed by Dawson's disciple, R. W. Dale, the Congregational Minister who had so profound an effect both upon the development of civic consciousness in Birmingham and upon the close relationship between religious idealism and secular municipal collectivism in the late-Victorian period. In his *The Laws of Christ for Common Life* (1884) Dale called for an 'Ethical Revival', which had at its centre the concept that local politics was a solemn and sacred calling: 'Civil authority – this is the main point I want to assert – is a Divine institution. The man who holds municipal or political office is a "minister of God". One man may, therefore, have just as real a Divine vocation to become a town councillor, or a Member of Parliament, as another to become a missionary to the heathen.' For Dale the municipality was the appropriate forum for 'the sacredness of what is called secular business':

> I sometimes think that municipalities can do more for the people than Parliament. Their powers will probably be enlarged; but under the powers which they possess already they can greatly diminish the amount of sickness in the community, and can prolong human life. They can prevent – they have prevented – tens of thousands of children from becoming orphans. They can do very much to improve those miserable homes which are fatal not only to health, but to decency and morality.

Like Charles Kingsley before him, Dale stressed that 'Medicine, and not the gospel only, is necessary to cure the sick', but whereas Kingsley put his faith in acts of Parliament and private, philanthropic activities, Dale stressed that those acts had now to be implemented and that the spirit which had prompted private efforts must now be transferred to local government. 'Municipal action, not the gospel only, is necessary to improve the homes of the poor', he argued, and, in a telling passage, he called for the earthing or grounding of the Christian ethic in municipal political life:

> The gracious words of Christ, 'Inasmuch as ye did it unto one of these my brethren, even these least, ye did it unto Me,' will be addressed not only to those who with their own hands fed the hungry, and clothed the naked, and cared for the sick, but to those who supported a municipal policy which lessened the miseries of the wretched, and added brightness to the lives of the desolate. And the terrible rebuke, 'Inasmuch as ye did it not unto one of these least, ye did it not unto Me,' will condemn the selfishness of those who refused to make municipal government the instrument of a policy of justice and humanity.[46]

Far more studies modelled on Hennock's scrupulous analysis are needed before we can say with confidence that mid- and late-Victorian sanitary improvements were the conscious products of a new, enlightened, civic ethos, but it is quite clear that the position of the 'economists' was undermined by more than just the pressing urban necessities of the day and that the tide of local opinion had, in community after community, turned against them.[47] By the 1880s advocates of sanitary reform were working in a much more favourable atmosphere and, aided by the support of the central government, by national organizations such as the National Association for Promotion of Social Science, by local sanitary aid societies, and public health groups, were no longer faced with such determined local opposition. They were also able to draw on local newspapers for considerable support.[48] Papers like the *Leicester Chronicle*, the *Flying Post* (Exeter), the *Warwick Advertiser*, the *Darlington and Stockton Times*, the *Leeds Mercury*, the *City Press* (London), the *Porcupine* in Liverpool and the *Town Crier* in Birmingham, and a host of other local newspapers were quick to publicize bad health conditions. They gave broad coverage to Privy Council or Local Government Board investigations and they often followed up these investigations with inquiries of their own. These journalistic forays into insanitary areas were designed to embarrass the local government into action, and if the local authorities remained apathetic or complacent the exposés were supplemented with skilful use of the Registrar-General's returns to stress the comparative insalubrity of the local area.[49]

In short, one cannot agree with the generalization offered by E. C. Midwinter that the newspapers were reluctant to present a detailed picture of the social abuses of the age for fear of offending their 'sheltered readers'.[50] If anything, stinks and vapours, noxious gases, filth, and fever made excellent copy and throughout the century papers found exposés profitable. In journalism, as in other areas, self-interest and genuine concern combined to form a powerful force for reform. Specialized journals such as the *British Medical Journal*, the *Medical Times and Gazette*, the *Lancet*, the *Builder*, the *Building News*, the *Charity Organisation Reporter*, the *Journal of the Statistical Society of London*, *Public Health*, and the *Sanitary Review* were powerful and informed voices of reform, but their readership was limited and in a sense they were preaching to the already converted. But their investigations and demands for sanitary reform were reported sympathetically in the national press such as *The Times*, the *Daily News*, *Reynolds' Newspaper*, the *Pall Mall Gazette*, *Pictorial World*, the *Star*, and in journals such as *Punch* and the *Illustrated London News*. Similarly, at the local level, it was the local press which made the public aware of the various Blue Books and the findings of the Registrar-General or of the specialized journals mentioned above.

An enlightened and informed public opinion and a civic consciousness which could promote social concern or civic pride were important contributing factors to the health of the nation: just as important was the impact of a group of professional sanitary officials, the MOH (in part the products themselves of that public awareness and evangelical commitment), upon the administration of local government. As we have already noted, the pace of reform varied so enormously from town to town that it is difficult to generalize about the rate of local improvement in public health.[51] Nevertheless, a somewhat clearer picture emerges when the role of the MOH is studied, for their success and failures serve as a microcosm of the attitude of local government to sanitary improvement.[52]

II

Public health codes might be devised and laws passed, local authorities might form boards of health or sanitary committees, but for much of the second half of the century the effectiveness of public health at the local level rested in the hands of the MOH. Communities could, it is true, lay sewers and provide pure water, pave streets and clean away filth, all without the help of a MOH, but preventive medicine in the broadest and most comprehensive sense, embracing pure food as well as water, houses fit for human habitation, rigorously applied sanitary by-laws, notification of diseases, clean air, the banning of 'offensive trades' and a host of other interrelated matters, was dependent on the appointment of a qualified medical officer. Thus nothing serves better as a barometer of general sanitary progress in Victorian Britain than the status of the MOH. Regarded by both fellow doctors and laymen alike as a 'distinctly separate caste', the MOH succeeded, against considerable odds, in involving the medical profession in the growth of community services, and in raising the health standards of the nation.[53]

In his *Report on the Sanitary Condition of the Labouring Population of Great Britain* (1842) Chadwick had relied heavily on the testimony of local doctors. His report and those of the Health of Towns Association and the Royal Commission of the Sanitary State of

Large Towns and Populous Districts (1844, 1845) had urged the appointment of MOH throughout Britain, and the *Lancet* had repeatedly called for MOH to help eradicate 'the insalubrity of streets and dwelling-houses.'[54]

But it was local communities and not the central government or the medical profession as a whole which took the initiative in the appointment of the first MOH. Leicester had appointed two MOH under the 1846 Nuisances Removal Act, but it was the selection, some three months later, of Dr William Henry Duncan in 1847 as Liverpool's first MOH, which caught the imagination of the nation.[55] Duncan was a medical man of considerable stature at the time of his appointment. He was physician of the Liverpool Infirmary, Lecturer in Medical Jurisprudence at the Medical School of the Royal Institution, and its past President, and his correspondence with Chadwick, Southwood Smith, William Farr and other sanitarians, his powerful pamphlet on 'The Physical Causes of the High Rate of Mortality in Liverpool', and his efforts on behalf of the formation of a Health of Towns Association in Liverpool, testified to his commitment to the cause of public health. His appointment served as an example and set the tone for other large towns.[56] Considerable thought had gone into the clauses of the private Liverpool Sanitary Act under which Duncan was appointed, and since they served as models for other communities they are reproduced here:

And whereas the health of the population, especially of the poorer classes, is frequently injured by the prevalence of epidemical and other disorders, and the virulence and extent of such disorders is frequently due and owing to the existence of local causes which are capable of removal but which have hitherto escaped detection from the want of some experienced person to examine into and report upon them, it is expedient that power should be given to appoint a duly qualified medical practitioner for that purpose:

Be it therefore enacted, that it shall be lawful for the said Council to appoint, subject to the approval of one of Her Majesty's principal Secretaries of State, a legally qualified medical practitioner, of skill and experience, to inspect and report periodically on the sanitary condition of the said borough, to ascertain the existence of diseases, more especially epidemics increasing the rates of mortality, and to point out the existence of any nuisance or other such local causes which are likely to originate and maintain such diseases and injuriously affect the health of the inhabitants of the said borough, and to take cognisance of the fact of the existence of any contagious disease, and to point out the most efficacious modes for checking or preventing the spread of such diseases, And also to point out the most efficacious means for the ventilation of

180

churches, chapels, schools, registered lodging houses, and other public edifices within the said borough, and to perform any other duties of a like nature which may be required of him; and such person shall be called the 'Medical Officer of Health for the Borough of Liverpool'; And it shall be lawful for the said Council to pay such officer such salary as shall be approved of by one of Her Majesty's principal Secretaries of State.[57]

The stress upon the prevention of diseases through frequent inspection and reports, the emphasis upon epidemics and the health of the poorer classes, and the role of the central government (as a confirming body, both for the appointment of the MOH and his salary) are all worthy of note, and it was suggestive that the wording of the Act cast the MOH initially in the role of *adviser* and *reporter* mainly, leaving prosecution and implementation of nuisances removal and other such legislation as then existed, at the discretion of the Council at large.

The following year, in 1848, the City of London was granted power, under the City Sewers Act, to appoint a MOH, and in 1855 the Metropolis Local Management Act made such appointments compulsory throughout London. The early work of John Simon as MOH to the City of London and of a remarkably conscientious and energetic group of MOH throughout London, gave ample evidence of the worth and importance of the MOH to the general health of the community. But although the 1848 Public Health Act permitted local authorities to establish local boards of health, few authorities chose to appoint MOH to them, and the examples set by Leicester, Liverpool, and London were not widely followed over the next fifteen years. In 1866, when the Privy Council conducted a survey of the adoption of public health legislation in England and Wales, it discoverd that of its sample of twenty-five major communities, only Cardiff, Leicester, Newport, Merthyr Tydfil, and Bristol had MOH, and only Leicester had had one for more than five years.[58] Leeds did not appoint an MOH until 1866; even more negligent were Manchester (1868), Wolverhampton (1871 and no full-time MOH until 1921), Birmingham (1873), West Bromwich (1885) and Smethwick (1884).[59]

The Royal Sanitary Commission in its report of 1871 (responding to pressure from both MOH and the Social Science Association) urged the appointment of MOH and, following its recommendations, the 1872 Public Health Act made the appointment of MOH obligatory for all local sanitary authorities throughout England and Wales. At that time there were, approximately, only fifty or so MOH throughout the country. It is thus from 1872, rather than from the more commonly accepted year, 1848, that we must date the adoption of preventive medicine in the cause of public health throughout England.

The next stage in the growth of the MOH did not occur until 1888 when the Local Government Act permitted the county councils, which were established under the Act, to appoint County MOH. The County MOH were content for the most part simply to send an annual *précis* of the local MOH's report to the Local Government Board, and their powers of inspection were severely limited by the size of their staff. The County MOH for the West Riding of Yorkshire, for example, had a staff of only five to help him in 1901, and only one of those was a sanitary inspector.[60] The County MOH did not form their own separate Association until 1902, but although their influence was limited in the Victorian period, they could at least offer encouragement and support to any MOH battling against their local authorities, and the very act of collecting and correlating local reports presented a clearer picture of the sanitary conditions prevailing throughout the country.[61] The appointment at the county level of an MOH brought prestige to the MOH in general, and although some MOH feared that their authority might be overridden by the new county MOH, they now were able to consult with and seek advice from a higher authority without having to go all the way to the Local Government Board's medical department.[62] The County MOH of the West Riding of Yorkshire was typical in regarding his principal functions as 'consultation, inspection, and familiarization', but in fact, like other county MOH, he also brought pressure on local authorities to implement sanitary legislation.[63]

Local authorities were slow to implement the compulsory legislation of 1872. In 1874 less than half the local authorities had appointed MOH.[64] In 1876 there were still only 828 rural and urban MOH, but by the end of the following year the number had jumped to 1,206.[65] By the end of the century there were over 1,770 MOH.[66] The increasing number of MOH offers a very rough indication of the rising concern for, and commitment of local governments to, the cause of public health. Measured in these terms, it was, alas, a very belated commitment.

The outline presented above of the appointment and total numbers of MOH offers only a shadowy indication of their importance; much more significant are their qualifications, aptitude for the job, functions, and relations with their local authorities. The 1875 Public Health Act required medical officers to be registered doctors and under the 1888 Local Government Act all MOH of districts over

50,000 in population had to be qualified doctors holding a diploma in sanitary science, state medicine, or public health, or have been an MOH of a district of at least 20,000 people for three consecutive years prior to 1892, or have been a MOH or inspector of the Local Government Board.[67]

How well-qualified to be practitioners of preventive medicine were 'duly-qualified' medical men? And how exacting was the Diploma of Public Health? The answer to the first question is, generally speaking, not very, for preventive medicine and sanitary science were not compulsory subjects in most medical schools, and the *Lancet* was certainly quite justified in pointing out in 1872 that many MOH were 'not much better informed than other persons on questions relating to public health'.[68] In 1878 Dr Buchanan spent much time at the Local Government Board in a 'critical reading' of MOH reports and concluded '. . . reports have been received that are quite perfunctory and without value, giving no evidence of sanitary science or acquaintance with the sanitary wants of the districts', and two years later he was still complaining that he was receiving reports from the local MOH 'which show very imperfect appreciation of sanitary science and which are recognizable as the production of medical practitioners who find themselves under the necessity of writing an essay on a subject to which they have devoted no special study.'[69] Throughout the last quarter of the century the Local Government Board tried to get the MOH to conform to a standard format (with an emphasis upon comparative statistics) for their annual reports.[70]

From the very outset of their appointment the metropolitan MOH were extremely anxious to improve their professional standing by introducing in the medical schools special courses for students interested in preventive medicine, and it was at their urging that St Thomas's Hospital created a Lectureship in Public Health in 1855 and appointed to it one of the leading authorities on preventive medicine, Dr Edward Headlam Greenhow, who later held a similar post at Middlesex Hospital.[71] But the uncertain nature of preventive medicine and the status of its practitioners may be gauged from the fact that the St Thomas's Lectureship was unpaid. As the local authorities slowly appointed MOH and their duties became more complex and demanding, and also better appreciated, so the need for specialized training became evident. In 1875 the first English Diploma in Public Health was established at Cambridge University (Trinity College, Dublin, had introduced the DPH into its curriculum in 1870), and several other institutions followed, so that in 1886 the General Medical Council

(the central superintending body in British medicine) formally registered the DPH as a medical degree; two years later the Conjoint Board
of the Royal College of Physicians and the Royal College of Surgeons
also granted the DPH, setting as a basic requirement one full year of
study after receiving qualifications to practise medicine. Between
1871, when Trinity College granted its first DPH, and 1888 nearly 400
legally qualified doctors received the DPH.[72]

By the final quarter of the century the requirements of public health
had become so complex and varied that highly specialized training
was obviously essential. In 1894, Dr Henry Armstrong, Newcastle's
MOH, accurately observed that within the profession, 'the ordinary
legal qualifications for a medical officer of health, *viz.*, those in
medicine, surgery and midwifery, have become generally recognized
as insufficient', and he added that 'the idea that the work of such an
officer [MOH] is widely different from that of the practitioners of
ordinary medicine, and demands different education and training is
now firmly established.'[73] Similarly, Arthur Ransome wrote that
although a general practitioner was probably 'well instructed in
physiology and general scientific medicine, and therefore might be
presumed to be acquainted with the subject of hygiene' that was not
enough, for

> such a man would probably be quite at a loss if he were called upon to
> decide how to deal with an outbreak of epidemic disease, to remove the
> causes of diseases of an epidemic origin, to protect the public from
> unwholesome food, to recommend, and see carried out, an efficient
> system of drainage, or to decide upon other methods of dealing with
> refuse material.

The average doctor might be 'quite competent to declare a house unfit
for healthy human habitation, or to condemn an unhealthy area', but
the MOH had to go beyond condemnation to 'point out the best
modes of reconstruction or rearrangement of such dwellings', and for
that the normal medical education was insufficient.[74] Hence the need
for MOH to take the course of study leading up to the Diploma of
Public Health.

The DPH guaranteed that the holder had some knowledge of
hygiene, sanitary engineering and preventive medicine in general, but
according to the General Medical Council at the end of the century
the quality of the Diploma varied greatly from institution to institution, and it complained that in general there were too many degree-
granting bodies to maintain a uniform standard of 'distinctively high
scientific and practical efficiency.'[75] The scope and breadth of the

MOH's specialized education can be seen from the Cambridge University DPH and the standard textbooks recommended for study for it. Part One of the examination for the Cambridge DPH examined candidates in physics and chemistry; methods of analysis of air and water; applications of the microscope; ventilation; water supply; drainage; construction of dwellings; disposal of sewage and refuse; and sanitary engineering. Part Two covered statutes regulating public health; sanitary statistics; the origin, propagation, and prevention of epidemics and infectious diseases; effects of overcrowding, unhealthy occupations, vitiated air, and impure water and food; nuisances injurious to health; water supply and drainage; the distribution of diseases within the country; and the effects of soil, seasons, and climate. The range of this examination was so extensive that it leads one to wonder just how deeply the candidate was required to go into any one subject, and this impression is strengthened by the bewildering variety of subjects covered in two of the standard texts – Louis C. Parkes's *Hygiene and Public Health* (1889) and A. Wynter Blyth's *A Manual of Public Health* (1890).[76] The chapters in Parkes's work, for example, covered water supply and purity; the collection, removal and disposal of excreta and other refuse; air and ventilation; warming and lighting; soil composition, drainage and building sites; climate and meteorology; exercise, clothing, and personal hygiene; food, beverages and condiments; infections; communicable diseases and their prevention and hospitals; maternity and child welfare; school hygiene; industrial and marine hygiene; disinfection; and statistics. The expansion of the MOH's duties can be quickly grasped by comparing the greater comprehensiveness of Parkes's coverage with the Cambridge DPH curriculum. Especially important were the new role of the MOH in maternity and child-care and the health of schoolchildren, and their growing duties of disinfection and isolation as a means of controlling infectious diseases. This formal training was often supplemented by an apprenticeship in public health; by the turn of the century most of the universities offering a DPH were requiring six months of laboratory instruction in methods of food analysis, meterological studies and general bacteriology, and the General Medical Council insisted that all candidates for the DPH should produce evidence of having studied for six months under the direction of a MOH of a county or large district.[77]

As important as their training undoubtedly was, an even more significant factor in the effectiveness of the MOH was their working relationship with their local authorities. In view of what has already been said about the strength of the ratepayer interest we should not be surprised that the status of the MOH was not as secure or as independent as they might have wished.

Duncan had been appointed by Liverpool at a salary of £300 pa, with the right to stay in private practice, but he quickly discovered that his official duties were too onerous for him to be part-time, and when shortly after his appointment, he insisted on becoming a full-time MOH, the Liverpool Corporation generously increased his salary to £750 pa.[78] Leeds paid its first MOH (Dr Robinson) £500 pa when it appointed him in 1866, but it was still £500 when he left in 1873 for a higher paid post. The Council replaced him with a MOH at £400 pa and somewhat predictably got a much less energetic, dedicated man.[79] Few local authorities were prepared to offer as much money as either Liverpool or Leeds. 'Economists' often had severe doubts about the need for a MOH in the first place. In Edinburgh the 'economists' almost succeeded in preventing the appointment of Dr Littlejohn and in other towns the cry for economy, combined with the general apathy or ignorance about public health resulted in salaries which were in many cases not much higher than those earned by the slum-dwellers visited by the MOH in the course of their duties. Several London vestries paid their MOH only £100 a year in 1856, but this must have seemed a princely sum to the MOH for Lincoln and Oldbury who received only £15 and £30 respectively for their labours.[80] As late as 1875 Hampstead's MOH received only £50 pa, and a number of rural MOH earned under £10 pa. In a large port like Southampton, where the MOH's work was even more arduous than usual, the MOH was paid only £150 pa in 1865. By way of comparison the salary for the Town Clerk at that time was £800 pa.[81] In Crewe, a town which doubled its population between 1861 and 1871, the MOH earned only £50 pa, and it was not until the Cheshire County Council offered to pay half his salary in 1893 that Crewe made a full-time appointment.[82]

Out of these meagre salaries many MOH were expected to pay for their own horses, gigs, grooms and staff.[83] By the end of the century salaries had greatly increased in London and the big towns in general, reflecting the rise in prestige and importance of the MOH and the increased value set on public health in local communities. In London for example most MOH were earning between £350 and £600 pa. Kensington paid its MOH £800 pa, as did the City of Westminster. The MOH for the City of London earned £1,500 pa.[84] Birmingham paid £1,000 pa, and Manchester £850. The County MOH for London received £1,000.[85] Nevertheless, at the close of the century twice as many MOH in England and Wales were earning under £200 pa as were earning £500.[86]

Given these salaries, only the best-paid MOH, about six per cent of the total, could afford to be full-time. Indeed, some MOH regarded the low wages as a deliberate policy on the part of the local sanitary authorities to force them to continue in private practice and thus keep them preoccupied.[87] Although the General Board of Health and the MOH's own association were anxious to have only full-time MOH appointed, the low salaries dictated otherwise.

The MOH were not only underpaid. They had, for the most part, the most uncertain tenure. The various general and private acts under which the MOH were appointed specifically placed their tenure and removal at the pleasure of the local authorities employing them. Complaints about the apathy or open hostility of the local administrations employing them run like a *leitmotif* through the literature of nineteenth-century public health.[88] John Liddle, Whitechapel's MOH, in urging that the MOH 'should be entirely free from local influence', was undoubtedly right to stress that many authorities would never have appointed a MOH had they not been compelled to do so.[89] The editor of the *British Medical Journal* observed that 'nothing is more anomalous in our present system of sanitary government than the position of the medical officer of health', while the *Lancet* acknowledged in 1868 that the MOH 'were in a very awkward position; if they conscientiously carry out the duties imposed, they can hardly fail to come into antagonism with the local authorities to whom they are subordinate', and, it sadly noted, the main impediment to reform was that the government had entrusted 'important sanitary powers to local authorities, constituted largely of a class against whom those powers ought frequently to be exercised'.[90] William Farr noted that active MOH were 'in great danger of dismissal', and *Public Health* put it in a nutshell in 1899: 'Sanitary officials, unfortunately for themselves, are obliged to interfere to a greater or lesser extent with the liberty of action and the privacy of the homes of their fellow citizens, besides calling upon them to open their purses.'[91]

We should perhaps not be surprised that one MOH was greeted on his appointment with the scarcely encouraging words of his vestry chairman, 'Now, doctor, I wish you to understand that the less you do the better we shall like you.'[92] The *Pall Mall Gazette*'s cynicism was perhaps not entirely misplaced when it commented sourly that to expect the London vestries to support and enforce sanitary legislation was akin to asking poachers to enforce the game laws![93] It was alleged in Bethnal Green that all doctors whose reports had been 'troublesome' and 'who are running about "stink-hunting" in the parish' were automatically excluded from consideration for the post of MOH.[94]

In his Seventh Annual Report as Medical Officer to the Privy Council (1865) Simon wearily wrote that 'Nuisance Removal Committees have continued in office in order to prevent nuisances from being removed' and he added that inspectors had been 'appointed on terms that implied a minimum of inspection to be required of them'.[95] The composition of local sanitary boards, and especially the presence on them of small property owners, prompted one of the commissioners on the Royal Commission on the Housing of the Working Classes (1884–5) to complain that their right to appoint MOH was rather like permitting wolves to appoint shepherds.[96] Of the 'wolves' the slum-owner was held by sanitary reformers to be the most vicious. At the height of the housing reform agitation of the 1880s the *Saturday Review* maintained that 'too frequently the owners of these rookeries are either members of the vestries or have influence with the vestries who should sweep the property away.'[97] And of course muck-raking reform journalists were fond of taking pot-shots at local officials whom they accused of being motivated by self-interest. George Sims, one of the most popular and influential journalists of the late 1870s and 1880s, writing in the *Daily News*, accused London vestrymen of being the 'owners of the murder-traps' of the slums, and insisted that 'much of the worst property in London is held either by vestrymen or by persons who have friends in the vestry.' The first thing, Sims claimed, that a purchaser of 'low-class and doubtful property' tried to do was to get elected to the local vestry.[98] George Haw, in his dramatic exposé, *No Room to Live: the Plaint of Overcrowded London*, which first appeared as a series of articles in the *Daily News*, wrote that there could be little hope of progress until a 'better class of men' got elected to local government. 'Property-sweaters, jerry-builders, rack-renting middlemen, and extortionate house agents', he declared, 'ought to be kept off the local boards altogether.'[99]

One should view these attacks upon local government officials somewhat cautiously, coming as they did from inflammatory journalists, but often the criticisms stemmed from men in a position to know, especially from MOH, who were not generally given to sensationalism or exaggeration. In the view of Dr Lankester, MOH for St James's, Westminster, and a man prominent enough to serve as President of the

Health Section of the Social Science Association, the 'ability [of many MOH] to act for the public good has been reduced almost to a sinecure', by their local authorities. At the least we can say that, in too many districts throughout the country, local government officials were considerably less enthusiastic about the growing sanitary code than were the MOH they appointed, too many who regarded such legislation as 'of rather too inquisitorial a character'.[100] The MOH hoped that they would have more freedom to act if sanitary laws were made obligatory for local authorities. The President of the Association of Medical Officers of Health argued in 1878 that 'the distrust which has been excited by the apathy of many local authorities' had 'strengthened the feeling of our profession that permissive legislation must, as regards sanitary measures, be replaced by paternal legislation.'[101] But given the vulnerability of the MOH, even where it was obligatory for the local authority to apply the law, it would have been a brave man indeed who would insist upon action. Several local authorities made their MOH read out their reports at a plenary session or before a sanitary committee and this must have further intimidated many MOH.[102]

In 1888 of 1,300 MOH only fifty-five were appointed on long-term contracts; more than 1,000 MOH were on annual contracts.[103] At the end of the century the *Lancet* was still insisting that without tenure the MOH could not use the extensive powers which, in theory at least, they possessed under the law. Above all his position was vulnerable, the *Lancet* wrote, because he often had to act against the direct interests of those who employed him:

> It is not an uncommon thing for a medical officer whilst endeavouring to have some insanitary property put in a proper state of repair to find that a quantity of it is owned by a member of the sanitary authority – i.e., by one of his masters, by one of the men who have absolute power to discharge him neck and crop without giving him rhyme or reason for their action.

The *Lancet* quoted, in part support of this assertion, the admission of one rural MOH:

> Well, up to three years ago I took a great interest in public health, gave up a lot of time to it, and really worked hard to effect some much-needed sanitary reform in my district – result, every year it was touch and go whether I was re-elected or not, consequently I decided to let the thing slide and now there is not a more popular official than myself; in fact, at the end of the year I shall almost certainly obtain a considerable increase in salary.

The *Lancet* concluded:

> That the medical officer of health is without security of tenure is, we
> hold, inimical to the well-being of the community; it retards sanitary
> progress, prevents the due administration of the Public Health Acts,
> and, lastly, places the medical officers of health in unfair, ambiguous,
> and in what in many cases have proven untenable positions.[104]

Although the Society of MOH, starting in 1865, had persistently
and repeatedly agitated for tenure, MOH in England despite the
urgent recommendations of the Inter-departmental Committee on
Physical Deterioration (1904) did not receive tenure until the Public
Health (Officers) Act of 1921. In Scotland the MOH enjoyed rather
stronger contractual rights, for there the central public health authority, the Board of Supervision, exercised a closer surveillance over local
authorities, and the Scottish Local Government Act of 1889 guaranteed tenure to all rural MOH.[105]

Just how precarious, in fact, was the MOH's position? *Public
Health*, the *Lancet*, textbooks (such as T. W. Hime's *The Practical
Guide to the Public Health Acts* (1901),[106] and the Society of MOH
were right to point out that in many cases the duties of the MOH and
the interests of members of their local authority were diametrically
opposed, but these journals, and sanitary reformers in general, tended
to exaggerate the venality, corruption, and inactivity of local
authorities. The resignation of a capable man like Dr Rendle, MOH of
St George's Southwark, 'in disgust that he was not allowed to carry
out the duties of office', received far more publicity than the dismissal
of a lazy, or incompetent MOH, like Dr Godrich (MOH, Kensington) for not doing enough.[107] One cannot help but be impressed by the
energy with which most large sanitary districts tackled their problems
of health from the 1860s onwards and the support which they gave to
the MOH. Yet no doubt many MOH diplomatically turned a blind eye
to insanitary dwellings or business premises they knew belonged to
board members or thought twice about advocating measures which
would increase the burden on the rates, and perhaps others were
forced by the delicacy of their situation to remain inactive. In 1899 the
Society of MOH learned of thirty-five recent dismissals for such reasons
as advocating a new water supply, suggesting sanitary improvements, calling for an isolation hospital, and, in one case involving
a MOH of many years' standing, for exposing the concealment of a
case of smallpox in the home of the chairman of the local authority.[108]

Thus, if the MOH was 'the pivot around whom the sanitary
administration of a district rotates, and towards whom the main

responsibility converges', he was, unfortunately, a somewhat insecure pivot.[109] Just as the nineteenth-century death rate is, in a sense, only the tip of the iceberg, indicating the enormous mass of disease, debility and discomfort beneath, so the number of actual dismissals serves to indicate the continuing widespread disagreement between the MOH and their employers, and the constraints and handicaps under which the MOH operated.[110] The Local Government Board occasionally objected to the dismissal of a MOH, but generally it gave the approval which was required for the appointment of a successor. Wherever it could, the Local Government Board tried to get local authorities to appoint for at least a three-year period, but it seemed more to fear the continuation in office of poorly-qualified men than the dismissal of good MOH. The criticism, which was voiced by sanitary reformers, of the Local Government Board's unwillingness to aid the MOH in their demand for tenure, is well deserved.[111]

The Royal Sanitary Commission, to whose enquiries both the Local Government Board and a national network of MOH owed their existence, had not urged the appointment of full-time MOH. Indeed, it had argued that MOH 'should not as a rule be hindered from the private practice of their profession', and although the Local Government Board was given authority to pay half the salaries of local MOH, it used this power only to recommend, not require, full-time appointments. Very occasionally, as in the cases of Portsmouth and South Shields, it was insistent on a full-time appointment, but in other districts, such as Merthyr Tydfil and St Helens it continued to pay half the salaries of part-time MOH.[112] One must conclude that the role of the Local Government Board in the professionalization and development of the MOH was not substantial. The relationship between the MOH and the medical departments of the Privy Council and Local Government Board was never intimate.[113]

If the Local Government Board was reluctant to put pressure on the local authorities to make full-time appointments, the local authorities, for their part, were suspicious of any suggestion of central government influence over their MOH.[114] The Birmingham Council, which had most reluctantly appointed a MOH after the passage of the 1872 Public Health Act, decided not to accept the Local Government Board's offer to pay half his salary because they wished, they said, to 'retain intact their power over the appointment, salaries and duties of their own Officers'. Leeds rejected the offer on the same grounds.[115] Nottingham was so concerned at possible centralization that it sent a circular to all the towns throughout the country urging them, in the name of local autonomy, to resist the temptation to turn to the Local Government Board for a subsidy towards the payment of MOH. Significantly, out of forty-four sanitary districts with populations of over 35,000, all but eight refused to accept the subsidy from the Board. The sentiment of local autonomy was clearly even stronger than the love of economy![116]

Given all that has been said so far – the miserable salaries, the attitudes of most local authorities, the lack of support from the central government, the onerous duties and the dangers to health implicit in them, and the fact that their appointments lay in the hands of the local governments – it would be reasonable to expect that the MOH would be of a very low calibre. The local authorities were often faced with a large number of applicants for the position, and here, as in so many areas of public health, they were called upon to make a decision for which they were poorly qualified.[117] Thus one perplexed ratepayer in Kensington asked how 'are we poor ratepayers or hardworked vestrymen, whose experience of medical men does not reach beyond the family doctor, to judge between scores of gentlemen, every one of whom bewilders us with an equal surface of close-printed assurances of his universal qualifications for the office?'[118] A letter to the press following the Metropolis Local Management Act of 1855 suggests the pressures upon the local governments to appoint local men:

> You, Sir, if you are not a vestryman, can form no idea of the excitement that prevails among those who seek the honour of being officers of health. Meddling mammas, flirting demure single ladies, young and old bachelors are canvassing for their doctors merely because he doctors them to their satisfaction; so that it is not improbable that a clever man who understands the constitution of the spouse of a vestryman may obtain the appointment.[119]

Sir Benjamin Hall, the President of the General Board of Health, wanted an examining body of qualified men to help the London vestries select the MOH, but his plan raised the spectre of government interference and, to a generation not yet used to the concept of specialized public health, and which had yet to receive clear proof of the superiority of medical men to general sanitary officials, it smacked of insufferable professionalization – the combination of bureaucratic interference and the mystique of medical science. Examinations, *The Times* criticized, would merely produce 'the wrangler in vital statistics, and first-class men in meteorology', and Simon, it drily observed, 'the best public health officer of our time, was not a child of the examination system'.[120] Despite widespread fears to the contrary, very competent, and in some cases outstanding doctors were selected as MOH. Of the forty-nine doctors first appointed in London, eleven were sufficiently prominent to be included in the *Dictionary of National Biography*, and of the forty-nine listed in the *Medical Directory* for 1857 seventeen were prolific authors and another ten had significant publications to their names.[121] Only Paddington it seems, submitted the candidates for interview by a panel of doctors and most vestries seem to have chosen their MOH in a casual manner. Just as in Edinburgh, the first MOH, Dr Littlejohn, the Police Surgeon, was meant to be a temporary appointment (he remained for forty-six years), so, in London, the vestries appear to have had few long-term plans when they selected their MOH. Most of the vestries left it to the new appointees to interpret their duties according to the guide-lines set by the General Board of Health; Wandsworth was exceptional in taking the time and interest to draw up a list of duties. Some towns took the appointment very seriously, however. When, very belatedly, Manchester decided it ought to have a MOH (1868), it instructed the Town Clerk to seek advice from Liverpool, Leeds, Glasgow, Hull and Bristol.[122] Elsewhere local doctors, and especially in rural areas, poor law doctors, held an advantage, and sanitary reformers were generally agreed that the smaller the sanitary district the lower the calibre of the doctor. George Bernard Shaw somewhat harshly generalized that in the combined rural districts MOH were 'only half Medical Officer, and the other half general practitioner [and] mostly third rate in both capacities . . .'[123]

In many cases the sanitary committees were only slightly better equipped than the local authority as a whole to comprehend the recommendations and work of the MOH, for, like the parent bodies, the sanitary committees very rarely had doctors or sanitary engineers on them and were composed mainly of the local property and business interests.[124] The medical officers, with their increasing professionalism, stood out in administrations which were largely amateur. As the century progressed, their specialized work – food analysis, or inspection for infectious diseases or insanitary housing, for example – called for both terminology and details which were generally beyond the comprehension of the men for whom they worked, and for the most part the MOH could expect little professional nourishment from their relationship with their local administrations.

For interchange with fellow professionals, men who could both understand and appreciate his work and the problems involved, the MOH had his own staff and the Society of MOH. Generally the MOH had one (or more, in larger urban districts) sanitary inspectors under him, and it was the inspector's duty to make house-to-house visits, either alone or with the MOH. This essential task was rendered even more important by the fact that the MOH could not rely upon complaints from tenants and neighbours (who were scared of being regarded as 'informers', or of eviction), but had to engage directly in house inspections if they were to ferret out sanitary defects and nuisances.[125] Although the office of an inspector of nuisances was essential to the efficacy of sanitary work, no qualifications for the office were set, and neither the 1875 Public Health Act, nor the Local Government Act of 1888, both of which established professional requirements for the MOH, did likewise for the inspector who carried out so many of the daily sanitary tasks. In 1876 the Sanitary Institute of London (later the Royal Sanitary Institute), was founded both to spread information about sanitary engineering and to act as a certifying body for surveyors and inspectors of nuisances, but throughout the nineteenth century its certificate remained an entirely optional, if highly desirable proof of competence. The Institute (which held its first certifying examination in 1877) served to bring together MOH, engineers, doctors and surveyors.[126] Much of the routine sanitary work in the MOH revolved around the concept of 'nuisances injurious to health', as defined in the various nuisances removal and sanitary acts, and the Sanitary Institute's courses, examinations, and annual congresses concentrated largely upon developing the inspectors' competence in detecting and removing such nuisances as insanitary dwellings, stagnant and foul pools, gutters and watercourses, broken and inadequate privies and ashpits, overcrowded or unhealthy cowsheds, workshops, private dwellings, and the like.[127]

Although as late as 1889 the Mansion House Council on the Dwellings of the Poor was complaining that there were among the inspectors too many 'men whose antecedents and technical knowledge are altogether inadequate for the important duties they are called upon to fulfill', there was a steady rise in professional standards, at least among the inspectors of larger urban districts. In rural sanitary districts, the Local Government Board complained, there were still too many grossly unqualified inspectors, among them watchmakers, grocers, dairymen, auctioneers, beershop-keepers, and publicans; in other areas they were recruited 'from the ranks of ex-sailors, ex-policemen or army pensioners'.[128] One vestry clerk expressed a view not uncommon among local government officials when he insisted before a Royal Commission that no special training was necessary for the inspector of nuisances: 'If a man was endowed with common sense I think it would be about as good a training as he could have.'[129] Unfortunately the nature of the job and the pay were hardly tempting to highly-skilled sanitary engineers; indeed, the pay was so meagre that in his textbook A. Wynter Blyth warned local authorities and MOH not to consider men over forty, for if men of that age applied for the job at the wages then prevailing 'they had obviously failed in other areas.'[130]

The inspectors of nuisances were right-hand men of the MOH, but until the end of the century there were simply not enough of them (especially in larger districts) to enable the MOH to conduct the extensive house-to-house visits upon which so much preventive medicine was dependent. In London, which was particularly ill-served in this regard, there was at mid-century only one inspector in St Pancras and one in Bethnal Green, districts with over 200,000 and 100,000 people, respectively. Progress, in London as elsewhere, was slow. In 1885 Islington had only one inspector for every 56,000 people, St Pancras one for every 59,000, Bermondsey one for every 86,000 and Mile End one for every 105,000.[131] But between 1885 and 1892 every district save two had doubled, trebled or quadrupled its staff of inspectors, and by the end of the century there was an average of one inspector for every 20,000 people in London, and an average of five inspectors for every MOH.[132] Given the slow growth of the staffs of the MOH in London and elsewhere it is all the more remarkable that the more energetic MOH were managing in the 1870s and 1880s to conduct five, six, and even seven thousand house visits a year.[133]

In the 1880s, with the widespread adoption in so many towns of modern forms of excrement removal and water supply, the prestige of engineers and their role in public health increased. This is reflected in the growing sense of accomplishment and purpose in the annual congresses of the Sanitary Institute of Great Britain and in the formation of both the Association of Municipal and Sanitary Engineers and Surveyors in the 1880s. MOH were prominent in the discussions of the annual congresses of the Sanitary Institute and they gave papers on a wide variety of subjects. Whatever the earlier rivalry and mutual suspicion between the medical profession and sanitary engineers over their roles in public health, cooperation and understanding had been achieved between the two groups by the 1880s.[134]

In their struggle to achieve professional standing the MOH were greatly aided by their Society. The metropolitan MOH had, immediately following their initial appointment in 1855, grasped the fact that they had many problems in common and that they stood a better chance of persuading their local authorities to adopt their recommendations if they banded together. Following a meeting of eight MOH in 1856, the Metropolitan Association of Medical Officers of Health was formed, and from this small beginning it grew into a national organization with several regional branches, and a membership of roughly half of all the MOH in England and Wales.[135] The organization changed its name several times – Metropolitan Association of Medical Officers of Health; Association of Medical Officers of Health (1869); Society of Medical Officers of Health (1873); and Incorporated Society of Medical Officers of Health (1891). An early proposal to change the name to The Society for the Promotion of Public Health was defeated, and it is clear that the Society wanted to remain a strictly professional organization rather than become a broad amalgam of reform interests (although it did occasionally give honorary membership to notable sanitary reformers, such as Dr Southwood Smith and Edwin Chadwick, and Major Graham of the Registrar-General's Office. From the national and regional organizations and their sub-committees (covering such areas as food adulteration, industrial diseases, trade nuisances, aetiology), the MOH developed the competence and awareness that comes with comparative analysis and frequent interchange of ideas and experience with fellow-specialists. Their meetings, published transactions and journal, *Public Health*, gave them an *esprit de corps* and an essential sense of their own importance at the national level. It also provided them with a forum in which to formulate reforms – such as the need for compulsory notification of contagious diseases, the establishment of isolation hospitals, the abolition of back-to-back housing, the regulation of overcrowding through a system of registration and by-laws, and, late in the century, a concerted effort to get at the root of the high level of infant mortality. The national Society helped in the drafting of the 1872 Public Health Act, assisted the Local Government Board in 1874 in drawing up model tables of vital statistics, gave valuable advice to local authorities on disease prevention (during the smallpox epidemic of 1876, for example) and on the control of measles among schoolchildren, helped remove the stigma of legal pauperization from those going into the Metropolitan Asylum Board's hospitals, joined the British Medical Association, the Social Science Association, and the National Health Society to achieve stronger laws governing the notification of diseases, and, in 1882, persuaded the Board of Education to draw up regulations for excluding from school children with highly infectious diseases.[136] The influence of the Society was always far greater than the total number of its members might suggest. Its meetings were primarily for the education of the members, but since the papers which were presented there were printed as pamphlets, the impact of the meetings went beyond the immediate confines of the Society.[137]

III

To be truly effective the MOH had to be integrated into the workings of local government, or at least, have *rapport* with it. This was often made difficult, even where the local authority was well-meaning and welcomed the MOH's appointment, by the incoherent and ill-organized nature of many local authorities. Dr Littlejohn in Edinburgh, for example, was responsible to the slow-moving Lord Provost's Committee and although both the Superintendent of Streets and Buildings and the Inspector of Cleaning and Lighting had public health duties there was no co-ordination between them and the MOH. Some ten years after his appointment, Edinburgh still had not established a coherent public health administration. But once a Public Health Committee was established (in 1872), it quickly saw to it that Littlejohn got two extra inspectors for working-class housing (up to that point he had had to make do with just one policeman and a clerk), and with the Public Health Committee behind him Littlejohn could at last embark upon much more vigorous and extensive work.[138] Similarly in Manchester, Dr Leigh discovered upon his appointment as MOH that his duties were scattered among nine separate committees of the city council.[139] The appointment of Leigh was an acknowledgement of the desperate need for a more rational and effective public health administration and the functions of all the committees were brought together in a Health Committee in the same year Leigh was appointed (1868). Two years later Manchester was divided into four sanitary districts, each with its own sub-committees, and it is from the date of the reorganization in 1868 that the improvement in the health of the city can be dated.[140] By 1890 the MOH's duties had developed to the point where he was complaining that there was all 'the confusion and overlapping of functions which must sometimes occur when identical duties are simultaneously discharged by several committees, acting independently of one another and with different objects in view.' His call for 'the simplification and co-ordination of modes and procedure' was met in 1890, and the work of public health was divided between two principal committees, the Cleansing Committee, responsible for scavenging and the disposal of refuse, and the Sanitary Committee, which was responsible for the cleansing of houses, the purity of food and the inspection of insanitary dwellings.[141]

But whether he worked in a newly organized administration or with old committees, the appointment of an MOH could often serve as a catalyst for reform.[142] Above all it is with the MOH that there appears for the first time the continuous and systematic course of *inspection* without which no public health reform could be truly effective. In his first report to the City of London Simon had stressed that sanitary reform rested upon 'inspection . . . of the most constant, most searching, most intelligent, and most trustworthy kind . . .'[143] It was a view which was shared and enthusiastically acted upon by scores of later MOH. Clause 19 of the 1866 Sanitary Act (which extended the definition of 'nuisance') and clause 20, which made it obligatory for local authorities to make inspections in their districts, were regarded by Simon, both at that time and at the end of the century, as absolutely crucial in the development of the nation's health.[144]

The MOH rarely undertook night-time inspection, but their day-time visits became a feature of working-class life and helped to break down the concept of the sanctity of private property and the axiom that an Englishman's home was his castle. Their daily inspections rendered the home in a sense no more sacred than the factory or workshop and helped to create a new sense of the responsibilities of property ownership.[145] It was a far cry from the 1840s, when the investigation of insanitary dwellings in Leeds was condemned as 'inquisitorial' and 'part of a Frenchified system, which was contrary to the principles and habits of Englishmen', or from the days when an 'economist' in Birmingham could denounce the Sanitary Committee's call for regular house inspections as 'unconstitutional and un-English' and a violation of 'that which has hitherto been held most dear to Englishmen – namely the sanctity of domestic life.'[146]

Their inspections served to persuade many MOH that the root cause of much disease was poverty. During the last two decades of the century, when they came to appreciate the extent of overcrowding and when they gradually developed an awareness of the need for higher standards of hygiene and nutrition, the MOH came to view their work as a frustrating battle against the all-pervasive influence of poverty.[147] In his textbook, *A Manual of Public Health*, Dr Wynter Blyth had urged his fellow MOH to keep their annual reports strictly objective and empirical and to avoid the temptation to 'ventilate therein the great social questions of the day'.[148] The statistical method employed by the MOH in their annual reports added to, and indeed formed the basic grammar, so to speak, of the growing science of preventive medicine. But the MOH went well beyond the minutiae and raw statistics of their local work, and the poverty which they encountered in their daily rounds forced them to rise above purely local considerations to wrestle with the social question on a broader scale. The work of the MOH brought the medical profession into close contact with the working classes and in so doing helped to keep it in touch with the realities of poverty and to humanize its responses. If the medical profession came to realize its social obligations in an increasingly complex industrial and urban society, it was in no small measure due to the MOH.[149]

While their increasing powers and professional standards reflect the development of both the public health movement and the medical profession in the nineteenth century, their choice of career and concern for improved living standards reflect the influence of Victorian humanitarianism on the world of medicine. It is fitting, therefore, to end this section with the words of Dr Young, MOH for Stockport, written in the year of Queen Victoria's death:

> In conclusion may I be allowed to say that the science of public health has both an objective and an ethical side. The former is represented by the routine work of a sanitary department – nuisances, drainage, infection, and their respective control. The ethical side is of infinitely greater importance, for it is more lasting in its effects, aiming as it does at the production of a cleaner, purer, and richer social life. . . . Local Authorities, by the organisation of measures for the improvement of the environment of the individual must eventually succeed in raising the standard of civilised life.[150]

The hostility of local authorities to central coercion, so evident throughout England, was also apparent in Scotland, where similar industrial and urban developments had created similar sanitary problems.[151] Scotland received a central public health authority in 1856, when the already existing Board of Supervision for the Relief of the Poor was given sanitary and health functions.[152] In all essentials the relationship between local health authorities and the Board of Supervision (which met in Edinburgh) was similar to that in England between local communities and the central government health agencies, although in Scotland the MOH were generally given greater support by the Board.[153] The generally stronger position of the Scottish MOH was reflected in the Scottish Local Government Act of 1889 which gave them tenure well before their English colleagues. Although under the Public Health (Scotland) Act of 1867 the Board of Supervision had the ability to enforce action on the part of local authorities, like its counterpart in England, the Privy Council, it preferred to 'stimulate to action' rather than to bully or coerce.[154] And like its English counterparts, the Board of Supervision was woefully understaffed. Dr Littlejohn, who continued as Edinburgh's MOH, was its only medical adviser, and his staff of just three inspectors also had poor law duties. Of necessity the influence of the Board (again like that of the Privy Council and Local Government Board) remained somewhat remote.[155]

Although Scotland received its own Nuisances Removal Acts in 1846, 1848 and 1856, the Board of Supervision complained that the legislation had been only sporadically employed, and that most authorities waited for an outbreak of epidemic disease before moving into action.[156] The reason is not hard to find. Scottish ratepayers were no different from the English – as one of Stirling's Police Commissioners, responsible for the town's health, expressed it, 'the great thing which the people of Stirling had to look to was that they be taxed as lightly as possible.'[157] It was argued north of the border, as well as south, that low taxation was essential for a town's success. In 1847, during the lengthy debate in Stirling to get a water-rate passed, it was argued that 'the privilege they now enjoyed of little local taxation had been a great means of bringing respectable inhabitants to the town, and they ought to take care how they encroached upon that privilege.'[158]

Not until the 1867 Public Health (Scotland) Act did Scottish towns have authority to levy a general rate for *public* health purposes (limited to 3d in the £ and to burghs with over 10,000 inhabitants). Until then the intensely localized rates stood as a barrier against sanitary progress. Thus in Stirling, where the sewers ran downhill, backed up, and came up through the drains into the roads, the residents of the upper town could not see why they should tax themselves for larger diameter sewers when the existing sewers were no problem in their part of town. In Stirling, as elsewhere, progress was made only after *general* rates could be levied following the 1867 Act. In the case of Stirling all it took was a 1d-in-the-£ addition to the rates for five years to build the required large-capacity sewers.[159]

It was partly because the local communities were rate-conscious that Scotland, despite its proud medical tradition, did not appoint local MOH any sooner than England. Edinburgh appointed its first MOH in 1862 and Glasgow followed a year later, both towns acting under private acts which were passed in the teeth of strong opposition, despite the clear need for more coherent and forceful sanitary administrations. It is true that in Scotland the local police commissioners had considerable public health duties concentrated in their hands, but they were generally not well equipped, either by training or temperament, to be vehicles for thoroughgoing reform, and most Scottish towns did not merge the powers of the police commissioners into the town council until the end of the century.[160]

As in England, progress in Scotland was partly associated with the greater borrowing powers local sanitary authorities enjoyed after mid-century. Between 1875 and 1899 Scottish authorities borrowed well over £2,000,000 for sanitary purposes, the greater part of it for new water schemes.[161] This flow of funds from the central government to local sanitary authorities was, as we have already seen for England, one of the most valuable contributions of the central State to the public health movement.

This applies equally to Ireland, where the local sanitary authorities borrowed over £4,000,000 from the British Government between 1876 and 1899, rising from a mere £7,587 in 1876 to £352,912.8.8d in 1894.[162] Ireland, of course, had a very much smaller proportion of her total population living in cities. Whereas in England in 1881 some 56.3 per cent of the population lived in towns of over 10,000 people, in Ireland the figure was only 16.3 per cent. Country living was undoubtedly healthier than urban, but in the country the administration of the public health acts was extremely lax. In the rural areas the poor law authorities served as public health bodies and they were extremely parochial in outlook and generally very reluctant to engage in sanitary work. In an effort to raise the level of sanitation in the countryside the Public Health (Ireland) Act of 1874 made all dispensary MOH *ex officio* public health officers at £10 pa salary, but they were not given much direction and it was observed some years later that they were paid 'to hold their tongues and take no notice of dirt and disease within their districts'.[163]

Ireland's sanitary code mirrored England's and thus expanded continuously from mid-century on.[164] But (as was so often the case in England) it was not until the appointment of MOH that an attempt was seriously made to apply the legislation. Dublin, for example, throughout the entire first half of the century lacked a civic body responsible for public health and as late as mid-century it had paved only thirty-nine of over a hundred city streets.[165] Not until 1879, when Dr Charles Cameron was appointed MOH, did a programme of reform begin. Before that date there had been almost no improvement in Dublin's large stock of sub-standard houses: only two hundred dwellings were closed over twenty-six years (1851–77). Over twice that number were closed by Cameron in 1881 alone, and between 1899 and 1913 another 4,263 houses and some 1,190 cellars were declared unfit for human habitation and shut down. The task facing Cameron and his staff was enormous, for in 1879 about one quarter of Dublin's tenements were considered to be unfit for habitation.[166] Cameron's staff was barely adequate under the circumstances, for he had a consulting MOH, a superintendent of disinfection, and two disinfectors with a 'variable number of whitewashers, two food inspectors, three constables acting as assistants to the meat inspector, and another fifteen officials for miscellaneous duties.' On paper this sounds like a large staff, but Dublin's health problems were enormous, and it is a measure of the remarkable growth in public health concepts that by 1914 Dublin's public health administration had grown to over a hundred officials. By this time annual expenditure on public health was over £24,000 each year.[167]

Where poverty was widespread dwellings tended to be insanitary and the risk of infectious diseases was higher, yet the total rateable value of the community, or its tax base, was often so low that it was difficult to raise commercial loans for improvements, or even qualify for low-interest government loans. Thus when in 1875 the Dublin Corporation was permitted by the Sanitary Act of that year to borrow money for main drainage, the Treasury refused to grant the loan on the grounds that the town's financial state did not permit it, and the completion of the city's main drainage was delayed until the 1890s.[168] Although Ireland followed England closely in her health codes and the general pattern of her sanitary administration, she was given a large measure of local autonomy in public health under her own Local Government Board. Only if one sees her continuing poverty in the nineteenth century as a legacy of British rule can one say that her problems of public health reflected her political subordination.

Within the ranks of those who, at the local level, helped by their actions or votes to promote the cause of public health, were many interests – religious men and women who took seriously the injunction that cleanliness is next to Godliness and who were convinced that there was a connection between physical and moral uncleanliness, businessmen and manufacturers, convinced that a healthy city made for economic growth, industrialists who regarded pure water supply or efficient waste disposal as advantageous to their business interests, men and women operating consciously or unconsciously under a Chadwickian impulse that regarded ill-health as inefficient and unnecessary, those who, while less than enthusiastic about reform were persuaded that it was in the long run cheaper than poor relief, and others whose main impulse was civic shame and its corollary, civic pride. And all these attitudes and impulses could be represented in one individual.

By the late nineteenth century the 'sanitary idea' had become an accepted part of local government, and local elections began to include, if not exactly revolve around, public health issues. In London a variety of groups, among them the Fabians, the Social Democratic Federation, and the London Trades Council included better public health on their election manifestoes, or drew up a series of questions, including aspects of public health, which local electors should put to candidates for local office.[169] Similarly in Leeds the local Sanitary Aid Society suggested that electors should obtain pledges from the candidates for municipal election in 1893 on four matters of public health — compulsory notification of contagious diseases, a slum clearance scheme, better street drainage, and the appointment of additional sanitary inspectors.[170] In fact the Leeds Liberals entered the local 1893 elections with a fully-developed municipal programme, which included 'the immediate clearing of insanitary areas' and rehousing for the evicted, the cleansing of the river Aire, and the further provision of public baths. Significantly at that late date, the Conservatives did not launch a criticism of the programme, but merely protested that the Liberals had stolen their platform from them.[171]

By the end of Queen Victoria's reign a remarkable improvement had been effected in the nation's health (see Chapter 12). As we have noted this was partly due to the decline in the virulence of certain diseases and to a general rise in the standard of living. But local authorities and their MOH could take much of the credit. The activities of the MOH clearly indicate the growing professionalism of public health administration as well as the growing complexities of modern life. In 1894 Dr John Sykes wrote that

> The medical officer of health, in addition to being well-grounded in physics, chemistry, and biology, and skilled in medicine in all its branches, especially in pathology (human and comparative), bacteriology, and etiology, is expected to possess also a knowledge of geology,

physiology, meterology, and climatology, of statistics, mensuration, and plans, together with a certain amount of knowledge of engineering, architecture, building, and plumbing, a little more of law, local government, sanitary jurisprudence, by-laws, regulations, procedure, and evidence, and a little more still of the industrial, scholastic, and other social conditions of life.

In addition Sykes wrote that the MOH should familiarize himself with the procedures of the magistrates' courts and the operations of water-works, sewage plants, mortuaries, and above all with isolation hospitals and disinfecting stations. It was a daunting list of requirements and expectations and certainly few MOH were skilled or competent in all these areas. Yet at the time Sykes wrote, the annual reports of the MOH indicate that their influence was making an impact on a wide range of community activities, for they were inspecting

common lodging-houses, model common lodging-houses, cellar dwellings, garret dwellings, stable dwellings, canal boat dwellings, tents, caravans, and sheds, and insanitary houses or areas, places where food is produced, prepared, or sold, as slaughter-houses, cattle, and other markets, retail premises, cowhouses, dairies, and milkshops, bakehouses, and school premises, various kinds of workshops, premises where the various offensive trades are carried on, nuisances, smoke, overcrowding, dampness, and many others too numerous to mention.[172]

The activities clearly indicate the growing complexities of modern life with which public health authorities had to contend. One could argue that they were slow to respond to the challenge, but by the end of the century it is clear that a firm commitment had been made to create an environment which would be fit for human habitation. One aspect of that physical environment – the air – provided a particularly difficult challenge, and it is to the threat of atmospheric pollution that we must now turn.

8

'The Black Canopy of Smoke':
Atmospheric Pollution

'And it is not a question of a few manufactories, but of industries all over
the country, which in relation to man are causing pollution of the air in
degrees sufficient to make them common law nuisances.'

John Simon, *PP*. XLIV (1878), 'Royal Commission on Noxious Vapours. II. Minutes of Evidence', p. 524.

Throughout this book both industry and its offspring, the industrial
town, have appeared almost in the role of villain, for many of the
problems so far discussed – high infant mortality, bad drainage and
sewerage, inadequate water supplies, the spread of infectious diseases
– have been placed within the framework of the manufacturing town,
and it has been argued that the urban setting aggravated problems
which, in the country, would have remained less pressing. Overcrowding and houses unfit for human habitation, the subjects of a later
chapter, also were most challenging to the nation's health when they
existed in the rapidly growing industrial towns.

That industrial growth exacerbated many of the social and related
health problems of the nation is certain. What is far more speculative
and much more difficult to prove is that had Britain *not* undergone an
industrial revolution the general death rate might well have been
higher. The pressure of population upon land and its resources may
possibly have brought to pass Malthus's gloomiest predictions of
famine and epidemics similar to those which so tragically devastated
Ireland at mid-century. The population explosion, combined with
rapidly diminishing returns from agricultural land and inevitably
lower nutritional standards, would have been accompanied by substandard housing, poor medical facilities, and over-burdened water
and sewer facilities – a predominantly agrarian Britain would have
provided the perfect nexus for recurrent and widespread epidemics.

That the agricultural districts generally enjoyed better health than
urban areas is not proof to the contrary, for the towns served as
essential purgatives, 'bleeding' the countryside of the population

which otherwise would have been a fatal burden. Industry, whatever the social and environmental ills to which it gave birth, provided jobs, higher living standards, employment for the entire family, and ultimately the exports which enabled England to pay for the imported food which was so essential to its health. Even those industries which polluted the environment and endangered the work-force played their part in helping to raise the standard of health. Alkali works, spewing forth their noxious gases, also helped to produce the cheap cleansing agents so essential to hygiene; the cotton mills, with their attendant occupational hazards, turned out readily washable and easily dried sheets and underwear; the glass furnaces gave rise to industrial diseases, but they also enabled houses to be fitted with inexpensive windows and so aided ventilation; and if the potteries were synonymous with ill-health they also manufactured the thousands of miles of cheap sewer pipes and bathroom appliances which did so much to halt the progress of epidemics.[1]

Having said this, it must still be stressed that the price exacted by the industrial town was high. As we have seen, its growth was too rapid and unregulated for public health measures to keep abreast and resulted, among other things, in the pollution of the atmosphere which is the subject of this present chapter. Economic progress thus had its attendant evils: 'industrial diseases' became a part of the Victorian vocabulary, air became smog, and rivers and streams turned into turgid, evil-smelling open sewers.

In an earlier chapter we described the barnyard smells of the Victorian town, but added to the pungent odours of dung and decaying vegetable matter was an assortment of smells peculiar to industry, a concoction of stinks as offensive as any produced malevolently by schoolboys in a chemistry laboratory. Each trade – tar works, jam factories, cement works, chemical works, glue factories, knackers' yards, tallow and candle works, tripe boilers, bone boilers, fell mongers, manure works, slaughter houses, and many more – had its own distinctive stench which either hung over a district giving it a unique and immediately recognizable odour, or mingled with others into an offensive mélange which pervaded the entire town. In Dublin, for example, it was the smell from the many tripe and gut houses situated throughout the residential area that assaulted the nose. 'In these dens', the Local Government Board for Ireland observed in 1902:

> the intestines of slaughtered animals are 'cleaned' and filled with a
> mixture of blood, milk, and herbs, and sold . . . The intestines, when

filled, are semi-cooked in open boilers, and the steamy stench and general surroundings of these places is most sickening.[2]

In Bermondsey, in London, the smells from the three tanneries, the breweries, the pickle, paper, and jam factories and from the hospital with its 'insistent, nauseating smells of chloroform', dwelt in the memory of Kathleen Woodward when she recalled her upbringing there. Of these, the 'abiding smell',

> the pitch and tone, was set by the breweries at the foot of London Bridge; and it was only after you had been long in the neighbourhood that you became aware, at intervals, of the smell of fruit fermenting, the odorous processes of tan, intermingled with the faint insidious waves of chloroform.[3]

While these all-pervasive smells, and the gases and smoke emitted by factories and workshops, were undoubtedly offensive to the senses, were they literally 'noxious'? Were they so harmful to health that they warrant inclusion in this book? As we shall see, it was extremely difficult to trace directly any illness to these outpourings of industry and it was partly for this reason that effective legislation to control them was slow in coming. But, as Simon insisted before the 1878 Royal Commission on Noxious Vapours, it was surely not necessary to prove that air pollution caused specific illnesses:

> To be free from bodily discomfort is a condition of health. If a man gets up with a headache, *pro tanto*, he is not in good health; if a man gets up unable to eat his breakfast, *pro tanto*, he is not in good health. States of languor, states of nausea, states of oppressed breathing, though not in themselves definite diseases, are *pro tanto* states of unhealth. When a man is living in an atmosphere which keeps him constantly below par, as many of those trade nuisances . . . particularly do, that is an injury to health (though not a production of what at present could be called a definite disease) . . . Every population includes a certain proportion who have sensitive *bronchi*; and such sensitive people are frequently much troubled with those vapours as an effect on health . . .

Simon rightly insisted that the quality of air was, indeed, very much within the province of those responsible for the nation's health:

> I think that those who are fighting for the interests of the public health may rightfully claim of the legislature that any such pollution of the common air as makes a common nuisance, either in acridity or in stink or in dust, shall be deemed a nuisance injurious to health, and shall as such fall under the ordinary nuisance provisions of the Sanitary Acts.

Simon pointed out that chemical works certainly destroyed plants and 'if trade effluvia are hurtful to vegetation, *a fortiori*, they are objectionable to man'.[4]

Nausea, vomiting, bronchial and respiratory complaints, poor digestion and lack of appetite, sleeplessness and a general feeling of malaise were some of the effects of smoke and gas emissions that were cited by health authorities. But perhaps just as important were the secondary or indirect effects, for in many towns the stench was so great that inhabitants were forced to keep their windows tightly shut, thus increasing the chances of infection, and while the soot constantly falling from factory chimneys onto the drying wash discouraged cleanliness it served to increase its necessity. As the Rev John Molesworth, Chairman of the Manchester Association for the Prevention of Smoke – one of many pressure groups for cleaner air – argued, smoke was indirectly harmful to health, for 'wherever cleanliness of the person is discouraged there is always an increased tendency to diseases'. This view was supported by Abraham Booth, a Professor of Chemistry: 'I think one great effect of the evil of smoke is upon the dwellings of the poor; it renders them [the poor] less attentive to their personal appearance, and, in consequence, to their social condition.'[5] In addition, smoke and smog could add to the burden of the family budget. In 1918 a study undertaken by the Manchester Air Pollution Board showed that 7½d a week more was spent by each family on fuel and materials for washing in smoky Manchester than in Harrogate.[6] Certainly in the nineteenth century many members of the working classes were too close to the poverty line to allocate the necessary additional amount for cleansing materials, and so smog and industrial grime continued to blacken their lives and no doubt to heighten their poverty in the eyes of their more affluent neighbours. Thus the very atmosphere contributed its baleful effect to the class divisions within Victorian society.

The Black Country was (and is) a term given to the industrial and mining parts of the Midlands, but in a sense wherever industry was located, the countryside was blackened. The French traveller, Leon Faucher, coming upon the 'most extraordinary . . . the most monstrous' 'agglomeration' of Manchester in the 1840s was so taken aback by the persistent 'fogs, which exhale from the marshy district, and the clouds of smoke vomited forth from the numberless chimneys' that he compared the town to an active volcano.[7] In Manchester at that time there were, according to an official report:

nearly 500 chimneys discharging masses of the densest smoke; the nuisance has risen to an intolerable pitch, and is annually increasing, the

208

air is rendered visibly impure, and no doubt unhealthy, abounding in soot, soiling the clothing and furniture of the inhabitants, and destroying the beauty and fertility of the garden as well as the foliage and verdure of the country.[8]

In Newcastle and its environs, the inhabitants 'were compelled to live under a black canopy of smoke'.[9] In Leeds, on close, heavy days, washing hanging out on the line was so befouled by the smuts from the chimneys that it had to be rewashed.[10] Indeed, cleanliness of linen became a rough indication of the cleanliness of the town, and according to Chadwick linen became as dirty after it had been worn for two or three days in Manchester as it did after a whole week in the London suburbs.[11] Not that London was a clean town, for with its thousands of small factories and workshops it was just as grimy as most towns with heavy industry. In the 1840s Dr Reid, who was in charge of the ventilation at the Houses of Parliament, conducted an experiment. He put up a veil 40 feet long by 12 feet high to check the dust and soot particles in the air and claimed to have captured in a single day some 200,000 visible particles of soot. Every Londoner, he told the Select Committee on Smoke Prevention, was familiar with 'these black

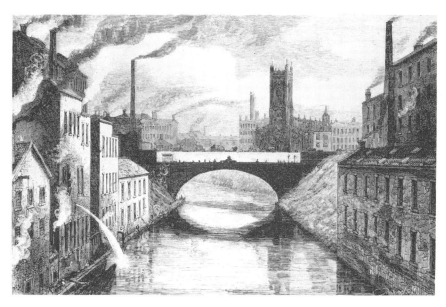

8. Air and water pollution in Manchester. Manchester in the 1840s was compared to an active volcano. It was clearly not much cleaner in the 1870s when this scene of Blackfriars Bridge over the Irwell appeared in *The Graphic*.

portions of soot'. At the Horse Guards the deposit of soot was so great 'that it formed a complete and continuous film so that when I walked upon it', he commented, 'I saw the impression of my foot left as distinctly on that occasion as when snow lies upon the ground.' In cold weather soot and frost mingled in an unholy alliance to form a strip under doors and windows 'bearing an exact resemblance to a pepper and salt grey cloth', and he concluded that the cost to society of the fall-out 'upon dress, upon buildings, upon comfort, upon washing, upon cleanliness, upon furniture, upon works of art, upon individuals going up and down the river' was surely much greater than any expense which would be incurred if manufacturers were obliged to install smoke-consuming devices. The fall-out in fact required a massive clean-up for the Great Exhibition of 1851, and *Punch* commented how 'every street is either whitewashing its face, or rubbing up its dingy complexion with a fine layer of Roman cement'.[12]

The Victorian parks were supposed to provide 'respirators' to help purify the lungs. As *Blackwood's* put it in 1842:

> Fresh air is a luxury to the Londoner. He drinks it up, when he can get it, as a coalwhipper inbibes strong beer. The air of the densely-populated parts of London — and what part of London is not densely populated? — surcharged with smoke and dust, and vomited forth once and again from a million and a half pairs of human bellows, becomes substantial vapour, gross and unpalpable. Sometimes you may smell it, oftener you taste it, and at intervals you may cut it with a knife. When you get into the Parks, clear of the dusty-town, your lungs at once inform you of the obligation you have conferred upon them by changing their diet; your muscular fibre, braced by the current of pure air, becomes endued with unwonted activity. . . .[13]

Yet even these 'lungs' were not always free of soot particles. The gardeners in Regent's Park claimed they could tell at a glance how many days the sheep had been pastured there by the blackness of their wool.[14]

London, affectionately known until recently as the 'old smoke', merited its name. In the 1840s a column of smoke extending for twenty or thirty miles hovered around it.[15] In Dickens's telling phrase smoke was 'the London ivy' which wreathed itself around every building and clung to every dwelling.[16] At Northfleet, down the Thames, the smoke from the neighbouring cement factories was so dense that it seriously interfered with navigation on the river and it was impossible on occasion to make out the bowsprit of one's own vessel. Residents of Northfleet complained that the smoke and smells from the factories caused 'considerable roughness in one's throat, irritation of the breathing organs, nausea of the stomach, and a feeling of sickness'.[17] In Battersea loss of appetite was attributed to the smoke and smell from the local sulphate of ammonia works, and as early as the 1840s the nurserymen in Chelsea were complaining that their crops were being damaged by the smoke pouring from London's factories and workshops.[18]

Much of the London fog, so beloved by Conan Doyle and countless of his Hollywood adaptors, was really smog, or as contemporaries called it 'artificial' or 'black' fogs. Although literary critics have rightly interpreted Dickens's use of fog in the opening pages of *Bleak House* as a metaphor for the legal obfuscation and opaqueness that is the book's theme, there is rather more to it than that; smog was, quite literally, London's dreary canopy. That the smog could occasionally give the city a romantic, Turner-esque light is clear from the almost spiritual Victorian paintings of St Pancras Station at twilight; those old enough to remember London before the clean air acts will recall its angry, brilliant, almost Dali-esque sunsets. But Dickens quite correctly saw in the murky and penetrating smog a vapour which polluted everything it touched and depressed the spirit. His picture is so evocative that it bears quoting in full:

London. Michaelmas Term Lately Over. And the Lord Chancellor sitting in Lincoln's Inn Hall. Implacable November weather. As much mud in the streets as if the waters had but newly retired from the face of the earth, and it would not be wonderful to meet Megalosaurus, forty feet long or so, waddling like an elephantine lizard up Holborn Hill. Smoke lowering down from chimney-pots, making a soft black drizzle, with flakes of soot in it as big as full-grown snowflakes – gone into mourning, one might imagine, for the death of the sun. Dogs, undistinguishable in mire. Horses, scarcely better; splashed to their very blinkers. Foot passengers, jostling one another's umbrellas in a general infection of ill temper, and losing their foot-hold at street corners, where tens of thousands of other foot passengers have been slipping and sliding since the day broke (if this day ever broke), adding new deposits to the crust upon crust of mud, sticking at those points tenaciously to the pavement, and accumulating at compound interest.

Fog everywhere. Fog up the river, where it flows among green aits and meadows; fog down the river, where it rolls defiled among the tiers of shipping and waterside pollutions of a great (and dirty) city. Fog on the Essex marshes, fog on the Kentish heights. Fog creeping into the cabooses of collier-brigs; fog lying out on the yards and hovering in the rigging of great ships; fog drooping on the gunwales of barges and small boats. Fog in the eyes and throats of ancient Greenwich pensioners, wheezing by the firesides of their wards; fog in the stem and bowl of the afternoon pipe of the wrathful skipper, down in his close cabin; fog cruelly pinching the toes and fingers of his shivering little 'prentice boy on deck. Chance people on the bridges peeping over the parapets into a nether sky of fog, with fog all round them, as if they were up in a balloon and hanging in the misty clouds.[19]

To Esther Summerson, newly arrived from the country, the London smog and smoke were quite overwhelming – 'The streets were so full of dense brown smoke that scarcely anything was to be seen', and her first question on alighting from her coach was to ask if there was 'a great fire' somewhere. 'Oh, dear no, miss', answered the man meeting her. 'This is a London particular.' But Esther had never heard of such a thing. 'A fog, miss', said the young gentleman. To which Esther could only answer, keeping her gloomy thoughts to herself, 'Oh, indeed!' Small wonder that she found everything initially depressing and strange – 'the stranger from its being night in the day-time, the candles burning with a white flame, and looking raw and cold . . .'[20]

Much of this smog, in London and elsewhere, was caused by domestic fires. As far back as the reign of Edward I (1272–1307) coal was being used as domestic fuel in London and apparently the air quality was so bad by the reign of Elizabeth that she issued a proclamation forbidding the use of coal while Parliament was in session. In 1648, when Parliament had weightier matters on its mind (Charles I was beheaded the following year), it was presented with a petition from the inhabitants calling for a ban on the importation of coal into the city.[21] Nothing, however, was done. By the 1840s Chadwick called for the use of anthracite to lower the pollution.[22] But the use of coal proceeded apace, and by the end of the century it was estimated that some 18,000,000 tons were being burned annually in London, of which only 7,000,000 tons were consumed in the production of gas and for manufacturing purposes.[23] In the United Kingdom as a whole some 110,000,000 tons of coal were being consumed annually. A city of Glasgow's size could burn up to 1,000,000 tons a year by the 1870s.[24] Even though Louis C. Parkes, Chelsea's MOH, writing in 1892, estimated that London consumed only 7,000,000 tons of coal a year, he gauged that over 200 tons of fine soot *every day* were escaping into the London atmosphere, and that 60,000 tons of carbolic acid thus vitiated the air every year. Ninety-five per cent of London's smoke, he estimated, was produced by domestic fires.[25]

Health reformers rightly regarded London's smogs as more than a nuisance. They were, they claimed, positively lethal. Thus in the fortnight ending 19 December 1891, when 'ordinary' atmospheric

212

conditions prevailed, the London death rate stood at eighteen (per thousand living). On 20 December, a dense fog descended and lasted to the night of the 25th. For the fortnight ending on 2 January the death rate had jumped to thirty-two, and a further 829 people, over and above the average, had died of respiratory diseases during that fortnight.[26] A dense fog could carry off some 500 to 700 people in a week in London, and in the view of the 1887 Select Committee on the Smoke Nuisances Bill, smog had increased significantly over the past few years in London. The issue was dramatized by the statement that during the great fog of 1886 the mortality rate rose to equal that of the worst cholera years and that fog was as lethal as any epidemic.[27] As we know from our own century, smog with its high sulphur and hydrocarbon content could be particularly dangerous for older people. In 1920 a parliamentary committee on air quality drew attention to 'the number of deaths from pulmonary and cardiac diseases' which 'increase in direct proportion to an increase in the intensity and duration of smoke fogs.'[28] There can be little doubt that smog greatly increased the chance of illness or death in a population which, as we shall see, was subject to a variety of pulmonary ailments caused by working conditions. Thus in London in 1886 – the year in which, during the dense fog of 9 and 10 February the mob took to widespread looting and threatened to take over the city – there were 11,213 deaths from bronchitis and another 480 from emphysema and asthma.[29]

As long as domestic fires were exempt from acts controlling smoke nuisances – and they were throughout the century – a pall was bound to enshroud all large cities and towns. The cost of converting domestic fireplaces to burn coal more efficiently was not high – somewhere between 10s and £1. It was estimated in 1887 that a London house with five fireplaces might cost only £3 for conversion.[30] While this represented only a minor expenditure for the upper and middle classes it was a deterrent for the working classes and for all rent-conscious owners of working-class dwellings. In any case, so long as there was no compulsory legislation demanding such conversions, or the use of anthracite instead of coal, little was achieved. And despite the very obvious smoke nuisance arising from domestic fires, Parliament was uninterested in passing such legislation. Partly it was a case of reluctance to interfere in what was regarded as the symbol of both the Englishman's castle and the revered family within it – the domestic hearth. Such controls would require a system of *domestic* inspection that was still most unacceptable to the majority of Victorians. To allow an inspector to examine external drains or water lines or to go into the dwellings of the poor was one thing: it was quite another to establish an inquisitorial inspectorate which would be free to wander through the homes of the middle and upper classes poking into every room, and quizzing scullery maids about their methods of stoking.[31] Widespread use of anthracite would have gone a long way to solving the problem of pollution from domestic fires, but anthracite was too costly to be used widely. In fact the process of converting coal to smokeless coke was in itself a great source of pollution. In Durham and Northumberland, where some 6,000,000 tons of coal were annually converted to coke, some 2,000,000 tons of volatile matter – carbonic acid, sulphurous acid, and nitrogen – were given off, and for much of the century these coke ovens remained unregulated.[32] In the countryside around the factories converting coal into smokeless coke in Northumberland and Durham and in South Wales, 'the growth of trees is checked or destroyed, fences are killed, crops of every description are injured, cattle suffer, and wool is made almost useless.'[33]

In addition to the pollution spewing forth from industrial and domestic chimneys there was in most towns a whole battery of small industries and trades which both offended the nostrils and threatened the public's health. These were the 'noxious trades', which included blood-boilers, bone-boilers, fell-mongers, soap-boilers, tallow-melters, tripe-boilers, blood-dryers, leather-dressers, tanners, fat-melters and fat-extractors, glue-makers, size-makers, and gut-scrapers. By the 1870s the Metropolitan Board of Works in London had made it increasingly difficult for these trades to exist within its jurisdiction and so they moved out just beyond its boundaries, spreading out eastwards along the river and causing much distress and anger among the middle-class residents of Blackheath, who discovered that while their houses, situated on higher ground, afforded them magnificent views and healthy winds, they were, alas, at just the right height to receive the full force from the offending chimneys of the many manure works, malt-roasting works, tar works, oil works, and sugar refineries and other 'noxious trades' situated along the Thames. Complaints were frequent, and capture some of the darker side of the supposedly salubrious and idyllic suburban life of the age. 'I am awakened in the night', stated one indignant Blackheath resident, 'with the house full of horrible smells and nearly choked, and I can have no rest.' While the smells may not have been, in themselves, permanently injurious to health, 'the intermittent discomfort, however, and interference with the ordinary enjoyment of life can scarcely be exaggerated . . .'[34] According to Dr Finch, the MOH for the Plumstead District Board of

Works, 'acid fumes . . . sulphuretted hydrogen . . . [and] a peculiar fetid smell of organic matter, a smell which one may describe as a watercloset smell' all combined to create a stench 'more nauseous than any in my experience' – far worse, he stressed, than that of any dissection or post-mortem.[35] Like so many residents of the inner city, dwellers in Blackheath had to shut tight their windows even on the hottest nights. Traditionally the flight to the suburbs in the nineteenth century has been viewed by historians in terms of escape from the epidemics, crowding, noise, and high land values of the central city, but in countless instances there is a simpler and more basic cause – one's nose, as much as any quest for respectability, or economic factors, dictated the decision. Dainton Lupton, the Mayor of Leeds, for example, fled from the smoke and stinks of his town to the suburbs: 'everyone does as I did a few years ago', he commented in 1845, 'I went out, I could not bear it any longer; and every one who can, is going out of town.'[36]

Given this great variety of forces contaminating the air and making life generally unpleasant and often hazardous to health, one might well ask why it was that the Victorians were so slow to rise to the challenge of deteriorating air quality. This is all the more remarkable in view of the fact that one might expect them to relate atmospheric pollution to their prevalent belief in atmospheric or pythogenic theories of disease generation. Here, after all, was a form of pollution that could be readily detected by the senses, that resulted in obvious, immediate discomfort and perhaps in the long run, in serious illnesses. And it was pollution which, while affecting most severely those who lived closest to the offending factories and workshops, knew no class barriers and extended out to the homes and gardens of the governing classes. A society which had shown such abundant good judgment and energy in rising to the challenge of sewerage might, after all, be expected to respond with equal determination to the challenge of air pollution. There are, however, many reasons why this was not so.

In their classic indictment of the ethos of the industrial revolution, Barbara and John Hammond wrote:

> Thus England asked for profits and received profits. Everything turned to profit. The towns had their profitable dirt, their profitable smoke, their profitable slums, their profitable disorder, their profitable ignorance, their profitable despair. The curse of Midas was on this society: on its corporate life, on its common mind . . .[37]

Whether smoke was ever profitable is debatable, yet the Hammonds were in a sense correct, for in the popular imagination smoke *was*

215

associated with full employment and with production, progress, and profits, rather than with pollution. Smoke was not only accepted as a necessary by-product of industry: it was even glorified as an outward symbol of social progress. Thus the essayist, W. Cooke Taylor, wrote of a valley near Bolton:

> The intervening valley is studded with factories and bleach-works. Thank God, smoke is rising from the lofty chimneys of most of them! for I have not travelled thus far without learning, by many a painful illustration, that the absence of smoke from the factory-chimney indicates the quenching of the fire on many a domestic hearth, want of employment to many a willing labourer, and want of bread to many an honest family.

And he added that rather than constituting a nuisance, the smoke added to the glory of nature: 'it produces variations in the atmosphere and sky which, to me at least, have a pleasing and picturesque effect.'[38]

Just as today, in the debate over 'alternative' sources of energy, the proponents of nuclear and coal-fired plants maintain that some danger of atmospheric pollution is a reasonable price to pay for full local employment, a higher local tax base, national strength and a growing economy, so, too, in the nineteenth century, similar, indeed identical arguments were put forward. In the nineteenth century, as today, the issue was often seen in simplistic terms to be one of a choice between economic stagnation or environmental pollution. Thus in Darlington, which was described in 1866 as 'a perfect forest of chimneys . . . daily belching forth their poisonous smoke', a member of the local board of health (who, together with another board member was a partner in the Banktop Brickworks, one of the worst offenders) argued in self-defence that the town would be definitely worse off without the smoke that was the inevitable by-product of industry:

> The question as I look at it is whether Darlington is to be a manufacturing town or not . . . If I go to Middlesbrough I see large works there – Snowdon and Hopkins for instance – sending out thousands and thousands of cubic feet of gas and smoke close to private residences. I ask the individuals who live there if they do not suffer in their health. They say 'No, it is all good for trade, we want more of it, we find no fault with smoke.'[39]

The theme, 'it is all good for trade', runs like a constant refrain through the debates on smoke pollution. Thus when the Earl of Derby complained in 1862 about the smells pervading St Helens from the local alkali works he was taken to task by the local newspaper:

> Noxious as are the vapours, St Helens cannot be said to be unhealthy.

The large amount of high-priced labour which these works provide would cause the inhabitants to rise as one man to resist by every legitimate means any attempt on the part of the legislature to pass any bill which would have the effect of crippling so important a branch of the trade of this district.[40]

The Royal Commission on Noxious Vapours (1878) ran into the argument that smoke and noxious vapours were the inevitable (and unalterable) cost of national prosperity: 'you cannot have manufactures carried on without suffering these disabilities', they were told, 'half or two-thirds of your incomes is derived directly or indirectly from manufacturing industry, and you must take the rough with the smooth.'[41] The Royal Commission concluded that this attitude was unfortunately shared by the local authorities who could therefore not be relied upon to enforce the nuisance laws or common law against the interests of 'their most important constituents.' Generally speaking, it declared:

> They will . . . do nothing which tends to discourage the establishment and extension of industries, which, although always offensive and sometimes injurious, contribute on the whole to local prosperity. They think it their duty, or for the interest of those whom they represent, to sacrifice the health and comfort of their constituents to the requirements of trade.[42]

Fear of the effect upon local industry thus served as a powerful deterrent to environmental improvement. Typically, when Dr Michael, the MOH for Swansea, tried to mount a campaign against the pollution from the local copper smelting and alkali works which, he claimed, was defoliating the countryside, he encountered the argument that his do-goodism would lead only to the total destruction of the town's economy. If he succeeded in forcing Swansea's industrialists to invest in smoke-consuming devices, 'the trade of the town was going to be shut up; [that] there would not be a single vessel coming to the port, and [that] all the people would starve.' Naturally, in the face of such dire forecasts, he was forced to back down.[43] Concern for local industrial interests always took paramount importance in the piecemeal legislation that was passed throughout the century to curb smoke and gas pollution. Typical of the cautious wording of such legislation and exemptions which weakened the impact of the law, was the clause in the 1875 Public Health Act which specified that while smoke was a 'nuisance' and that furnaces should be built to consume their own smoke, this was to be done only 'as far as practicable, having regard to the nature of the manufacture or trade . . .'[44]

Local authorities were, quite understandably, reluctant to enforce legislation that would drive industrialists to relocate in districts where more lax attitudes prevailed. It was basic economic commonsense to avoid any action that might weaken the local tax base. Thus when the Select Committee on Noxious Businesses (1873) examined the tallow and soap workshops of St George's-in-the-East (later Stepney Borough), they were told that while these were doubtless causes of pollution, 'It [St George's] is a very poor parish . . . it [cannot] afford to get rid of its large ratepayers.'[45] To this, a kind of law of inertia was added, which stated that as long as a town was not demonstrably worse than the average there was no reason why it should take any steps to be better than average. No town was about to pioneer by-laws handicapping its own industry to the advantage of rival towns. Thus this law of inertia served to keep most towns in a bad state simply because they considered others to be in just as bad a condition. And the argument was constantly heard that while smoke and gases were no doubt an annoyance they could not be proved to be actually harmful to health. Men apparently lived and thrived – or at least they did not drop and die like flies – in the vicinity of smoking factories. It was even argued that some fumes, such as those from the gunpowder at Woolwich Arsenal, acted as disinfectants against disease![46] In 1845 the Select Committee on Smoke Prevention asked George Smith, a London manufacturer, if he considered 'the emission of large volumes of smoke' to be a nuisance. No, he stoutly replied,

> I do not consider it a nuisance; it is a question certainly of a degree of dirt, and soils everything that stands around it, no doubt; but, as regards an inconvenience, a person who has been in London all his life, as I have, makes up his mind to a certain amount of inconvenience.

When the Committee persisted and commented that they had received evidence from several doctors that smoke affected the health, Smith smugly countered by offering himself as an example to the contrary:

> I should take even the opinion of physicans on a point of that matter with a good deal of caution. I believe, for the last 30 years, no person has been out of London as little as myself, and I enjoy the most perfect health.[47]

It has been observed that the Victorians were remarkably responsive to hard evidence, especially if it could be presented in statistical form. The response to the appalling evidence of the connection between 'fever' and insanitary conditions, gathered by Chadwick's researchers and supported by the Registrar-General's and the Privy

218

Council's statistics of mortality, is just one case in point. Clearly no such statistical connection between air pollution and mortality or even sickness could be made, and in its absence and in view of all the considerations mentioned above, the legislature was reluctant to impose restraints upon industry. Had they done so early in the century, or even at mid-century, when timid smoke abatement acts were first tentatively passed, they would have met widespread opposition. Even as late as 1878, some half-century almost after the first factory inspectorate was established, a spirited resistance was encountered by the Royal Commission on Noxious Vapours when it explored the idea of broad government rights of inspection of all factory furnaces and chimneys. Hussey Vivian, the owner of copper-smelting works in Swansea – one of the industries held responsible, as we have just seen, for pollution in the area – told the Commission that such inspection would violate English principles of liberty:

> I need not say that there is and must be a great dislike upon the part of any manufacturer to have inspectors running over his works with power to go where they please, and spy into everything they like. I for one, as a free Englishman, object to that on principle to the greatest degree . . . No one has a right to come into our works. I want no one to come into our works unless I choose to allow him!

Indeed, Vivian had the effrontery to argue that all legislation 'in respect of manufacturers is extremely dangerous. I am one of those who believe that a good deal of the present frightful condition of trade in this country is due to the legislation of the past 20 or 30 years. . . .'[48]

In view of all these arguments obviously it was impossible to introduce sweeping reforms and compulsory legislation overnight. What was needed was slow, piecemeal, persuasive legislation, calling upon industrialists to co-operate and proceed at a reasonable pace. In the face of all the opposition and prevailing attitudes it is perhaps remarkable that so much legislation was attempted and that so much voluntary action was taken. To say that it was all insufficient – a case of too little too late – would be whiggish. Yet when the next section on legislation is read it should be borne in mind that, at best, all it accomplished was to turn the urban skies of Britain from a gritty black to a dull grey. In an earlier chapter we saw how prevalent rickets was in industrial cities, and in part that was due to the inability of the sun to break through the canopy of urban smog. It was left mainly to our own century to clean up the skies over industrial regions: but it was the Victorians who took the first important steps in that process, experimenting in environmental protection in the name of good health.

II

As early as 1819 Parliament had appointed a committee to investigate whether users of steam engines and furnaces ought to be compelled 'to erect them in a manner less prejudicial to Public Health and Public Comfort'.[49] Nothing came of the Committee and it was not until 1843, with the appointment of the Select Committee on Smoke Prevention, that serious attention was given to air pollution. The Committee discovered what thousands of town dwellers already knew only too well – that nuisances arising from smoking factory chimneys were widespread. The Committee, however, was cautious, and drew back from advocating legislative measures which would force the factory owners to install smoke-consuming devices and filters on their furnaces or chimneys. Yet it argued that 'smoke, which is the result of imperfect combustion, may in all cases be much diminished, if not entirely prevented', and at a trifling cost to the manufacturers.[50] It was, at best, a polite request to industrialists to undertake some kind of voluntary improvement.

Rather than national legislation it was left to local by-laws and nuisance acts to point the way towards purer air in the 1840s and 1850s. London operated mainly under two acts: the Smoke Nuisance Abatement (Metropolis) Act of 1853 (16 & 17 Vict.c.128) and its amendment in 1856 (19 & 20 Vict.c.107). The 1853 Act covered 'every furnace employed or to be employed in any mill, factory, printing-house, dye-house, iron foundry, glasshouse, distillery, brewhouse, sugar refinery, bakehouse, gas works, waterworks, or other buildings used for the purpose of trade or manufacture within the Metropolis.' The 1854 Act repealed the exemption, contained in the earlier Act, of glass and pottery works and extended the Act to vessels on the Thames. The Acts were administered through the Home Office, which appointed an inspector of nuisances who worked in consultation with the Metropolitan Police. By 1887 there were ten full-time and forty part-time police engaged in the detection of smoke nuisances. Although the Home Office thought that on the whole the Acts were well-applied, it pointed out that one result had been that several industries guilty of pollution had simply relocated just outside the Metropolitan area and that as a consequence London was now ringed with polluting factories. We have already seen the effect of this upon life in suburban Blackheath. The Home Office also thought that since the Acts did not touch domestic fires the quality of London air was still dangerously low.[51]

In London the low fines (£5 maximum for the first offence and £10 for the second) and the wording of the Acts, which requested that factories consume their own smoke only 'as far as possible', coupled with the difficulty of pinning pollution down to any one factory or workshop, resulted in only minor and painfully slow improvement. The same, unfortunately, is true for the provincial towns. In 1866 the Home Secretary sent out questionnaires to several important industrial towns and the answers he received indicate how much more still needed to be done to control air pollution. Birmingham, Derby, Huddersfield, Leicester, Sheffield, Stoke-on-Trent, and Worcester, all operated under the Towns Improvement Clauses Act (10 & 11 Vict.c.34, sect.108).[52] Birmingham also operated under a local improvement act (1851) as did Leeds (1856), Newcastle (1853) and Sunderland (1851). In theory the combination of acts should have been sufficient to effect improvement, but the number of convictions under the various acts was not impressive. Birmingham prosecuted only three offenders in 1854 and not until 1859 were there more than thirty convictions: but the fines were only 40s a day! In 1861 it imposed seventy-two fines, and fifty-nine and fifty-two fines in the following two years. Despite the low fines Birmingham claimed in 1866 that 'almost all furnaces are fitted with some method for consuming the smoke produced. The effect has been greatly to diminish the quantity of smoke within the borough, and the atmosphere is rendered purer than before.' Derby had issued only nine convictions since 1860 and admitted that 'from carelessness or other causes, the law is not so generally observed as it ought to be.' Leeds' record was not terribly impressive either, for it never issued more than nine convictions in any single year between 1857 and 1866 and under its local laws, dyeworks, ironworks and brickworks were excluded. Leicester, too, did not resort to prosecuting manufacturers, but it claimed in its own defence that 'the diminution of the smoke nuisance has been very great, and the small amount of smoke, considering the number of long chimneys, is the subject of observation to all strangers.' Manchester, Newcastle, Liverpool (where the maximum fine was £5, 'however often the person may have offended'), and Huddersfield, all claimed to have effected considerable improvement. In Sheffield the smoke was 'to some extent diminished, but manufacturers generally evince reluctance to comply with the by-laws.' Stoke-on-Trent, a notoriously smoky town, admitted that there had occurred 'no perceptible' improvement. Sunderland confessed that 'the enforcement of the law has been very partial, which is not surprising since it did not push for convictions but preferred to rely on the goodwill of manufacturers. Wolverhampton prevaricated by stating that 'it is difficult to say' whether there had been any improvement, although it claimed, somewhat vaguely, that higher chimneys had 'in some instances' helped. If the experience of the alkali industry is any indication though, higher chimneys generally served only to spread pollution even further on the prevailing wind currents! Swansea refused to answer the questionnaire.[53]

What is clear from these returns is that while many manufacturers could be relied – or prevailed – upon to improve their furnaces, significant improvements could be effected only by the introduction of comprehensive, compulsory, legislation backed up by a system of rigorous inspection. Local acts, such as Manchester's Borough Police Act of 1844, generally contained a clause to the effect that manufacturers were obliged to install smoke-consuming furnaces only 'where the same shall be practicable', and this element of practicability was, of course, open to generous interpretation and made prosecution very difficult. Liverpool's Sanitary Amendment Act of 1854, for example, exempted all manufacturers who had done their best to consume smoke and it would be a foolhardy individual or council member who would run the risk of incurring costs by prosecuting any manufacturer he thought guilty of pollution. Thus even though Manchester had appointed a smoke inspector in 1847 who, by 1850 had served some eighty-seven firms with notices to improve their furnaces, it was still thought that the existing legislation was very inadequate.[54] Similarly, the Leeds Improvement Act of 1866 contained the usual clause 'as far as practicable' and there were so many industries exempt from the Act – dyeing, iron-ore smelting, refining processes, conversion of coal to coke, and brick-making, among them – that, despite claims to the contrary, the improvement in the quality of air left much to be desired.[55]

This is all the more to be regretted since the technology existed for inexpensive improvement. By the 1850s the Juke's furnace had proved very successful as a smoke-consuming device, and a similar furnace had been patented by Bodmer as early as 1834. The Bodmer device had been installed by Truman, Hanbury, and Buxton in their brewery in Spitalfields, and they claimed that not only had it resulted in the control of pollution from their fourteen furnaces but that it had also led to an annual saving in fuel of about £7,000. According to the General Board of Health most of the smoke-consuming devices that had been installed had led to savings to the manufacturer as a result of the more efficient combustion.[56] In London by 1861 there existed some 7,875 smoke-consuming furnaces, and another 397 in the City.[57]

The basic trouble with local acts is that they were regarded as punitive and grossly discriminatory when neighbouring towns or towns with similar industries did not impose similar restrictions. What was required was central or national legislation with some teeth to it. But when in 1875 the Public Health Act (38 & 39 Vict.c.55) consolidated the existing nuisances acts, it again considerably weakened the impact of smoke control by stressing that no offence was to be construed if

> fireplaces or furnaces [were] constructed in such manner as to consume *as far as practicable*, having regard to the nature of the manufacture or trade, all smoke arising therefrom, and that such fireplace or furnace has been carefully attended to by the person having the charge thereof.[58]

Although the Local Government Board could force local authorities to take action, this clause vitiated the Act, and in any case, once again, several important industries were granted exemption. And although under the Act local authorities were empowered to sue outside their own district, the expense involved was enormous and this, together with numerous adjournments generally ordered by the judges, placed yet another barrier in the way of progress. Greenwich, for example, tried to use the Act, but soon learned, literally to its cost, that it had no powers of inspection outside its boundaries and that, in any case, magistrates placed a very lenient construction on the phrase 'as far as practicable'.[59]

In 1884 the National Smoke Abatement Society complained that there were too many fines of 2/6d to 10s and that three-quarters of all the fines for negligence in London were below the legal minimum. Thus low fines and the high legal costs to authorities combined to give a quasi-immunity to polluting industry. The fines rarely covered legal expenses.[60]

Effective central inspection was urgently needed, and as early as 1854, quite seriously it would seem, the General Board of Health had suggested that special constables should be stationed as smoke observers at the top of the Monument to report on all smoking industrial chimneys in London: literally a tall order, nothing came of it. Similarly, when in 1878 the Royal Commission on Noxious Vapours called for four special units of inspectors to control smoke pollution, no action was taken.[61] The suggestion in fact led to quite a heated exchange among the witnesses about the merits of central inspection. Somewhat surprisingly, John Simon and Dr Edward Ballard told the Royal Commission that they were opposed to a central inspectorate. Perhaps they felt that the Local Government Board had enough on its plate without undertaking further work for which it was inadequately funded. Simon who came out of retirement to appear before the Commission, emphasized that the Local Government Board should be a body that persuaded rather than dictated. It should, he said, serve as a 'sort of cyclopaedia' to guide local authorities and to direct national legislation. But it should not attempt to act as an inspectorate in the first instance: 'I want to see the works watched by the general nose of the public. I want the public to be the inspector of the first instance.'[62] Ballard supported this very limited view of the Board's role, even though he admitted that local authorities had displayed an appalling ignorance about noxious trades and that their inactivity could in part be explained by the fact that 'in the manufacturing districts the manufacturers themselves not unfrequently constitute a large proportion' of the sanitary authority.[63]

Although the Royal Commission on Noxious Vapours condemned the local authorities for their inactivity, their pleas for a strong central inspectorate went unheeded, and the quality of the nation's air down to the end of the century was left a matter of negotiation between local authorities and local manufacturers. Both groups varied enormously in efficiency and goodwill. But over much of urban England the quality of the air was still sufficiently bad in 1904 for the Inter-Departmental Committee on Physical Deterioration to condemn it as one of the several causes of the nation's low standard of physical health. The Committee concluded that the main factors leading to the continued pollution of the air were the non-enforcement of the smoke-abatement laws, the incomplete system of inspection, the failure to regulate domestic smoke and the absurdly low penalties imposed or threatened. Rather like the parking fines which are of little consequence to the rich today, so with the smoke nuisance fines in the late nineteenth century – one Manchester resident indignantly told the Committee that 'there are people in Manchester who systematically pollute the air and systematically pay the fine – the ridiculous fine that is imposed; it is a mere bagatelle.'[64]

Where industrialists discovered for themselves or where they could be persuaded that industrial waste products could be turned to profit, or that more efficient furnaces could save money on fuel, self-interest achieved what government persuasion or local smoke abatement societies found so difficult. This took place in several industries as the century progressed but never on a broad enough scale in towns with a wide variety of trades to affect significantly the quality of air. There was, however, one industry where improvements on a major scale were made and it is one which attracted such attention in the nineteenth century that we must examine it briefly before we leave this discussion of air quality and turn our attention to river pollution. That industry was alkali.

Alkali works were defined as all works where the manufacture of sulphate of potash, involving hydrochloric acid (HCl), occurred. HCl was 'a clear, colourless, fuming, poisonous, highly acidic, aqueous solution of hydrogen chloride.'[65] The manufacture of alkali began in the mid-1820s and by 1862 it was employing 19,000 men and producing finished goods worth £2,500,000 annually.[66] The extent to which the fumes from the alkali works were noxious was open to considerable dispute, but there could be no doubting that they constituted a major 'nuisance', for the sulphuretted hydrogen which escaped into the air had the odour of rotten eggs and spread a pall over the countryside around the factories. Major James Cross, an alkali manufacturer and a member for seven years of the Widnes Local Board of Health (and for five years its chairman), admitted to the Royal Commission on Noxious Vapours (1878) that he could not deny the 'damage done in past years to properties adjoining the works, nor the occasional destructive escape of gases in recent years, nor the frequent – almost continuous – violation of the Acts by some manufacturers, up to the present time.' The Commission, quoting his evidence, reported:

> He states, 'I think most distinctly that Sir. R. Brooke's case is about the worst that I know in the whole country, for it is a sad thing to see an old ancestral seat like his being to all intents and purposes destroyed by smoke from those towns (namely) Widnes and Runcorn. In 1872, 1873, 1874, he says, the gases killed all the fruit and fruit trees round his own house . . . He attributed the damage done in these years 1872–3–4, to one or two works hastily constructed to meet a large rise in the market, and carried on in the most reckless manner.'

Thus much of the blame was transferred from the industry at large to badly managed or designed works and to accidents – but as the Commission pointed out, 'an accident that was happening too often at these works'. Cross admitted that under cover of night alkali manufacturers allowed much gas to escape and that there were several manufacturers 'on whom you could not rely upon their doing what is right. . .'[67]

Rather like the modern debate over the near-disaster at the Three Mile Island nuclear plant in Pennsylvania, human error and poorly-operated equipment, rather than the basic dangers of the industry itself, were pointed out by defenders of the industry, and it was also stressed that generally where alkali was produced there was also considerable production of coal and that it was difficult to tell which of the two processes was responsible for the undoubted pollution of the air. Thus in the Widnes area alone (a large alkali-producing region) over 1,000,000 tons of coal were consumed annually and around St Helens (another district of alkali manufacturers) over 1,500,000 tons of coal were burned each year.[68]

Whatever the causes, there could be little doubt that the countryside around alkali works had, in the words of one historian, 'undergone melancholy transition to the drab lifeless grey of industrial waste-land'.[69] Contemporary descriptions of the countryside where alkali works were situated suggest a landscape resembling a World War One Flanders battlefield, with once luxuriant trees browned and bare and the fields taken over by stunted elder bushes or deadly nightshade.[70] This was Blake's vision of England's once green and pleasant land in the grip of dark, Satanic forces, with a vengeance! The 'forest of chimneys' was belching forth its 'destructive clouds of acid' at such a rate that 'at least 13,000 tons of commercial acid were being distributed over the north country at the whim of the prevailing winds'.[71] Near Widnes, trees some six miles from the nearest alkali works were 'prematurely stag-headed' (i.e., with bare branches) and oak, ash, beech, birch and conifers were all damaged. On Sir Richard Brooke's estate, mentioned in the testimony of Major Cross, quoted previously (an estate which was unfortunately situated three miles from the Widnes works and two and a half miles from alkali works at Runcorn), 3,000 trees were so damaged that they would have to be felled, and, the Royal Commission was told,

> The hedges are destroyed, and must be replaced by fences at great cost. He (Brooke) has hardly a shrub. Away from the Runcorn and Widnes sides the shrubs are green, on the other sides they are quite brown and bared. When the vapour has gone over his farms it is just as if a fire had been over them; they are perfectly burnt, and become perfectly yellow.

Wheat was affected and the horses refused to eat the hay.[72]

Again, somewhat like the modern nuclear industry, the alkali industry was accused of being potentially a double polluter, for not only did it permit gases to escape which could be carried from its chimneys even by 'gentle winds' some eight or nine miles, but it was accused of dumping its byproducts on stinking and dangerous waste-heaps.[73] In 1875 the Local Government Board was informed that the main source of pollution was no longer the hydrochloric acid from chimneys but the sulphuretted hydrogen from the sulphide waste heaps at the alkali works – and these heaps were not controllable under the existing alkali acts.[74] The alkali works situated by the Tyne were dumping their wastes into the sea, much to the harm, it was claimed, of the local fishing industry.[75]

The effect of all this pollution on the health of local residents was, it was argued, considerable. The MOH for St Helens suggested that it might be a contributing factor to the high local infant mortality rate and that it was 'the cause of many epidemics of infectious diseases assuming a malignant type'. Alkali gases were blamed for their 'lowering effect on the breath of those breathing it' and for causing 'malaise, general depression, and even sickness'.[76] Several witnesses from alkali-producing districts gave evidence before the Royal Commission on Noxious Vapours of the effect of the pollution upon their health, complaining of difficulty in breathing, constant coughing, nausea, and 'prostration'.[77] One of the by-products of alkali, chlorine, which was used widely in the bleaching of flour, bleaching powders, dye-works, and paper mills, also added to discomfort of workers in the industry, and it was held to be the cause of much distress, including choking, coughing, smarting of the eyes, and nausea.[78] The amount of pollution from alkali works in the mid-1870s was closely related to the general physical state of the plant, and the Royal Commission discovered that while many factories were well-designed and efficiently-run, others were positively frightening: 'in some [plants] the walls were cracked, the towers out of perpendicular, the joints of pipes leaked, the furnace walls emitted gases, and the general appearance of the works betokened an insufficiency of means to carry on the work efficiently . . .'[79] Again, the parallel with the modern nuclear industry suggests itself.

And, like the modern energy industry, alkali in the nineteenth century was vital to the national economy. It contributed well over £1,000,000 pounds to the total income from trade in the country. It was 'obviously a duty of the legislature', as the Select Committee on Noxious Vapours (1862) pointed out, 'to be very cautious in dealing with a trade which [employed] so large a portion of the manufacturing industry of the country.'[80] But on the other side was the indisputable pollution, and since the main sufferers were property-owners in the vicinity of the alkali works, it was bound to attract the attention of a legislature that had been sensitive throughout the century to landed interests. On the one hand it was argued that the industry gave rise to local employment which in turn made the land more profitable as housing and business sites, on the other that pollution led to a disastrous decline in agricultural rents.[81] The House of Lords Select Committee on Injury from Noxious Vapours (1862) had among its members great landlords – Lord Stanley, the Duke of Richmond, Lord Derby, the Earl of Shaftesbury, Graham, and Grey, and they were naturally all concerned with the effect of industrial pollution upon land values.[82] Certainly the protection of private property, rather than the protection of the nation's health, was the underlying motive behind the early investigation of the alkali industry.

The 1862 Select Committee heard evidence from two eminent scientists, Edward Frankland and Lyon Playfair. What emerged from their and other testimony was that some means of control, through condensation of muriatic acid, was possible, but that industrialists had little incentive for improvement and that the old nuisance laws and common law were both inadequate and costly. The Committee had considered the extension of the Smoke Prevention Acts to the alkali industry but manufacturers had effectively argued that theirs was a special industry requiring special legislation. In view of 'the noticeable want of unanimity among the scientists present' the Committee did not recommend any specific process for pollution control, but it did call for inspectors free from local control. However, the Bill which emerged after the Committee's deliberations established a fixed standard of 95 per cent condensation of gases, with penalties of £50 for the first offence and £100 for subsequent offences, and it called for inspectors to be appointed by the Board of Trade. The manufacturers for their part called for moderation, arguing that it was only very recently that technology had become available for dealing with the pollution from alkali works.[83]

The Alkali Act which passed in 1863 (26 & 27 Vict.c.124) was for a five-year test period only. It enacted the 95 per cent condensation level and imposed the fines mentioned above but perhaps its most important feature was that it established an inspectorate. A Chief Inspector, Robert Smith, was appointed with four sub-inspectors under him. Smith's technique was to work closely with the manufacturers, using persuasion rather than force, and to convince them that the condensation of gas and control of pollution was in their own economic interest. In this he and his sub-inspectors (operating from Glasgow,

Newcastle, Manchester and Liverpool) were remarkably successful, and Roy MacLeod, in his study of the Alkali Acts Administration concludes that under Smith's guiding hand 'optimism pervaded the industry, and enthusiasm for inspection increased with the appearance of Smith's suggestions for new and profitable ways to transform the formerly wasted hydrochloric acid into hydrochlorite and commercial bleach for the textile industry. The first flush of success brought cheers from Lord Derby and growing demands for technical advice from the manufacturers.' In this first, highly successful period of control, Mac-Leod states, 'Almost unintentionally, the Inspector was becoming the manufacturers' best ally; almost unconsciously, the State was providing a service to industry which would ultimately reverse the relative economic importance of hydrochloric acid waste and alkali product.'[84] In the five-year period of experimentation the average escape of hydrochloric acid fell significantly, but the large increase in the number of alkali works meant that the air was still being polluted, and in 1872, the year in which the Public Health Act transferred the inspectorate to the newly created Local Government Board, Smith called for new legislation to provide stronger powers of inspection. In 1874 the Alkali Act (1863) Amendment Act set a volumetric standard of hydrochloric acid gas escape (0.2 grains per cubic feet), extended inspection to wet copper works where salt and hydrochloric acid were involved, and required all alkali works to use 'the best practicable means' to prevent the escape of other noxious gases.[85]

By 1876 most alkali works were employing their own chemists to help them comply with the acts and to seek profitable uses for their waste gases and products, and the *Chemical News* wrote, with justifiable elation, 'If the Act is successful the result is mainly due to his [Smith's] zeal, tact, and intelligence. His method has been to lead, not to drive, the interests affected. He does not seek to lay down at once a hard and fast line, but as a truly practical man he aims at and effects gradual improvement.'[86] While there were grounds for congratulation and optimism there were, however, still many complaints from local landowners and pressure groups, such as the Lancashire and Cheshire Association for Controlling the Escape of Noxious Vapours and Fluids, and since, in the period 1862–76 the annual value of the alkali works had trebled, its capital expenditure increased fivefold, and its production doubled, the growth of the industry had, as Smith frequently pointed out, seriously increased the total amount of gases escaping over the countryside.[87] The Royal Commission on Noxious Vapours arrived at the same conclusion in its report (1878) and going against the recommendations of the Local Government Board, supported Smith and his central inspectorate and called for more inspectors with increased powers, and for the extension of the Alkali Acts to all noxious works. This legislation was provided by the 1881 Alkali Works and Regulation Act which provided that 95 per cent of the hydrochloric acid gases and vapours had to be condensed and placed stricter controls on the amount of sulphuric acid that could escape into the air. Included in the Act were salt works, cement works, chemical manure works, nitric acid works, ammonia works, chlorine bleaching, and gas works.[88] The Local Government Board's concern for economy was met by the introduction of registration fees for all works included in the Act and by the payment of local inspectors' salaries by the local authorities. Smith was promoted, his staff was doubled and given higher salaries, and the number of works brought under the Alkali Acts quadrupled to just under 1,000.[89]

The regulation of the alkali industry has been treated here at some length because it was indicative of several important facets of nineteenth-century air pollution. It reveals that progress could be achieved when industrialists could be educated to explore the profitability of better combustion of furnaces or condensation of gases and utilisation of waste products. As early as 1869 the Weldon process of chemical conversion of alkali waste to bleaching powder suggested that self-interest and national interest could coincide, and under Smith's patient guidance the profit motive was made to serve in the community's interest.[90] After 1887 the Chance process for the recovery of sulphur from alkali waste resulted in a new source of sulphuric acid and an additional source of industrial profits from a former nuisance.[91]

Secondly, the Alkali Act, as Dr MacLeod has pointed out, demonstrates the nature of much Victorian administrative reform − less philosophical or Benthamite than pragmatic and professional. It indicates that the 'intolerability thesis' does have validity; in the case of alkali pollution, the quality of air was demonstrably and measurably 'intolerable'; that resulted in an inspectorate, and the inspectorate worked patiently and consistently towards more effective legislation and close liaison with industry. What, in the history of public health, is perhaps unique with alkali control, is that the issue was somewhat removed from popular passions and even interest, and so could remain in the hands of scientific experts like Smith. Unlike the control of water pollution, the alkali pollution was subject to accurate chemical measurement and technological innovations that could result in industrial profits. When these were indicated by an understanding and dedicated inspector the result was significant improvement.[92] The Alkali Acts indicate the importance of quantification to Victorian social reform. 'Intolerability' was bound to remain a subject of dispute and personal interpretation so long as it was unmeasurable. The career of Smith reveals how important the scientist could be if he had a strong administrative base. Even though Smith and Lambert, his chief at the Local Government Board, did not always agree on the best way to handle those alkali manufacturers who were guilty of pollution (Lambert eventually lost patience with Smith's techniques of gentle persuasion and education), Smith was able to present convincing scientific data for legislative standards of pollution levels.[93]

Unfortunately the Alkali Acts also reveal that private property rather than public health was the main concern of those determined to reduce pollution levels. In 1878 the Royal Commission on Noxious Vapours stated, somewhat in surprise, that apart from the Salmon Fishing Acts, the Alkali Acts 'were the first and only Acts which sanction the expenditure of public money on inspection in cases where the object of such inspection is simply or at any rate mainly the protection of private property.'[94] Smith was anxious to develop his chemical analysis into a sweeping study of 'chemical climatology' that would bring a degree of scientific exactitude to all pollution studies, but though such a study of the quality and composition of air would have been of great service to public health, he got no support from Simon or the Local Government Board in general, and although Smith was also made Chief Inspector of Rivers Pollution in 1876 he was unable to realize his 'broader climatological schemes' of chemical analysis. Thus the general quality of air and water at the end of the century was still, with the exception of alkali effluents, a matter of inexact and largely impressionistic debate. This was one important area of public health that did not catch Simon's imagination.[95]

Thus air pollution remained to the end of the century subject to the vagaries of a wide range of smoke abatement, public health, and local nuisances acts, most of which were rendered inoperative by their 'best practicable means' clauses and by the system of local inspection and high legal costs. Modern experience with urban traffic congestion and the resulting pollution has indicated how vital an influence the quality of air is, especially for older people and all those suffering from respiratory or heart problems. The impact of air pollution upon the health of Victorian Britain can only be guessed at. Perhaps ultimately it must be seen rather in terms of massive discomfort, of smarting eyes and foul smells, of hastily-closed windows, withered vegetation and begrimed curtains and clothing rather than in terms of specific diseases and mortality. The remarkable growth of industry in the nineteenth century was simply too rapid and widespread to result in anything other than an increase in the distress and discomfort we have described in this chapter. Even Smith's optimism was flagging by the 1880s in the face of the growth of the alkali works. Progress and growth thus had their effect, for good and evil, upon the quality of life. William Morris's vision of the ideal factory of the future was one which would 'make no sordid litter, befoul no water, nor poison the air with smoke'.[96] It was, alas, only a vision at the end of Victoria's reign.

9

'Reservoirs of Poison': River Pollution

'. . . the growth of manufactures, the accumulation of wealth, and the increase of population . . . are intimately connected with the abuse and pollution of . . . rivers.'

PP. XXXIII (1867), 'Third Report of the Royal Commission . . . the Pollution of Rivers. I. Report', p. xi.

Just as industry polluted the air Victorians breathed, so industry and urban growth polluted their rivers. Industrial growth and the development of sewerage systems transformed the rivers into open sewers or brackish, turgid streams, evil smelling, offensive to eye and nose, fatal to fish, and noxious to man. As this chapter heading suggests, river pollution seemed to be the price that an industrially advanced society paid for progress. Rivers are 'polluted in proportion to the extent of local manufactures', the 1867 Royal Commission on the Pollution of Rivers declared, and 'if no precautionary measures are taken to prevent or diminish pollution, it will go on increasing, with the growth of local trade.'[1]

Although it is difficult to imagine, the rivers were as filthy and smelly as the dirtiest industrial towns. The Thames was described in an official report in the following terms:

> Throughout the whole course of the river from Cricklade to the point where the Metropolitan Sewerage commences, fouling of the water by sewage from cities, towns, villages, and single houses, generally prevails. The refuse from paper mills, tanneries, &c. passes into the stream. There is no form of scavenging practised for the surface waters of the Thames, but carcasses float down the stream until wasted by corruption. The river receives unchecked the whole of the pollution, solid and fluid, of the district; and this same water, after it has been so polluted, is abstracted, sand-filtered and pumped into the Metropolis for domestic use.[2]

Towns, the names of which perhaps conjure up visions of quiet cloisters or pleasant riverside retreats – Oxford, Windsor, Eton – were systematically dumping their untreated sewage into the river, and the

233

great irony of the Chadwickian revolution was that as they became 'more fully sewered and drained [they] pour out continuously a much larger proportionate volume of sewage.'[3] Oxford, in the view of one don, committed 'as great an outrage as can be' on the Cherwell and Isis. At Reading 'human ordure' rested for days on the surface of the Kennet. At Kingston 'the daily discharge of the sewage of several thousands of persons renders the banks and streams in the vicinity disgusting to the sight and frequently offensive to the smell.' At Windsor the castle sewers overflowed after heavy rains and the lawns along the river were strewn with sewage and so were 'most offensive and putrid'.[4] Before London embarked on its great sewerage scheme in the late 1850s some 250 tons of faecal matter daily found their way into the Thames; at the end of the century Bazalgette's sewers were pouring some 150,000,000 gallons a day into the river at the outfalls at Barking and Crossness, constituting about one-sixth of the total volume of the river water.[5] That the Thames, like other rivers, also served as a convenient depository for the victims of murder and infanticide, and for suicides, hardly contributed to their purity: A government return discovered that eighty-five bodies had been found in London's river Lea in 1882 and 1883; another 236 bodies were fished out from the Lea and 226 bodies from the Regent's Canal between 1877 and 1881.[6]

Compared with all the ebb and flow of human excrement, dead cats, and flotsam and jetsam of discarded objects, the industrial pollution of rivers was understandably not seen as a major problem. It was after all, just one of many polluting agents. Nevertheless it was a particularly noisome and visible one. The paper mills along the Thames spewed forth carbonate of soda and lime, as well as the wash from old rags and bleaching powders and the Royal Commission on the Pollution of Rivers described how the Lea had become blackened with industrial wastes:

> Large quantities of various metallic salts, dye-stuffs, brimstone, and other objectionable, and, in some cases, poisonous materials are, after use in the processes of cleansing, bleaching, and dyeing of the goods, discharged into the stream from which water for the domestic use of a large portion of London is drawn.

And to this at various stages along the river was poured sheep wash, which contained arsenic.[7]

Much the same depressing state of affairs existed throughout the nation. The Irwell at Manchester was so silted up with filth that it was claimed in the 1860s that the river bed was rising at the rate of two or three inches a year.[8] At St Helens a brook was described as 'an open sepulchre full of pestiferous odours', and the Tees, which was used for drinking water by 250,000 people in Darlington, Stockton, Middlesbrough, and other large towns, was condemned as an open sewer by the Local Government Board – 'Seldom, if ever', it wrote in 1893, 'has a case of the fouling of water intended for human consumption, so gross or so persistently maintained, come within the cognizance of the Medical Department.' The result inevitably, was endemic enteric fever.[9] The Trent, flowing through five counties, was at the end of the century 'almost from its source . . . polluted with sewage' in the opinion of the Local Government Board. Along its course the Potteries added to the general turgidity of a river already in a deplorable state from barge-loads of 'night soil'.[10] The Aire, dramatically described in 1840 as 'a reservoir of poison carefully kept for the purpose of breeding a pestilence in the town', was indeed composed of a disgusting array of lethal ingredients:

> It was full of refuse from water closets, cesspools, privies, common drains, dung-hill drainings, infirmary refuse, wastes from slaughter houses, chemical soap, gas, dye-houses, and manufactures, coloured by blue and black dye, pig manure, old urine wash; there were dead animals, vegetable substances and occasionally a decomposed human body.[11]

Through Leeds the Aire took on the appearance, according to the Royal Commission on River Pollution, of 'a black and greatly polluted stream'. The human and industrial waste products of Bradford, Keighley, Skipton, Leeds, Halifax, Huddersfield, and Wakefield, all found their way into the Aire and Calder and their tributaries and these, according to an earlier report,

> are abused by passing into them hundreds of thousands of tons per annum of ashes, slag, and cinders from steam-boiler furnaces, iron works, and domestic fires; by their being made the receptacle to a vast extent of broken pottery and worn out utensils of metal, refuse bricks from brick yards and old buildings, earth, stone and clay from quarries and excavations, road scrapings, street sweepings, &c.; by spent dyewoods and other solids used in the treatment of worsteds and woollens; by hundreds of carcases of animals, as dogs, cats, pigs, &c., which are allowed to float on the surface of the streams or putrefy on their banks; and by the flowing in, to the amount of very many millions of gallons per day, of water poisoned, corrupted, and clogged, by refuse from mines, chemical works, dyeing, scouring, and fulling, worsted and woollen stuffs, skin-cleansing and tanning, slaughter-house garbage, and the sewage of towns and houses.[12]

The Mersey, near Warrington, was described as 'black as ink at most times, and most offensive in smell; the Wear at Durham was 'simply a gigantic cesspool . . . emitting a stench vile enough to generate a pestilence . . .'; the Bourne, where it emptied into the Wear, was 'at times . . . as yellow as ochre and as thick as glue . . .'; and the Worth, which had a bed some 5' or 6' higher in 1870 than the level forty years earlier, was infested with rats which fed off the dead carcasses in the river; it could be smelled some half-mile away.[13]

The textile industry, which was dependent upon pure water, was in fact one of the worst polluters. Bradford Beck, for example, was clear above Bradford, and abounded in fish, but below the town it was scarcely distinguishable from an uncovered sewer, the inevitable consequence of receiving the untreated waste of 168 woollen mills, ninety-four stuff mills, thirty-five dyeworks, seven size works, ten chemical works, three tanneries, and three grease-extracting works. In Yorkshire, 'as polluted as Bradford Beck' became a common saying and served as a basis for invidious comparison. Indeed, the Bradford Beck Canal was so polluted that the gases which it emitted could even be ignited.[14] The Royal Commission concluded in 1867 that 'with very few exceptions the streams of the West Riding of Yorkshire run with a liquid which has more the appearance of ink than water.'[15] At the time of the Commission's report wool was still often washed in human urine and treated with pig's dung or salts of ammonia, and the wash, or 'scour', was thus discharged as a 'yellowish, glutinous, stinking liquid' into the streams around the woollen towns. But that was only the first stage of pollution, for generally the same river would serve dye-works, with their colourful pollutants, and fulling works which discharged large amounts of soapsuds into the river. Add to all this the thousands of gallons of human sewage, and one has arrived at a partial chemical analysis of the composition of the rivers of the West Riding. Around Leeds some 2,750,000 hides were processed by the leather industry, and the chemicals which were used to scour the hides of their salts and oils were also poured into the rivers and streams.[16]

Industrial growth might be measured by economists in terms of productivity, net profits and the like, but for local inhabitants a rough measure of productivity was the volume of pollutants pouring into the rivers from which they drew their drinking water and, where still possible, their fish. Thus the largest carpet works owned by the Henderson Company in the 1870s was discharging into the Wear some 2,745,000 gallons of liquid refuse, 225,000 gallons of soapsuds, and the excrement of 530 workers a year. Industrial deposits turned the Irk at Manchester 'black and foetid', and the Don, which was relatively free of trade effluents, was nonetheless polluted from the wash from mines, and down to Sheffield had a dull ochre colour.[17]

Typical of the situation in the country as a whole in the mid-Victorian period was that prevailing in Leeds:

> The whole of the becks flowing through the town are faded with waste refuse from dyeworks, tanneries, and the various other manufactures, from their source beyond the municipal boundaries to the Aire, which river is also polluted along both margins. Carcasses of dead animals float down until intercepted by shoals and banks, where they remain to become putrid and most offensive. No adequate form of water conservancy is exercised either within or beyond the area of the borough.

Indeed, fifty carcasses of dogs, cats, and even pigs, were removed every day from the Aire![18]

One can gauge the amount of sludge which was deposited into the rivers which flowed past large towns when one considers the case of Birmingham, which at its outfall works at Saltley filtered some one hundred tons of muck every day. This was dug into the soil and soon covered an area of seven acres to a depth of four feet. The liquid filth passed through the sodden land and, thus somewhat filtered, entered the Tame. What Birmingham took the trouble and expense to process (under the threat of action in the Court of Chancery it enlarged its tanks, increased their number and added to the size of its sewage farm), many towns allowed to slide untreated into their rivers.[19] The Royal Commission on River Pollution in 1867 painted a grim picture of cattle diseased from drinking river water, declining prices for houses with water frontage, and of manufacturers deserting the rivers along which they had built their mills and factories and being forced, at great expense, to seek pure water from farther afield:

> Manufacturers pollute the water for each other until the streams have to be abandoned for all but the coarsest purposes of trade, and clean water has to be purchased from waterworks companies, or must be sought at great cost in well-sinking and boring, to which must be added the charges for extra steam-power. In some cases the manufacture and dyeing of finer sorts of goods has been necessarily abandoned . . .

The Commission expressed grave concern for the future supply of water for drinking and industrial purposes.[20]

In Scotland conditions were perhaps better due to the value of salmon fishing to the economy, but just as it had some of the freshest water in the British Isles – the Dee and Upper Tay, for example – so Scotland had some of the filthiest – the Dighty, Esk, Almond, Gala, Kelvin, and the lower Clyde. Both Glasgow and Edinburgh had polluted rivers.[21] The Welsh rivers were, if anything, worse than England's. At the end of the century practically the whole liquid sewage of Ebbw Vale was discharged without any filtration or treatment into the river. Swansea's river Tawe was polluted, well before it flowed through the town, by a variety of 'alkali works, copper works, collieries, sulphuric acid liquid, sulphate of iron from tin-plate works, and by town sewerage, slag, cinders, and small coal' and other deposits. Bridgend's Ogmore was similarly polluted and Cardiff's Taff was filthy from the town's sewerage and the liquid refuse of chemical, iron and other factories. It was just as well that most Welsh towns could turn to mountain streams for their drinking water.[22]

The reader might well ask at this stage why this state of affairs continued. How was it that public health reformers, who were so effective in attacking a variety of urban abuses and health hazards, were so ineffective or perhaps uninterested in protecting the environment? Why, in short, did England, a nation of nature lovers, permit such a desecration of the natural environment? For the paradox is glaring – Englishmen prided themselves on being a nation that had undergone massive urbanization but had not lost touch with the countryside; yet for all this, and despite the fact that they lay no claim to a special urbanity, the Victorians were probably far more successful at improving their urban, than in protecting their natural environment.

The answer lies partly in the dilemma which faced them. Like so much else that governs the action of men, whether social, political, economic, or, as in this case a mixture of all three, it was largely a question of priorities, of *values*, when faced with severe challenges. The prime challenge was the alarmingly high death rate. The response was water-borne sewers. As human and industrial filth piled up on land so the rivers offered themselves as an easy solution to a mounting problem. Conveniently located, running down to the sea, involving no construction costs, constantly moving, and, at least theoretically, self-cleansing, they seemed to be in every sense the natural way to get rid of human and industrial waste. This attitude of mind was cogently captured by Lord Salisbury in 1875 during a debate on river pollution. The 1848 Public Health Act, he commented, called upon local authorities to introduce an efficient system of drainage. The result was predictable:

> Drainage must be put somewhere. You could not put it in the air; you could not always put it on the land; and when you could not put it on the land, you necessarily put it into the river. Concurrently with this process there had been an enormous growth of manufactories of all kind . . .

238

The result was 'a fearful condition of pollution'.[23] Educated or compelled by the public health laws not to allow great mounds or pools of human filth to lie above or below ground, local authorities had yet to be convinced that there was anything wrong with using the rivers. As late as the beginning of the new century the Clerk of the West Riding of Yorkshire Rivers Board sadly reflected that among the public there remained 'the still lingering belief born of long usage that the flowing streams are the natural means for carrying away the off-scourings of the population.'[24]

Chadwick, though not unaware of the potential problem, tended to underestimate the effect of water-borne sewage on water pollution. 'The chief objection' to flushing excreta into sewers, he wrote,

is the pollution of the water of the river into which the sewers are discharged. Admitting the expediency of avoiding the pollution, it is nevertheless proved to be of almost inappreciable magnitude in comparison with the ill-health occasioned by the constant retention of . . . pollution [i.e. excrement] in the most densely-peopled districts.[25]

Chadwick's solution was to urge sewer farms, which he hoped would pay for themselves (see Chapter 4). But these, as we have seen, required large financial outlay and advanced technology and prejudice against them was, in any case, slow in dying. Despite the work of Snow on water-borne cholera and the connection that was made later in the century between typhoid and polluted drinking water, the fact remained that death rates *were* declining and so polluted water did not appear to be particularly hazardous. In the ten years before the completion of Cardiff's sewer system the average annual death rate had stood at 30.1 per thousand; in the ten years after its installation it was only 22.5. That the Taff was now hopelessly polluted did not seem, in the larger scheme of things, too great a price to pay for so dramatic an improvement.[26] Given the nature of the challenge can we say that the Victorian response was wrong? The effluvia or miasma theory of disease demanded immediate and quick removal of filth, common sense dictated it, countless reformers and public servants enthusiastically advocated it.

The benefit of hindsight might encourage us to condemn the Victorians for polluting their rivers, but water, after all, runs silent and deep and, although it also was beginning to run turgidly and polluted as early as 1860, the danger to health was not imminent. It seemed clear that on balance dumping sewage into the rivers saved far more lives than it took in the occasional outbreak of typhoid or the even rarer cases of cholera. Thus a Glasgow chemical manufacturer might concede in 1876 that 'it would be certainly a great boon to be able to look down on it [the Clyde] from the bridge and see it bright and clean, and to be able to sail down it without being annoyed by the stench', but, he insisted, 'There is no proof that, in an improved state, it would do anything to improve the sanitary state of the city.'[27] That, unfortunately, was the dominant and typical attitude of mind. Bailie James Bain, Deputy Chairman of the Clyde Trustees, railed in vain against it. 'Surely', he argued, 'it is not necessary to kill a man right off before it will be allowed that he has suffered injury', and he cited as evidence the fact that passengers on the Clyde steamers had occasionally become so overwhelmed by the 'stench of the river' that they had to be led ashore, although no doubt cynics responded that that was due to sea-sickness.[28]

Only very rarely did fatalities stimulate a debate on river pollution and expedite sanitary reform. A dramatic example is the disaster which took place on the Thames in 1878. In September of that year the excursion steamer, the *Princess Alice*, collided with another boat near the Metropolitan Board of Works' sewer outfalls at Barking and Crossness. Several of the passengers drowned, and of the 130 survivors, fourteen eventually died. For some time the Thames Conservancy Board and the Metropolitan Board of Works had been feuding about the amount of sewage and the consequent pollution from these two outfalls (eleven and thirteen miles from London Bridge), and some newspapers carried lurid reports of the victims of the disaster having died from choking on the floating sewage. This was obviously an exaggeration but what was more probable was that the victims had died from poisoning by the sewage. The dramatic accident and the deaths of those who had been saved from drowning served to publicize the state of the river and to strengthen the argument of the Thames Conservancy Board and others critical of London's sewerage system that the outfall works were no longer adequate. But the incident soon blew over and it is significant that the debate revolved not so much around issues of public health as around the effect of the sewage on the river bed, its banks and navigation. Not until the last two years of its existence (1887–8) did the Metropolitan Board of Works agree to improve its outfall works and contract to carry the sludge out by boat to sea.[29]

Although the general attitude that utilization of the rivers for industrial and human waste removal prevented far more deaths and illnesses than it could possibly cause was a powerful deterrent to reform, an even stronger deterrent lay in the cost to the ratepayer and to industrialists of the improvements called for by environmentalists. The waters of the Spennymoor were polluted where they entered the Wear, but, according to a local resident,

> No one in Spennymoor will say a word. They prefer being poisoned to the chance of having a rate to pay for the improvement of the drainage of the district; and I fear the medical men, who are painfully aware of the fatal character of the effluvium arising from this Stygian stream would probably be afraid of giving offence in certain quarters by giving evidence.[30]

As for the industrialists, they insisted that there was no other way to get rid of their waste-products. And while smoke-consuming devices were relatively inexpensive or offered additional benefits in the form of saving on fuel or marketable by-products, there were no such immediate benefits to be had from the control of river pollution. Thus the hard realities of costs and profits confronted the reformers. The 1867 Rivers Pollution Commission was told that if the Leeds tanners were deprived of their river outlets, 'it would shut up the entire trade, and throw perhaps 20,000 people out of work'.[31] Similarly, the terrible pollution of the Tyne and Wear could have been tackled, however partially, by existing fishing acts, but the Commission was told that 'the inhabitants derive so much benefit from manufactories that they are very much disinclined to interfere.'[32]

Thus there was raised the familiar cry that control of pollution might lead to severe economic dislocation. When at the turn of the century effective pressure was brought to bear on the manufacturers they immediately raised the cry that if pollution was bad where they were it was even worse elsewhere, and that they were being singled out in a manner damaging to local industry. In 1876 a Scottish industrialist argued that legislation designed to make the Clyde 'pure and limpid' would be grossly discriminatory and a 'kind of luxury', for the state of the Clyde 'is not so bad as that of many of the rivers of England. Things might go on as they are for fifty years, and it would not be as bad as the Irwell in Manchester or the Aire in Leeds are at the present time.'[33] When in 1892 a special Rivers Pollution Act was passed for the Mersey and Irwell, industrialists in and around Manchester protested that it had effectively imposed a tax of £300,000 a year on the local industries, and in 1901 a commission reported that the manufacturers in the area 'feel very strongly . . . that it is only fair that manufacturers all over the Kingdom should be compelled to treat their trade waste in the way that those in Lancashire have been compelled to.'[34]

Throughout the last quarter of the century, the slowly developing legislation to control river pollution reflected sensitivity to manufacturing interests, and was based upon the government's perception that 'any measure absolutely prohibiting the discharge of . . . refuse into rivers . . . might [not] be remedying one evil at the cost of an evil still more serious in the shape of injury to health and damage to manufactures.'[35] Indeed, the Rivers Pollution Prevention Act of 1876, for example, categorically stated that the Local Government Board would not sanction the control of rivers by any local authority

> of any district which is the seat of any manufacturing industry unless they are satisfied after due inquiry . . . that no material injury will be inflicted by such proceedings on the interests of such industry.

It was not until the 1892 Act which governed the Irwell and Mersey that this clause was omitted. Up until then clear water took second place in national priorities to industrial interests and municipal finances. And of course both industrial and municipal interests were in a strong position to resist the efforts of reformers. As Lord Salisbury somewhat gloomily pointed out in 1875, Parliament was confronted by two conflicting property interests:

> On the one side, the rivers had been so absolutely polluted that the rights of the riparian owners had been virtually ousted and destroyed . . . On the other hand, the owners of great pecuniary interests – extensive manufacturers employing large numbers of people and carrying on manufactories essential to the prosperity of the country – had set up their works all along those streams.[36]

Of these two interests (and it is worth noting that the general health of the public was at that stage, 1875, not regarded as an 'interest') the later interest was not only well organized, it was also represented in local government boards of health.[37] Local boards could hardly demand of industrialists what they were themselves so reluctant to do. In most cases industrialists did not have to lobby or influence local boards, for maintenance of the *status quo* served the interests of one just as it did of the other. Thus the forces for continued dumping far outweighed the voices of reform.

II

From the above description of things one might mistakenly assume that the Victorians evaded the problem of river pollution. It is true that *effective* legislation was slow in coming. But that was certainly not for want of public debate and the Victorian statute book is peppered with well-intentioned, if weakly enforced, legislation on the subject. The history of legislative control of river pollution is a long one, stretching back to 1388, when an act was passed prohibiting the casting of animal filth and refuse into rivers or ditches.[38] Throughout the nineteenth century river pollution was, technically speaking, a nuisance in common law even before it was condemned by specific legislation. But common practices and attitudes far outweighed common law in this matter and the costs involved in prosecuting in the common law courts were prohibitive. Only a foolhardy man would risk those costs when it was generally impossible to pinpoint the blame for pollution upon one offender or even group of offenders. Looking back over the course of the century Alfred Adrian, Assistant Secretary to the Local Government Board, saw three main phases in the public's attitude towards the pollution of rivers. In the first, roughly from 1842 (Chadwick's report) to 1857, the dominant concern was for the immediate removal of all sewage from the centre of towns. This quickly came to mean wholesale dumping of wastes into flowing streams.[39] In the second period, from 1858 to the 1870s, the fear of disease being engendered by land irrigation sewerage systems gradually weakened, and was accompanied by an awareness that sewage could be treated successfully (although expensively) by land filtration and chemical means. In the third period, from 1870 or so to the end of our period, the conviction gradually developed in Parliament and among sanitary and environmental reformers that the prevention of river pollution should be (to use Adrian's phrase) 'an indispensable requisite of every system of sewage disposal which can lay claim to efficiency'.[40] It was not until the final phase that the issue was faced squarely and a belated effort was made to bring the principal rivers of Britain back to something approaching their natural state of purity.

The legislative tone of the first period was set by the 1847 Towns Improvement Clauses Act, which permitted local authorities to pass their sewage into rivers or the ocean, and this permission was unfortunately not confined to tidal waters. The Public Health Act, passed the following year, did not improve matters, for it encouraged local authorities to construct sewerage systems 'to communicate with and be emptied into such places as may be fit and necessary'. Lord Salisbury rightly saw the beginnings of massive river pollution in this Act, and although the General Board of Health and the Privy Council's Medical Department advocated sewage farms, they still preferred to see sewage poured into the rivers than have it accumulate in heaps outside houses, or in cesspools underneath.[41]

The second period dawned in 1859 when Greenhow engaged in a series of studies, on behalf of the Privy Council, into diarrhoea, the conclusion of which was that *'in the districts which suffer the high diarrhoeal death-rates, the population either breathes or drinks a large amount of putrefying animal refuse'* (Greenhow's emphasis). To Greenhow it was certain that deaths from diarrhoea were intimately connected either with atmospheric or water pollution.[42] These findings, summarized by Simon in the same report as the 'putrefactive pollution of the system', were an indication of a growing concern with the problem. In 1861 the Local Government Act Amendment Act required local authorities to purify sewerage before discharging it into natural watercourses, and the 1865 Sewage Utilisation Act gave authorities power to proceed against the polluters of rivers. This Act was the first fruit of the Royal Commission on the Prevention of River Pollution, which had been created in 1864, and which was to sit, on and off, for nine years, and issue several lengthy and largely repetitious reports. Perhaps its ultimate significance lay in its finding that everyone was blaming everyone else! Local authorities claimed it was futile for them to make improvements when other local authorities upstream from them did not. They argued that in essence their reforms benefited inhabitants downstream and not their own ratepayers. As for industrialists, they, too, pointed accusing fingers upstream or argued that conditions were worse elsewhere. The Commission did, however, gather enough evidence to indicate that drastic measures had to be taken. Unfortunately the Commissioners disagreed as to the appropriate course of action, and were divided on the issue of leaving controls up to local authorities or establishing river conservancy boards with broad powers. Nothing much, for the moment, came of their long deliberations.

The Commission's reports did, however, provide a powerful indictment of the existing system of sewerage and also of the existing system of laws governing river pollution. It concluded that 'the right way to dispose of town sewage is to apply it continuously to land, and it is only by such application that the pollution of rivers can be avoided.' It left little doubt about the relative merits of land and river disposal of sewage:

> We have never taken a sample of effluent sewage that has been subjected on a working scale to any other cleansing process [than land irrigation], which was not still so highly charged with putrescible animal matters as

to be utterly unfit for admission into running water. Irrigation is the only process of cleansing sewage which has stood the test of experience and unless it be extensively adopted there is but little hope of any substantial improvement in our own sewage-polluted rivers.[43]

As for the law, the Commission was equally clear in its message:

The law, as it at present exists, is only applicable to local and individual cases. There is no power of general application. One town or one manufacturer may be proceeded against, but there is no authority having the means and the power to deal with nuisances throughout an entire drainage area.[44]

Under the existing laws, the pollution of rivers was considered to affect only private rights, and so only individuals could sue, either in the common law courts or by filing a bill in Chancery for an injunction. Both methods were expensive and the plaintiff was required to prove that the nuisance was caused wholly or in part by the defendant. This was generally very difficult, for as the Commission noted:

besides the defendant there is probably a multitude of manufacturers who, at various points higher up the stream, cast in liquid refuse from their works; these impurities are carried down by the current, and by the time that they reach the plaintiff . . . they are all mingled confusedly together, and the offence of the defendant has ceased to be distinguishable. The plaintiff accordingly fails to establish his case.

The Commission complained that manufacturers could easily avoid litigation 'by simply removing the discharge' downstream from the plaintiff, and it indignantly pointed out that, in effect, manufacturers remained free to pollute the rivers since, in addition to all the other difficulties faced by a plaintiff, it was necessary to prove that a 'public nuisance' had actually occurred. Plaintiffs, the Commission noted, were most unlikely to get support from local authorities, since

principal offenders are the governing bodies of large towns. These do not prosecute one another for the reason that each is guilty of the same offence towards his neighbour, and they are rarely prosecuted by private persons because few are willing to bear the expense and odium of acting as private prosecutors . . . Accordingly, whatever the inconvenience to the public, the nuisance continues unabated. Rich and poor alike submit to it as to a sort of destiny.[45]

Occasionally bizarre legal situations could arise. The Bradford Canal Company, for example, was successfully sued in Queen's Bench for creating a nuisance. In fact the real offender was the town itself. It dumped its sewage into the Bradford Creek from which the canal company drew its water. The company did not have the financial resources to fight the town and so had to close down.[46]

One very prominent cause for the growing awareness of both the inadequacy of existing laws and the increased pollution was the mounting concern for the industry and sport of fishing. Indeed, just as property rights rather than health stimulated concern for air pollution, so fishing rights as much as public health occupied the attention of the various river pollution commissions. The 1866 Commission's minutes of evidence are full of complaints from professional and amateur fishermen that their livelihood or sport was endangered. Henry Bohn, representing the Thames Angling Preservation Society, maintained that at low tide, when the mouths of sewers were exposed, the fish spawn died and that spawning was in general severely harmed by sewage. Tench, apparently, were the hardiest of fish and they managed to survive in the polluted waters, but salmon, which hitherto had been caught, some weighing thirty pounds, at Marlow, had now completely disappeared. The Medway had once been teeming with salmon, but these had vanished by the 1870s, perhaps understandably since that river, according to the *Sanitary Record*, consisted of 'immense sheets of dirty white froth, which float like icebergs down the river and at times accumulate into vast sheets . . . [and] hillocks of floating foam-like pollution.' A Salmon Fishery Act had been passed in 1861 which forebade the putting of sewage into waters containing salmon but it was difficult to enforce, since the plaintiff had to prove that the effluents actually 'poison or kill' fish and that the defendant had not used 'the best practicable means within a reasonable cost' to avoid polluting the river. Both the Tyne and Wear, for example, should have been protected by the salmon fishing acts, but as we have seen they continued to be among the most polluted waters in England. There was in fact considerable disagreement concerning the effects of industrial and human waste upon fish. Witnesses before the 1866 Commission argued that some fish actually went to the mouths of the sewers to feed, and apparently thrived on the effluents. One witness maintained that 'the sewage is good food for fish and that many fish live on it.' Roach, dace, barbel, chub, perch, jacks, and even a few trout were apparently thriving in the murky Thames waters in the mid-1860s. Others insisted that trout, once among the most prolific and valuable of all Thames fish, had been harmed. On the one hand it was argued that the water around the sewer at Hampton Wick was 'quite black with fish', on the other that fish had all but disappeared. In this, as in other respects, the testimony of fisherman was not the most reliable.[47]

Timidity of legislation continued throughout the 1870s. The draft legislation of the Public Health Act of 1872 would have permitted local authorities to group together for the control of river pollution and it proposed pollution standards which would have obliged the authorities to take water samples for analysis. But these measures were discarded in the final act and a wide gulf remained between the Commission's recommendations and the laws. The 1875 Public Health Act, however, made it easier for local authorities to build sewage farms and permitted them to become shareholders in private sewage treatment plants. The Act also made it illegal for local authorities to pour 'sewage or filthy water' into any watercourse (including canals, ponds, and lakes), unless the effluents had been 'freed from all excrementitious or other foul or noisome matter, such as would affect or deteriorate the purity and quality of the water...' Yet once again, this Act, like others, was considerably weakened by the need on the part of anyone determined to sue to prove that the 'best and available means' had not been used by the accused party. It was also easy for industrialists to get exemption from local authorities, and these authorities could proceed only when they had convinced the Local Government Board that the manufacturers being prosecuted would not suffer financial hardship.[48]

The failure to meet the challenge head-on was again demonstrated when Disraeli's administration followed up the final report of the Royal Commission on the Pollution of Rivers with a bill on the subject. Once again the recommendations of the Commission were passed over, and although the original bill was in some respects imaginative, it became steadily emasculated as it was debated and amended through its passage. The debate, led by Lord Salisbury, reveals an impossible striving for compromise between industrial and ecological interests. Salisbury, in introducing the Government's bill, had asked his fellow-peers to recall the Great Stink of 1858 and to multiply that indescribable stench by thirty-six in order to get some idea of the pollution of the nation's major rivers. Strong words, indeed, but the tone of the debate was set by the Earl of Morley, who conceded that there was obviously the need to do something:

> but the subject was one of great complexity and great difficulty, and the Bill before their Lordships would affect a very large number of manufactories, and consequently very large manufacturing and commercial interests ... their Lordships must not lose sight of the fact that any legislation would affect most materially a vast amount of industry.[49]

As the bill progressed so the industrial interest took precedence over the interests of public health and conservation. The original bill, for example, called for some central controls to ensure uniformity, but this was quickly attacked, and control of pollution was placed in the hands of county court judges who, besides being already overworked, were hardly equipped to decide on the technicalities of pollution. Had the judges been given a set of chemical standards for purity and pollution levels perhaps they would have been effective, but the chemical standards which some members of the Royal Commission had urged were quickly brought into ridicule in Parliament. Indeed, the uncertainty of the Commission on the subject of chemical standards, was cited by Morley;

> Two sets of experts usually come to opposite conclusions, and, instead of helping the tribunal before whom they appear to form a sound judgment, they only increase its embarrassment, and the general result is either that the Court, rejecting altogether the conflicting scientific evidence, arrives at what it considers a common-sense conclusion, or by some ingenious and fallacious process contrives to twist the discordant statements sufficiently into harmony to afford some justifications for conclusions thus apparently based upon them.[50]

Distrust of 'expert' scientific advisers, forsaken in the case of the alkali industry, dominated the legislative mind when it came to rivers. As Salisbury pointed out, 'people who had noses had proved to be well able, by the old and well-known process, to decide what was a stink.' In the same way he believed 'the County Court Judges would be able to decide, by common sense, what was the pollution of a river.' He conceded that they could not altogether do without the opinion of experts, 'but he hoped we should have as little as possible to do with them'.[51] Instead of definite standards, the old phrase 'best practicable and available means' was again introduced. When confronted with the argument that the phrase offered a licence for continued pollution, the Lord Chancellor somewhat weakly conceded that 'it was difficult to decide what were the "best practicable and available means", but the Government had not been able to devise anything better than this interest.'[52]

The bill was held up in the 1875 session by more pressing business, and when, the following year, it was reintroduced, it was in a form 'carefully framed to escape the wrath of the manufacturing interests'.[53] The final bill was characterized by Lyon Playfair as 'so little in the interests of the public and so vastly in the interests of polluters', that he could see little purpose in voting for it.[54] During the final reading, the bill was described as a 'manufacturers' bill', and though it passed, it was totally without enthusiasm or optimism on any side. One Member summed it up in terms that read almost like a forecast of its certain ineffectuality:

> The idea was that, much as they desired the purity of the river, they considered that the welfare of the great manufacturing interests, by which the people lived, ought not to be lost sight of, and was of greater national importance than even the purifying of the streams.[55]

The 1876 Rivers Pollution Prevention Act enabled the Local Government Board to direct local authorities to take action against polluters. The Board was hardly encouraged to be a strong directing force, for it was required to 'have regard to the industrial interests involved in the case and to the circumstances and requirements of the locality', and it could not permit legal proceedings

> by the sanitary authority of any district which is the seat of any manufacturing industry, unless they [local Goverment Board] are satisfied, after due inquiry, that means of rendering harmless the poisonous, noxious, or polluting liquids proceeding from the processes of such manufactures are reasonably practicable and available under all the circumstances of the case, and that no material injury will be inflicted by such proceedings on the interests of such industry.

Although the Act made it obligatory for local authorities to allow manufacturers to make connections to their sewers, the authorities could refuse to make such a connection if they thought it would overload or harm the sewers. This led to considerable squabbling and it was not until 1898 that the matter was finally settled in favour of the local authorities.[56]

Not surprisingly, in view of the many inadequacies in the Act, it did not accomplish much and, as we have seen, river pollution proceeded apace. A government return of 1885 disclosed that since 1876 there had been, on average, only nine prosecutions a year; when the century ended not a single prosecution had taken place in Ireland, although its rivers were being polluted.[57] In 1898, W. S. Curphey, the inspector for Scotland under the Act, sadly commented that it had received 'but limited application'. Perth was dependent on the Tay for its drinking water, yet before it reached Perth the Tay received the sewage of an estimated 45,000 people. The Gala, Tweed, Devon, and Clyde were also all seriously polluted by domestic and industrial wastes.[58] By the 1880s several lochs had become polluted, and their banks transformed from firm sand to slimy mud; a greasy film floated on their surface, and they had become so smelly that they discouraged bathing.[59] At the beginning of the present century an official report concluded that, throughout Britain,

> the Rivers Pollution Prevention Act, 1876, has not resulted in the general purification of our rivers. This is partly due to the reluctance of the authorities to put the Act into force, but partly also to the difficulty which a sanitary authority experiences in proving that the pollution within its district comes from the district against which, or the person against whom, action is taken. An authority wishing uniformly to enforce the Act in its own district has no security that the authorities above and below it on the stream will do the same, and it is therefore naturally disinclined to take action.[60]

What was desperately needed as a first step in the control of river pollution was to take matters out of the hands of local judges and local authorities and place them in those of bodies which could regulate, and impose uniform standards on, an entire river basin. The establishment of general boards had been recommended, with monotonous regularity, by the various commissions on river pollution. In 1857 it had been argued that 'the abuses and nuisances which have now grown up with the growth of towns and manufacturers urgently demand some available law for the conservancy of rivers from their source to their outfall,' and in 1865 it was recommended that 'the whole river be placed under the superintendance of one governing body.' The 1865 Commission called for 'a central authority or board' and its Chairman forcefully stated that the 'total disregard of mere legal enactments . . . the constant evasions of obligations imposed by law dictated the formation of an

> authority superior to all these local municipalities, embracing in its scope the whole area of the watershed sub-divided among these bodies, and to confer upon such authority powers differing both in kind and degree from that exercised by ordinary municipalities . . .[61]

In 1867 the Royal Commission on River Pollution was told by a Wakefield worsted and woollen manufacturer that the imposition of controls to prevent river pollution would not be regarded as a hardship 'if all we manufacturers were put on the same footing we should get it out of the public in the end' – that is, pass the costs along to the consumer. What worried them was locally applied legislation that put them at a comparative disadvantage. But while legislation which was imposed on Wakefield alone and not on Yorkshire as a whole was regarded as discriminatory, as soon as more sweeping legislation and general conservancy boards were suggested, the cry of central tyranny was immediately raised. On the one hand local laws were said to impose a handicap on local manufacturers, but on the other, central boards were a violation of local autonomy![62]

The first step in the effective control of water pollution was taken in 1888 in the Local Government Act of that year. The new county councils were given the authority to enforce the 1876 Rivers Pollution Act and on application from interested counties the Local Government Board was empowered to establish joint committees to represent and co-ordinate the efforts of all bodies along the entire length of any river and its tributaries. For the first time, therefore, general legislation was passed, which placed river pollution control in hands other than those of local bodies. As we shall soon see, by the end of the century three such boards had been established – the Mersey and Irwell Joint Committee, the Ribble Joint Committee, and the West Riding Rivers Board.

A prototype for these river boards lay in the Lee and Thames Conservancy Boards. The Thames Board had been established under a local act in 1857 and the Lee Board in 1864. These boards had been established for a whole range of duties and purposes that went far beyond overseeing the purity of the river water, but they did possess the right to make by-laws governing pollution and fishing rights. The impurity of the Thames and its tributaries, much publicized in the Great Stink of 1858, when the windows of Parliament had been hastily closed, had not been solved by the extensive sewerage system undertaken by Bazalgette for the Metropolitan Board of Works, and throughout the period of the Board (1855–88) there were complaints about the back-flow of sewage up the Thames from the outfall works. The Metropolitan Board of Works was generally very sensitive to these complaints and did everything it possibly could to improve the situation. Usually the Thames and Lee Conservancy Boards did not play a prominent part in bringing complaints either against the Metropolitan Board of Works or against industrialists, or in seeking improvements.[63]

If the Thames and Lee Conservancy Boards set a precedent it was one which was unfortunately not followed until the last decade of the century. When in 1891 a Joint Committee for the rivers Mersey and Irwell was formed, it was in response to a realization that these rivers had become a national disgrace and that the 1876 Act had remained 'practically a dead letter'.[64] Interestingly, it was now the local authorities themselves which decided to take the initiative by petitioning the county councils of Lancashire and Cheshire to approach the

251

Local Government Board on the subject. At the local inquiry, held by the Local Government Board, local manufacturers supported the idea of a joint board, partly because by this late date they had become painfully aware that the local rivers were so polluted that they would soon be forced to go far afield for the pure water on which their manufacturing processes depended, partly because they strongly felt, as they had all along, that 'individual cases ought not to be taken indiscriminately, or dealt with separately, without some assurance being given that others in the district, in competition, would be treated on the same principle.'[65]

The Mersey and Irwell Joint Committee, like the central government, did not attempt to set rigid standards for pollution levels, for it rightly argued that conditions varied enormously from district to district. As its Chief Inspector explained:

> Where works are situated in the country, with plenty of vacant land around, good tanks and filters can be built, and a high standard of excellence attained; but when a works is situated in a town, with no available space beyond a yard, or perhaps a tank under the floor of the works, the difficulties are very much increased.[66]

Once again that vague and generous phrase, 'the best practicable and reasonably available means', was used by the Committee's inspectors as a criterion for prosecuting or for leniency. The Committee's hands were considerably strengthened by the Mersey and Irwell Act of 1892 which was an important departure in two ways. First, it went well beyond the 1876 Act by making it an offence to put *all* solid matter into the two rivers and, secondly, it was no longer necessary to prove that the solid matter or sludge interfered with the flow, or increased the pollution of the rivers. Also, and most important, the new Act omitted the phrase, which, in the 1876 Act, had provided a built-in excuse for inactivity – 'The said Board [Local Government Board] in giving or withholding their consent, shall have regard to the industrial interests in the case, and to the circumstances and requirements of the locality.' Also omitted from the 1892 Act was the clause prohibiting the Local Government Board from giving approval to any local proceedings which might result in 'material injury' to industry.

Armed with this stronger legislation and the threat of coercive action which it contained, the Mersey and Irwell Committee in fact preferred to work closely with manufacturers (perhaps indirectly influenced by the example of Smith in his administration of the Alkali Acts), and to hold frequent conferences with them. The manufacturers' need for pure water was a factor in its favour and between its

252

formation and 1901 the Committee had to take only some twenty-one proceedings. Although it applied to the Local Government Board for another thirty-nine proceedings, it was quick to point out that it had encountered 'no organised opposition' to its activities.[67] Nevertheless local manufacturers did complain that they were expected to meet standards not enforced elsewhere in the kingdom.[68] Although the progress was slow, there was ample evidence of changed attitudes, and by the end of the century, the Mersey and Irwell Joint Committee, with jurisdiction over a wide area which included the towns of Bolton, Bury, Manchester, Oldham, Rochdale, Salford and Stockport, was expressing cautious optimism.

In 1893 the West Riding of Yorkshire Rivers Board, with powers over an area which included Bradford, Halifax, Huddersfield, Leeds, and Sheffield, and a total population of almost 2,500,000 people, was established. In the view of its clerk, it was formed in response to the 'exceedingly foul state of the rivers of the Riding', which had become 'the scavenging agency for the solid and liquid filth of the towns and villages', and in respose to 'an increasing public opinion in favour of purer and more sanitary waterways'.[69] As with the Mersey and Irwell Committee, the West Riding Board operated under specially-created legislation – the West Riding of Yorkshire Rivers Act of 1894 – which enabled it to take speedier action and no longer required it to furnish proof that effluents were causing pollution – the very fact of the entry of solid waste into the rivers was enough in itself for legal action. Unlike the 1876 Act, the Act of 1894 provided for the right of entry into factories to take samples of trade effluents. The Board had a Chief Inspector with nine inspectors under him, and spent about £6,000 a year in its investigations. Its task was made considerably more difficult by the fact that in 1901 only about half the 230 or so sewage works in its district operated on a land filtration system. The others used the rivers. Only about one-fifth of Bradford's sewage, and the same proportion of Huddersfield's, was treated by land filtration. Though the Board was energetic, its Chief Inspector, H. Wilson, argued that industrial development and the increased use of water closets made its task increasingly difficult. His report to the 1901 Commission was full of descriptions of outworn systems or new systems inadequately designed. Thus Huddersfield's works, constructed in the 1890s, had been designed to handle 4,000,000 gallons of sewage a day but it could barely handle half that amount efficiently. Yet at the end of the century it was receiving 10,000,000 gallons of sewage daily and it had no option but to pour much of it into the river. Compounding the difficulties was the expansion of industrial towns, which were 'constantly taking-in parts of the rural districts around or absorbing urban districts . . . but they have not been increasing their sewage works'.[70]

The third joint board, the Ribble Joint Committee, formed in 1891 over an area which included Blackburn, Burnley, Preston, and Wigan, did not apply for a special act, but unlike the other joint boards, tried to operate under the 1876 Act. Similarly a Joint Committee, without special statutory powers, was established in 1894 for the upper waters of the Tame, a tributary of the Trent.[71]

Although these joint boards represented an important advance, there were still too many factors operating against a speedy or effective improvement in the state of the nation's rivers. Among these none was more important than the continuing ambiguity of the law. Officials in 1901 were still complaining of the 'composite character' of the existing laws and of the absence of 'a precise code of rules'.[72] It was still uncertain at the end of the century if local authorities were under the obligation to provide sewer connections for all the factories in their district. Typical of the confusion was the case which arose between a tannery and a local authority in 1901. The tannery sued the local authority for not allowing it to link up with its sewer system. The local authority claimed that the effluents from the tannery destroyed the bacteria which got rid of the impurities in the sewage. 'Expert witnesses' unfortunately supplied totally contradictory evidence on whether this was the case, and it was only after the local authority and tannery had run up legal costs of £6,000 and £1,000, respectively, that the case was finally settled in favour of the latter.[73] At the turn of the century, in the West Riding, twenty-nine local authorities still refused to accept trade effluents into their sewers. One could hardly blame the local authorities for their reluctance to accept the outpourings from the factories, for these trade effluents amounted to torrents of filth. The carpet mills of Firth & Sons each week discharged 18,000 gallons of soap suds, 10,000 gallons of dye, and between 180,000 and 200,000 gallons of effluents from their print works, into the Clifton Beck, a tributary of the Calder. C. J. Hirst & Sons, woollen manufacturers in Huddersfield, discharged between 400,000 and 500,000 gallons of trade effluents each week into the Longwood Brook, a stream which, as the director of the company not surprisingly admitted, was 'at the present moment in a very foul condition'.[74]

Far from improving significantly, the pollution of the rivers continued to such an extent that by the end of the century the unimaginable had come to pass and the ocean waters were beginning to become polluted. Partly this was due to coastal towns directly discharging their sewage into the ocean, but it was also due to the industrial pollution of the rivers which flowed into the sea. As with river pollution, one of the main stimuli for reform lay in the concern for the fisheries, and especially for shellfish. The 1876 Act specifically exempted tidal waters, and although the Local Government Board issued orders extending penalties for pollution to tidal waters, almost no improvement was made in this direction.[75] Sea fish, including shellfish, were theoretically protected under the Sea Fisheries Regulations Act which prohibited the discharge of solids and liquids detrimental to fish into the sea, but a government inquiry in 1904 discovered that 'sewage and trade effluents from towns on tidal rivers and the coast are usually discharged in an unpurified state into tidal waters.'[76]

Oyster and mussel beds around England were becoming seriously threatened, and outbreaks of typhoid and enteric fever were traced to the eating of shellfish. In Brighton one-third of all the cases of enteric fever was blamed on contaminated shellfish. In Manchester, between 1897 and 1902, 274 cases of enteric fever were traced to contaminated shellfish, and it was claimed that in London at least eight per cent of all the cases of enteric fever were traceable to the same source. In 1902 guests at two mayors' banquets, in Winchester and Southampton, came down with the same illness after dining on oysters.[77] Apparently England's moat against 'the envy of less happy lands' had fallen victim to pollution.

In 1865 it had been forecast that unless something was done on a national scale there would take place 'the intersection of the island in all directions with a net-work of open and noxious sewers instead of the former pure and wholesome streams.'[78] As we have seen, nothing was done on a *national* scale and even the new efforts on a wide regional scale, embracing whole river basins, which were commenced in the 1890s, were only partially effective. No standards were set, through chemical analysis, for acceptable levels of pollution, no compulsory sytem of land irrigation and filtration was introduced, no precise legal definition was given of either polluting effluents or of water pollution, no substantial penalties were placed on offenders. The cost of land, and its scarcity, and the technical difficulties and costs involved with sewage farming, account for its slow and halting adoption, and in view of all the difficulties we must sympathize with municipal authorities which, beleaguered by so many new demands and new sanitary codes, took the easy way out and used the convenient rivers as an integral part of their sewerage systems. Nor can we be too critical of those authorities which were reluctant to add to the volume of the discharge into the river, or risk their costly sewer or filtration systems by accepting trade effluents. And while chemical analysis at the furnace or chimney was possible to ensure cleaner air, there were more variables where water pollution was concerned. The objection was frequently raised that pollution levels varied with tidal flows, rainfall, and other factors. During the first three-quarters of the century the pollution of rivers proceeded largely unnoticed, insidious and silent. When attention was drawn to the situation in the 1870s, it had become a problem much too widespread to allow for easy solutions, and the voices of reform were not powerful enough to convince a public which either accepted the inevitability of some pollution or simply calculated that it was better than urban sewage problems, evil-smelling sewage farms, or industrial hardships. In the last quarter of the century water pollution seemed the unavoidable price to be paid for all the social and economic benefits of industrial and urban growth. Cholera was now a thing of the past and a nation that had lived through its ravages mistakenly believed that it could take in its stride the occasional, confined outbreaks of typhoid and enteric fever. The pollution of rivers called for a degree of administrative centralization and professionalization that the nation was not yet ready to accept: central boards for the entire watershed of rivers were late in coming, and in 1914 the government was still trying to determine if it could accept the evidence of experts and establish chemical tests for standards of water purity.[79] The prevention of river pollution must be viewed, therefore, as one of the least satisfactory chapters in the history of Victorian public health.

10

'The Canker of Industrial Diseases'

'... the canker of industrial diseases gnaws at the very root of our national strength.'

John Simon, *PP.* XXVII (1862) 'Fourth Annual Report of the Medical Officer to the Privy Council, for 1861', pp. 31–2.

In an earlier chapter it was suggested that many men and women who survived the debilitating or fatal diseases of the day probably did so with constitutions ill-suited to stress or challenge. Yet many hundreds of thousands of working men and women did in fact pass the greater part of each day working under stressful and hazardous conditions. For industrial workers (and by mid-century the majority of Englishmen were so employed) the working day meant early starts, long hours, and often physically demanding labour in conditions that would have challenged even the strongest constitutions. To start work at 6 am, perhaps after walking through sleet or rain, and to continue at it all day in over-heated, drafty, or ill-ventilated work rooms meant for many a slow process of physical decline or a life lived continuously on the brink of exhaustion. For those workers already weakened by the insidious effects of the urban and domestic environment, working conditions could literally mean the difference between life and death.

When Kathleen Woodward, in her autobiographical *Jipping Street*, recalled her life as a young girl in an Aldersgate shirt-collar factory, the enduring memory was of utterly deadening fatigue. Although work did not begin until 8.00 am, she had to work until well after 7.30 pm, when, after all the other girls had left, she remained to sweep up, 'weeping impotently as I swept'. She recalled:

> The tiredness, the sheer physical exhaustion that came upon me at this time of day . . . I could have slept as I stood. To this day I cannot look at Jewin Street [where the factory was located] without being overwhelmed with the tiredness I there knew – an aching tiredness, drawn out by the knowledge of a to-morrow which would surely bring with it the same inexpressible fatigue.[1]

Factory labour provided the perfect nexus for aggravating or accelerating ill-health. In 1884 a government report on the health of cotton operatives pointed out that:

> It seems to be evident that these conditions are not such as to prevent that large proportion of workpeople whose constitutions are naturally vigorous from following their calling without serious inconvenience. But there remains the proportion, also very considerable, who have a constitutional tendency to one form or other of rheumatic, phthisical or dyspeptic ailment. Such tendencies cannot fail to be intensified by working continuously in an ill-ventilated atmosphere, whether pervaded by mineral dust or rendered artificially damp.[2]

The generally debilitating, as well as the specifically lethal effects of factory work were also stressed by John Simon in 1862. He pointed out that sedentary indoor labour was 'in some cases combined with an almost deforming constraint of bodily posture' and that 'the working day thus spent is commonly of at least ten hours duration, and sometimes extends to 12, 14 and even 16 hours.' These conditions, when combined with 'scanty . . . bodily exercise', made the workers' health 'necessarily low' and particularly vulnerable to tubercular disease. Simon rightly regarded industrial conditions as falling within his duties as a public health officer, and he sadly reflected that 'gigantic branches of our national industry', textiles, earthenware and china, steel and iron, posed a considerable threat to the health of the nation. Among the many 'aggravating circumstances' he argued that 'none is so effective as the bad ventilation' of workplaces, for he maintained that for the greater part of the day the workmen of England were breathing air that was filled with 'finely divided metal, grindstone, flint, clay, shell, ivory, bone, charcoal, wool, cotton, flax, silk . . .' With his customary fervour Simon concluded that 'to be able to redress that wrong is perhaps among the greatest opportunities for good which human institutions can afford.'[3]

The task before Simon was, however, enormous, for manufacturers and the general public were not well-informed about the long-term effects of industrial work upon health, and the worker himself, as Simon was at pains to point out, was hardly in any position to 'exact his sanitary rights', partly because of his insecure position in the labour market, partly because he was fatalistic and there existed a widespread belief that wages represented danger money and that if conditions improved wages might fall.[4]

The movement for better factory conditions and shorter hours embraced far more than the health of the workers, although implicit in that movement and in the government factory inspectorate which was established under the 1833 Factory Act was the physical well-being of the labour force.[5] The history of the factory reform movement has been analyzed in great detail many times and it is not necessary here to recount the many legislative enactments which, by improving the factories and shortening the hours of labour, made the lives of the workers healthier. This chapter is concerned only with the specific industrial processes that were harmful to health and which came under the observation of the public health authorities. While hours and conditions of labour, and industrial accidents belong more properly to economic or social history, industrial diseases are specifically related to public health, that is, to the history of community action to prevent disease.[6] Surprisingly, occupational diseases have been ignored by most historians of public health, yet they commanded the attention of Simon and other reformers and prompted a legislative response, although a factory medical department, comparable in strength and expertise to the medical departments of the Privy Council and Local Government Board, was not established until the very end of the century.

The early writers on factory conditions, among them J. P. Kay (*The Moral and Physical Condition of the Working Classes employed in the Cotton Manufacture in Manchester*, 1832), P. Gaskell (*The Manufacturing Population of England, Its Moral, Social and Physical Condition . . .*, 1833), and C. Thackrah (*The Effects of the Principal Arts, Trades and Professions, and of Civic States and Habits of Living, on Health and Longevity*, 1831), were all concerned with the effects of factory work upon health. Although they tended to concentrate upon the health of children, arguing that the period of physical growth should not coincide with hard manual labour, and, to a lesser extent, upon the health of women, their works did much to draw attention to the physical (and, as important to contemporaries, moral) environment of the factory. Historians still argue about the accuracy of these and other reports.[7] But what is important for us here is not the question of the accuracy of their observations but the material they provided for the factory reform movement which developed in the decades of the 1830s and 1840s. While there was no attempt to pinpoint the incidence of occupational diseases, a powerful, emotion-filled and generalized indictment of the factory environment was stamped upon the public mind, and the factory system, both in popular works of fiction and protest literature, became something of a whipping boy for all the social and moral ills of society. The detrimental effects of closed windows, high humidity, long hours, and arduous labour upon children and women became an equation which needed no scientific support or close medical evidence to sustain it in the popular imagination. As Leon Faucher, viewing Manchester in 1844, wrote: 'The operatives are pale and meagre in their appearance, and their physiognomy has not the animation which indicates health and vigour.' To Faucher it was self-evident that 'the race is degenerating', and, he added, placing his finger on what he thought was the cause, 'factory labour must ever be incompatible with health, so long as the working hours are not curtailed.'[8] Similar indictments and conclusions were published in the *Lancet*, which called for legislation and gave prominent and favourable reviews to the work of Thackrah and the other reformers. Similarly, the London Medical Society passed a resolution in support of a ten-hour day for children in 1833.[9] As early as the 1802 Health and Morals of Apprentices Act, factories which fell within the provisions of the Act were to be whitewashed twice a year and the windows were to be large enough to provide adequate ventilation. The thrust of the 1833 Factory Act, which resulted from the reform agitation, was in a different direction (limiting of hours), but it did introduce the novelty of a state inspectorate. It did not, however, take up the lead of Thackrah, who had examined in considerable detail the hazards associated with various industries and had, among other things, advocated the watering down of rocks and coal during the cutting process, and urged periodical health check-ups for miners, frequent baths, proper exercise, and fresh air.[10]

The literature on industrial diseases was not significantly supplemented until 1843 when Dr Holland published his *Diseases of the Lungs from Mechanical Causes and Inquiries into the Condition of the Artizans exposed to the inhalation of Dust*, in which he argued that the dry grinding process used in the manufacture of Sheffield cutlery caused many respiratory and pulmonary diseases, including phthisis.[11] The next year Chadwick in his *Report* drew attention to the connection between overcrowding in tailors' workshops and consumption and to the abysmal conditions in the workshops of the handloom-weavers of Spitalfields. The workers, he wrote in considerable disgust, were 'decayed in their bodies; the whole race of them is rapidly descending to the size of Liliputians,' and, he added, using an argument that he hoped might prove effective, 'You could not raise a grenadier company among them at all.'[12] Piecemeal information continued to be gathered, and the census of 1851, as Farr wrote, 'gave us an opportunity for the first time of determining the influence of occupations on sound principles, that is, by a comparison of the living at each age and the deaths at each age.' Using comparative statistics, Farr argued that the high mortality from pulmonary disease of miners in Cornwall, and in northern England and northern Wales, was due to their occupations. [13]

Certainly enough scattered evidence had been compiled by mid-century to indicate the need for an official government inquiry, and industrial medicine was placed firmly on the agenda of public health by Simon in his preface to his *Collected Sanitary Reports*, published in 1854. In what his biographer has described as 'a sort of personal programme and a public manifesto', Simon called for 'a general law, that every establishment employing labour be liable to inspection and regulation in regard to whatever acts and conditions are detrimental or hazardous to life', and specific regulations 'for those who labour with copper, mercury, arsenic, and lead . . . lest they be poisoned! For grinders, lest their lungs be fretted into consumption! For match-makers, lest their jaws be rotted from them by phosphorus!'[14] Simon was instrumental in bringing this 'manifesto' closer to reality in legislation when in 1856 he secured the post of the first Lectureship in Public Health in Britain (at St Thomas's Hospital) for his close friend, Dr Edward Greenhow. Greenhow almost immediately, and with every encouragement from Simon, set out to interpret and correlate the statistics that had been gathered by the Registrar-General. The result, *Papers Relating to the Sanitary State of the People of England*, was published by Simon as a Blue Book in 1858. Among other things, Greenhow used the comparative statistical method to demonstrate convincingly that one of the reasons why mortality rates fluctuated widely from district to district was to be found in the lethal nature of certain occupations. [15]

From his position as Medical Officer to the Privy Council Simon was able to build on Greenhow's research to bring the subject of occupational diseases to the attention of the government. In the years 1860 and 1861 he had Greenhow carry out a massive investigation for the Privy Council of thirty-three industrial towns. Among the occupations and towns inspected were silk, flax and wool in Preston, Blackburn, Macclesfield, Leek, Coventry, Bradford and Leeds, hosiery at Leicester and Nottingham, earthenware and china in Stoke-on-Trent, tin-mining, copper-mining, coal-mining, iron-mining, and lead-mining at Redruth, Penzance, Wolverhampton, Merthyr Tydfil, Abergavenny, and metal-smelting and instrument-making at Wolverhampton, Sheffield, Birmingham, Merthyr Tydfil, and Abergavenny. [16] The years 1861 and 1862 saw Simon directing inquiries into the use of arsenic, phosphorus, lead, and mercury in industry and their effects upon the health of the workers.[17] These inquiries were both detailed and sophisticated in their method. Greenhow, for example, had discovered that the pottery workers in Stoke-on-Trent and Wolstanton had a far higher mortality rate from phthisis and other respiratory and pulmonary diseases than the local population in general. He cautioned that factors other than industrial conditions might be partly responsible – the Stoke pottery workers were, for example, notoriously heavy drinkers. But he noted also that their hours of labour were, relatively speaking, quite short (generally from 7 am to 6 pm), and that their houses were generally quite sanitary. The fact that many of the workers had been employed in the Potteries from the tender age of seven and that the workmen refused to open the factory windows, no doubt aggravated their condition: chronic bronchitis was common among the workers.[18]

Armed with all this information Simon set out in his annual reports to build up the case for legislation. In his *Third Annual Report* (1861), Simon had suggested, in rather vague terms, that 'in proportion as the male and female populations are severally attracted to indoor branches of industry, in such proportions, other things being equal, their respective death-rates by lung disease increased.'[19] In his *Fourth Annual Report* (1862) he was now able to be much more explicit, and his tone took on the urgency and indignation which was characteristic of his style:

> The results of this very large inquiry are, in one sense of the word, satisfactory. They answer the question which claimed investigation. They establish in detail what had appeared generally in the statistics. They explain how it is that the inspected occupations are so hurtful to those who follow them – how it is, that, in much of our best national industry, the workman, by reason of his work, loses some considerable part of his life.

Simon stressed that in most of the inspected industries there was inadequate ventilation and that the industrial processes involved 'in some gigantic branches of our industry', textiles, earthenware and china, steel and iron, caused the workforce to 'break down prematurely with lung-disease, under pressure of the mere dustiness of their occupation.' Similarly, miners 'break down prematurely with bronchitis and pneumonia, caused by the atmosphere in which they labour'.[20] Simon was far too experienced in the ways of politics to let the case for reform rest in the pages of his annual reports. In 1862, for example, at the annual meeting (held in London) of the Social Science

Association he chaired a session on 'the effects of occupation upon health'. The main speaker was Greenhow, who gave a clear summary, with statistics and case-studies, of his earlier investigations and successfully moved a resolution for the extension of the factory acts to cover industrial diseases and unhealthy working conditions.[21]

Not until two years later, however, did Simon's efforts produce legislation.[22] The 1864 Factory Act was the first to put a major emphasis on proper ventilation, stipulating that 'every factory to which the Act applies shall be kept in a cleanly state and shall be ventilated in such a manner as to render harmless so far as is practicable any gases, dust or their impurities generated in the process of manufacture that may be injurious to health.' In 1866 the Sanitary Act extended the definition of 'nuisances' to all factories and workshops not covered in the 1864 Factory Act, and these two acts were supplemented by legislation passed in 1867 (the Factory Extension Act) which protected women and children from certain harmful industrial processes and required extractor fans in factories where grinding, glazing, or polishing were carried on, in 1875 (the Public Health Act) and in 1878 (the Factory and Workshops Act).

Somewhat understandably, but rather prematurely, Simon rejoiced that, with these Acts, 'proper protection was at last constituted for the special sanitary interests of the artisan population' and that they guaranteed good ventilation, cleanliness, control of dust and other impurities, and, at least for women and children, protection from certain dangerous industrial processes.[23] Unfortunately, as with so much sanitary legislation, effective inspection and implementation lagged behind, and the Acts were not rigorously enforced. The early factory acts, for example, had stipulated that youngsters employed in factories had to have certificates testifying to their age and health, but although the Association of Certifying Medical Officers of Great Britain and Ireland was formed in 1868 and it was dedicated to collecting all possible information about industrial diseases, there was little unity of purpose at the centre. There were two Chief Inspectors of Factories, one in Birmingham, the other in London, but neither was a medical man and their staff was totally inadequate for the inspection of the 110,000 factories and workshops which were theoretically under their control in 1871.[24] Not until 1896, with the appointment of Dr Arthur Whitelegge as Chief Inspector of Factories, and, two years later, the appointment of T. M. Legge as the first Medical Inspector of Factories, was any concentrated emphasis placed upon industrial diseases as opposed to general sanitary conditions within the factory.

Whitelegge had been MOH for Nottingham (1884–9) and County MOH of the West Riding of Yorkshire (1889–96) and he brought to his new post (which was administrative and non-medical) a knowledge of public health that was lacking in his predecessors. Thus it was not until the very end of the century that the central government introduced a central administration that finally applied to the study and control of occupational hazards some of the expertise and purpose of mind that had borne such fruit in other areas of public health. Unfortunately, the 1891 Factory Act transferred the sanitary control of workshops from the factory inspectors (where it had been placed by the 1871 Factory Act) into the hands of the already overworked local authorities. In Sheffield, for example, there were at least 2,000 workshops, an impossible number for the local sanitary officials to inspect adequately.[25]

Although working hours were made shorter, ventilation improved, protective guards around dangerous machinery introduced, and factory toilets and washrooms brought under inspection, the quite specific industrial diseases were not subject to any effective control until very late in the century. The 1891 Factory Act enabled the Chief Inspector of Factories to require special provisions to be applied to any factory where harmful trades were carried on, and the 1895 Factory and Workshop Act required the notification of industrial diseases for the first time: lead, arsenic, and phosphorus poisoning, and anthrax were listed as notifiable diseases, and a Home Office Dangerous Trades Committee was established to examine actual or potentially harmful industrial processes.[26]

II

In the nineteenth century industrial diseases were simply an accepted part of working life, as inevitable and as unpleasant as the long hours or uncertainty of employment. Miner's asthma, or, as it was more graphically called, 'black spit', potter's asthma, or 'potter's rot', brass-founder's ague or 'Monday fever', matchmaker's necrosis, or 'phossy jaw', cutlery grinder's asthma and chimney sweep's cancer, or 'soot wart' – these and many more were all part and parcel of the Victorian vocabulary. One did not have to possess the penetrating acumen of a Sherlock Holmes to detect the specific trade of various working men. The tailor was betrayed by his concave chest and stooped shoulders, the file-maker by his paralyzed wrist or thumb, the matchmaker by his (or her) teeth or jaw, the miner by his calloused knees and elbows and bad eyes, the potter by his asthma, the lead worker by his paralyzed wrist, the brass worker and copper worker by the tell-tale greenish tint of the hair, teeth, and clothing, the pottery and earthenware worker by his blue gums, the worker handling mercury by his 'trembles', and the confectionery worker by the skin boils which were the first sign of arsenical poisoning. Industrial diseases thus further accentuated the different physique and appearance of the working classes.

Among the occupational diseases which attracted the attention of the government was anthrax. Although it occurred also among furriers, tanners, and upholstery workers, anthrax was primarily a disease of wool workers, and was known in France as the 'maladie de Bradford'. First isolated in England in 1847, after the importation of alpaca, camel hair, and mohair, it became endemic in the cloth industry. In 1880 there were outbreaks of fatal anthrax in Bradford and Leicester, in 1882 in London, again in Leicester in 1886–7, and again in London in 1893. In 1899 the Chief Inspector of Factories and Workshops reported that anthrax was still a problem in the cloth industry; in that year seventeen cases of anthrax had been reported.[27] Rather like cholera, another disease which originated in Asia, anthrax (which was always endemic in Siberia), was greatly feared partly because of the speed with which it killed, and because there was no known defence against it. A woolworker might complain of 'increased oppression of breathing, giddiness, shivering, drowsiness, sore throat and vomiting', one day, of 'terrible prostration' the next, and be dead on the third. Some workers were dead within a day of first complaining about feeling ill or showing any symptoms noticeably different from the 'flock fever' or 'shoddy fever' that were endemic to workers in the cloth trades. Other workers who contracted anthrax escaped with their lives but suffered disfiguring skin blisters, paralysis of the fingers, and fevers which might last several months. Simon and the Local Government Board's medical department could do little more than to report outbreaks and to urge a close examination of wool and hair from abroad. Anthrax remained a much-feared and bewildering scourge of woolsorters and wool and hair workers into the present century.[28]

Unlike anthrax, which affected only a handful of workers, arsenical poisoning was widespread in Victorian Britain. The Medical Society of London discovered that arsenic was used in a remarkable variety of consumer products, among them:

265

paper, fancy and surface coloured, in sheets for covering cardboard boxes, for labels of all kinds; for advertisement cards, playing cards, wrappers for sweetmeats . . . for the ornamentation of children's toys; for covering children's and other books; for lamp shades, paperhangings for walls and other purposes; artificial leaves and flowers; wax ornaments for Christmas trees and other purposes; printed or woven fabrics intended for use as garments; printed or woven fabrics intended for use as curtains or coverings for furniture; children's toys, particularly inflated india rubber balls with dry colour inside, painted india rubber dolls, stands, and rockers for rocking horses and the like, glass balls (hollow); distemper colour for decorative purposes; oil paint for the same; lithographers' colour printing; decorated tin plates, including painted labels used by butchers and others to advertise the price of provisions; japanned goods generally; venetian and other blinds; American and leather cloth; printed table baizes; carpets, floorcloth, linoleum, book cloth and fancy bindings. To this list may be added coloured soaps, wafers, sweetmeats, and false malachite.[29]

Working with arsenic usually resulted in severe dermatitis, eczema, and other skin diseases, including skin cancer, and workers suffered from boils and pimples, itching rashes around the nostrils, and 'irritating eruptions' around the genitals.[30]

Green arsenites, which were extensively used in lithographic printing and in the tinting of wallpaper and wrapping paper, were also used to colour the paper used for American 'greenbacks', and it was reported that 'the frequent handling of these paper notes by clerks at banks, and their occasional contact with the lips, is recorded to have produced symptoms of arsenical poisoning.'[31] Although direct contact with arsenic caused the severest skin problems and the occasional death, it could also be breathed into the system, leading to headaches, vomiting, and severe bronchial and laryngeal irritations, and it was here that the factory acts enforcing better ventilation and exhausting of fumes had a beneficial effect upon workers using arsenic. Nevertheless one is left wondering how many of the general malaises, especially headaches and sense of nausea, of which Victorians complained, were due to the leaching of arsenic from consumer items. In one experiment, some ten grains of white arsenic were extracted from fifty leaves of artificial flowers and a hundred grains from twenty yards of a green ball gown![32]

Attracting more widespread attention than any other occupational disease was phosphorus poisoning and its effects upon the thousands of factory and domestic workers in the match industry. Throughout the century the industry employed women and children, often in a domestic setting – a classic cottage, or to be more accurate, garret and cellar, industry. Safety matches used red or amorphous phosphorus which was harmless to workers involved in their manufacture. But while several European nations permitted the manufacture of only safety matches, their sale was not great in England, and, quite remarkably, the government was slow to ban the use of the dangerous, or white, phosphorus, in the manufacture of matches. Indeed, despite mounting evidence of phosphorus poisoning, and what amounted to a public scandal concerning 'phossy jaw', it was not until 1910 that white phosphorus was finally banned. The trouble, and indeed, blame, lay partly with the English public, which rejected the safety match (Bryant & May had taken out a patent on safety matches as early as 1855). 'Most people', it was claimed, 'seem to prefer to carry loose matches about with them in their pockets, and ignite them on the walls of rooms, or their trousers, or on the furniture . . .' The widespread belief that a match placed in the hollow of a tooth was the best cure for a toothache doubtless increased the risk of phossy jaw.[33]

This reluctance to use safety matches led to untold discomfort and disfigurement for many match-makers. The 'suffocating effects of the phosphorus' given off by some of the workers at the Bell and Black match works, wrote two factory surgeons, 'have been so powerful as to cause quite a feeling of stifling and faintness, and we have been obliged to leave the door open for a considerable time [after the match workers left their surgery] . . . to air the room.'[34] Dr George Cunningham, the Senior Dental Surgeon to the London Hospital, made something of a speciality of phosphorus poisoning, and discovered that phosphorus could be absorbed in three ways – by inhaling it, by transferring it from hand to mouth, or by skin absorption. But whatever the process, the result could be terrifying. Cunningham stated that often a patient would first complain of a tooth-ache:

The wound in the gum, however, was found not to heal; offensive matter would begin to ooze from it, and ere long a portion of the alveolus [the tooth socket in the jaw bone] became exposed. Occasionally the portion of the bone thus denuded came away, bringing with it, perhaps one or two of the neighbouring teeth, and the disease made no further progress. More frequently, however, the disease continued to spread; and sometimes slowly, sometimes rapidly, more and more of the jaw-bones became denuded, the gums grew spongy, and retreated from the alveoli; the teeth got loose and fell out, the fetid suppuration became more and more copious, the soft parts around grew swollen, tender, and infiltrated, and often the seat of sinuses. And thus the disease continued to progress, till in the course of six months, a year, two years – it might be even five or six years – the patient sank from debility, or from phthisis, or from some other consequence of the local affection; or, having lost piecemeal, or in the mass, large portions – one half, or even the whole – of the upper or lower jaw, returned to his original state of health, but the victim of a shocking and permanent deformity.[35]

Contemporary medical descriptions of necrosis have something of the tone of a horror story about them – it was an industrial disease that could transform one rapidly from a Jekyll into a Hyde: when the 'inflammatory symptoms are at their height', according to one dental textbook (*Dental Pathology and Surgery*, 1874), 'the whole head, except the summit of the scalp, is involved – the eyes are closed, the nose, and even the forehead, swollen; the cheeks, lips, neck, and throat, are one continuous area of florid intumescence.' The skin emitted 'an ichorus pus, ragged or irregular on its surface, and of a dirty, blackish gray colour'. During the early stages of the diseases the patient was likely to have an intense fever 'with delirium and agonising local sufferings . . . interfering with or altogether suspending the action of the mouth, and, by the secretion of foul and fetid pus, producing nausea, ructus, vomiting.' Thus the victim was transformed into some ghastly reminder of plague victims of a by-gone age.[36]

This then was hardly a disease which worked insidiously and in a furtive manner! Nor was it an industrial disease which failed to attract medical attention. As early as 1847 Dr Samuel Wilks at Guy's Hospital had issued a report on phossy jaw and in 1861 John Bristowe at St Thomas's Hospital had studied the effects of phosphorus in fifty-seven match-factories in England and had concluded, rather too optimistically, that necrosis could be prevented by the introduction of sanitary and precautionary measures. Yet it is very revealing that Simon did not give as much attention to this industrial disease as to others and in fact does not make any special mention of it in his massive survey of public health, *English Sanitary Institutions*. Even as late as 1892 in his published Milroy lectures, *The Hygiene Diseases and Mortality of Occupations*, J. T. Arlidge, an expert on industrial diseases, argued, not for the banning of red phosphorus, but for greater sanitary precautions. He maintained that '. . . even match-making is not incompatible with a good share of health, and with life of average duration, provided always', he added, 'the workpeople are sound when they take up the occupation, and that they rigidly attend to cleanliness and work in well-ventilated rooms.'[37]

That medical authorities were not calling for an immediate ban at this late stage is quite incomprehensible, especially as there was good evidence that it was not only workers with bad teeth or in bad health who could fall victim to the dreadful effects of necrosis.[38] Although the 1878 Factory Act banned children from the dangerous dipping process and women and children from eating where any dangerous process was carried on, there was little concerted effort on the part of the government to wipe out necrosis in the match-factories. Perhaps it was thought that the Act, backed up by regular inspection, and the trend towards fewer, but larger, match-factories would accomplish the desired effect.[39]

If so, it was a mistaken belief, for between 1894 and 1898 there were thirty-six cases of necrosis reported among factory workers, and that must surely have been just the tip of the iceberg, for there were still many match-makers employed as outworkers in their homes, whose physical condition was not included in government statistics.[40] The conditions prevailing in the domestic manufacture of matches were revealed in a Salvation Army survey. In one case a mother and her two children, both under the age of nine, were working sixteen hours a day to turn out 1,000 matchboxes for a combined pay of just 1s 3¾d a day, out of which they had to provide their own paste. The chances of contracting necrosis were greatly increased by the practice of feeding the children bread as they worked. Colonel Barker of the Salvation Army gave further publicity to these conditions by taking newspaper reporters and members of parliament on tours of the homes of the domestic match-makers, and, in a dramatic and macabre demonstration, would turn off the lights to show how the workers' jaws gave off a greenish-white glow like a spectre's. The Salvation Army's solution was to open its own factory in 1891 in the East End for the production of their 'Lights in Darkest England' matches of red phosphorus.[41]

The domestic manufacture of matches continued throughout the Victorian period, and even when in 1892 the manufacture of lucifer matches by any other means than red phosphorus was certified as a 'dangerous process' and brought under stricter controls by the Home Office, little was accomplished within the factories. A government report at the end of the century lamented that it was still a matter of too little, too late:

> it cannot be said that due diligence has been generally exercised, either in observing the letter and spirit of the existing rules, or in introducing the improvements and precautions which have been brought forward, to some extent, in this country, but more extensively abroad, since the rules were framed.

The *Report* went on to criticize especially the slow substitution of machinery for hand labour, the inattention to workers' teeth, and especially the negligence in 'reporting known cases of phosphorus poisoning, or even watching for their occurrence', amounting, in some instances 'to deliberate and long-continued concealment.'[42]

One cannot conclude other than to indict the late Victorian governments for persistently placing their trust, against all the evidence, in sanitary improvements and factory regulation, rather than in the outright banning of white phosphorus and the prohibition, or strict regulation, of all domestic manufacture of matches.

Far more widespread than necrosis, and of much greater concern to the governments of the day, was lead poisoning, or lead colic, which caused constipation and eye problems and could lead to encephalopathy, that is convulsions, delirium and coma. Printers, painters, glaziers, and those working in the paper-colouring, linoleum, and floor-covering industries, and of course all those working directly with lead, were all in danger of contracting lead poisoning, or 'plumbism' as it was more commonly called.[43] It was particularly prevalent in the 'lead counties' or Durham and Cumberland, especially in those districts where the workers lived in ill-ventilated and over-crowded dormitories close by the factories. The seepage of lead from the factories was so bad that it was claimed that cattle grazing in adjoining or neighbouring fields died from the contaminated grass. Women were widely employed in the especially dangerous white-lead industries, and many miscarriages were attributed to lead poisoning.[44] In the 1864 Factory Act it was laid down that no meals could be taken by women and children in the 'dipping houses' or drying rooms of earthenware factories where white lead was used in the glazing process, but not until the Factory Act of 1878 were children and women under eighteen banned completely from work involving the use of white lead, and not until 1880 were special orders issued by the Home Office requiring special dining rooms in factories where white lead was employed.[45] Three years later the Prevention of Lead Poisoning Act, 1883, set standards of ventilation, lavatory accommodation, meal-rooms, baths for women, protective clothing and respirators, for all white-lead factories.

By the end of the century the more responsible manufacturers were providing protective clothing and bathing facilities. It seems, however, that there was considerable reluctance on the part of the work force to take advantage of the clothing. Perhaps understandably, the wearing of respirators during the long hours of labour did not go down well with many workers, and it was claimed that the 'capacious blouses and overalls ... petticoats and trousers', provided for the female workers, 'are tossed aside because they hide the charms of the wearers, or for some equally cogent reason.'[46] One suspects that all too often the precautionary measures and protective clothing and respirators were introduced without adequate education or preparation of workers to ease their acceptance.[47] Not until 1898 did lead poisoning become a notifiable disease, and some measure of the efficacy of earlier acts is indicated by the fact that within a year over 1,000 cases were reported.[48]

As serious as lead poisoning was, it was neither as widespread nor as debilitating as the respiratory and pulmonary diseases associated with other metal industries, especially file-cutting and cutlery-making. 'Grinder's asthma' was widespread in Sheffield, Birmingham, and other centres of the metal industry for much of the century. It was an industry that employed large numbers of men – at the end of the century there were about 4,000 workers employed in file and rasp manufacture in Sheffield alone, all engaged in various hand-processes. 'Grinder's asthma', a severe form of bronchitis, was caused by the fine particles of steel dust and cuttings that the worker breathed. In addition file-making was done with a chisel and hammer, and the hand holding the chisel rested constantly in the dust from the filings, and since the file cutters were continually moistening their thumbs to get a better grip on their tools, they ingested the cuttings in addition to breathing them in. The work not only led to paralysis of the wrist and thumb (partly due to lead poisoning, partly due to the fact that, according to the size of the file being cut, the workman had to wield a hammer of up to 9lbs all day long), but, more important, to chronic and indeed fatal bronchial troubles.[49] Dry-grinders were more affected than wet-grinders, but in many processes the two worked side by side, and the minute particles of steel and stone, dust and sand, thrown off by the grindstones, pervaded the atmosphere.[50] The early warning signs of constipation, indigestion, and bodily weakness, 'long antecedent to the development of more alarming maladies' were noted by Dr Sinclair White, the Lecturer in Public Health at the Sheffield Medical School, and in a random survey of a hundred metal workers, he discovered that seventy-four had lead line on their gums, twenty-eight had lead colic and twenty suffered from paralysis of the thumb or wrist. Alarming as these figures were, White concluded that they hardly told the whole story 'because file cutters, when they become seriously paralyzed in the wrist, are unable to follow their

271

employment, and either take to some other calling or too frequently become a burden to the community, until a life of decreptitude and disease terminates in premature death.'[51] The high death rate among file and cutlery workers can be readily grasped by the tables on pages 280–1 and 282. Dreadful as the *overall* death rate in the cutlery industry was at the end of the century, even more appalling was the death rate earlier in the century among those who worked exclusively at dry-grinding, such as the fork-grinders. In 1843 Dr Calvert Holland, a Sheffield physician, conducted a survey which he published as *Diseases of the Lungs from Mechanical Causes*. He discovered that of sixty-one fork-grinders who had recently died, no fewer than forty-seven died under the age of thirty-six, and thirty-five died before reaching their thirtieth year. Not one of them lived beyond fifty.[52]

The principal cause of death among these workers was grinder's phthisis, or, as it was commonly known, 'grinder's rot'. In the workshops it was common to see and hear the workers caught up in a helpless fit of coughing, which expelled 'black, hard masses, in appearance accretions of dust, varying from the size of a pea to that of a small marble.' Dr Holland's well-publicized report was followed by others, notably reports by another Sheffield physician, Dr Hall (in the *British Medical Journal* in 1857), and by Dr Greenhow for the Privy Council (1860–1). Although the various factory acts should have improved conditions of ventilation and cleanliness, file- and cutlery-workers were still working in lethal surroundings in 1899. A government investigation that year revealed that their general working surroundings had 'remained practically unaltered' over the past thirty years. The trouble lay in the nature of the industry and its organization, for it was common practice for the workers to provide their own tools and work in tiny 'shops' or huts, tiny, cabin-like 'hulls', as they were called, barely large enough to house the grinding stone. 'Most of these shops', the Report of 1899 commented, 'are of such a rude and primitive description that they appear not to have been built for the purpose, and to have been simply out-houses in the yards belonging to dwelling-houses'.[53] These workshops escaped the inspection that had been introduced by the factory acts and while the owners argued that it was the workers' responsibility to improve the ventilation and general working conditions of their hulls, the workers, for their part, apparently revelled in their sense of independence and were hostile, probably for monetary reasons, towards all outside efforts to enforce sanitary improvements. Thus right down to the end of the century there was no general provision for file-cutters to wash before eating, and even if there had been it would probably not have made a great deal of difference, for it was a common practice for the workers to leave their lunch on the dust-laden work benches. Thus deaths among metal workers remained high. In Sheffield alone between 1885 and 1896 there were ninety-one recorded deaths from lead-poisoning (the great majority of which were file-cutters), and in those years the death rate from diseases of the urinary system was over twice that in the country at large. In the nation as a whole at the end of the century cutlery- and scissor-makers had a death rate from respiratory diseases over four times that of agricultural workers, and three times greater than that of coal miners.[54]

III

Thus throughout the century industrial hazards caused countless discomfort, disfigurement, and loss of life. As dangerous to health as was the smoke-laden air of industrial towns, the atmosphere of factories in a wide variety of industries presented even greater health hazards right down until the final third of the century, when ventilation fans and extractors were widely introduced. For ten or more hours a day the workers were in a sense consumers also – consumers of fine particles of the materials on which they were working. Particularly affected in Simon's opinion were the grinders and polishers of steel, china-scourers, carding-room operators in cotton works, and flax-workers.[55] In 1861 Simon discovered that about three-quarters of the flax-workers he examined had severe bronchial disorders, and of these about one-quarter had some haemorrhaging of the lungs. Others had stomach or eye troubles caused by the fine dust.[56] Several years before Simon brought the condition of cotton-factory operatives to the attention of the nation, Elizabeth Gaskell had done so in her *North and South* (1854–5). Bessy, one of the characters in the novel described how in the carding-room the 'fluff got into my lungs', and, she added matter-of-factly, 'poisoned me':

> Fluff . . . little bits, as fly off fro' the cotton when they're carding it, and fill the air till it looks all fine white dust. They say it winds round the lungs, and tightens them up. Anyhow, there's many a one as works in a carding-room, that falls into a waste, coughing and spitting blood, because they're just poisoned by the fluff.

Although some carding-rooms had extractor fans, they were unpopular with the majority of mill owners, because they cost 'a deal of money', and 'brings in no profit', and with workers 'because they said as how it made 'em hungry', since they had become accustomed to swallowing the fluff. According to Bessy it was for that reason that the operatives wanted higher wages in mills which had installed fans![57]

Even worse in terms of air quality was the pottery industry. In 1898 Dr J. T. Arlidge wrote:

> This manufacture stands foremost among those wherein the employment is distinctly chargeable with the production of disease; and the principal materials to which its unenviable character is due are the clays and the flint used in it. However these mineral substances are not the only agents that render the fictile [pottery] trade one so highly injurious to health; for lead also is largely used for glazing and colour-making, and is a frequent cause of plumbism among the artisans.[58]

Pottery workers inhaled dust from siliceous and common clay, flint, plaster of Paris, calcined bones, and felspar. In addition 'they also get an abundant share of coal-dust and coal-smoke – the firing of pottery calling for a profuse use of coal – far too much of which is thrown off from the ovens in the shape of dense black smoke, intermingled with the gases of combustion.'[59] The amount of exposure to the dust varied enormously from process to process: perhaps the most vulnerable workers were the china-scourers, 'always women, belonging usually to the rougher, more ignorant, and reckless of their sex', whose task it was to brush and beat off the dust from the finished chinaware and whose lot it was to spend their long working hours in 'clouds of dust'.[60] Although long hours of labour around very high-temperature ovens and drying stoves resulted in the rheumatism, lumbago and sciatica which were characteristics of the pottery workers' constitution, it was 'potter's asthma', or 'potter's rot', resulting from the fine dust from calcined bones, flint, and clay, which presented the greatest health hazard to the thousands of workers employed in the china industry. As early as 1860 doctors in the pottery towns were beginning to talk in terms of race degeneration and the Physician to the North Staffordshre Infirmary, in Stoke-on-Trent, wrote that

> The potters, as a class, both men and women, represent a degenerated population both physically and morally. They are as a rule stunted in growth, ill-shaped and ill-formed in the chest. They are certainly short-lived; they are phlegmatic and bloodless ... of all diseases they are especially prone to chest diseases, to pneumonia, phthisis, bronchitis, and asthma. One form would appear peculiar to them, that which is known as potter's asthma or potter's consumption.[61]

One problem in the pottery industry was that, for most of the century, it was conducted completely with hand labour, and protective equipment and adequate ventilation were introduced only very late in the century. Even then workmen viewed these improvements 'with astonishing indifference: they accept their fate of chronic disease and shortened days . . . Plans introduced from time to time to amend their conditions of labour have oft been frustrated by negligence or willfulness.'[62]

The tables on pages 280–1 and 282 below clearly indicate the disastrous effects of working conditions in the Potteries. Apart from inn-keepers, pottery and earthenware workers had the highest mortality rates of any occupational group at the end of the century and a death rate from respiratory ailments some four-and-a-half times greater than that of agricultural workers. Their life expectancy was, at 46 years and six months, some seven-and-a-half years less than that of non-pottery workers living in the Stoke-on-Trent area; while 27 per cent of all deaths in the Stoke area resulted from respiratory ailments, for potters the figure was 60 per cent.[63]

If potters had their inevitable asthma, brass-founders had their own peculiar ague, a chronic bronchitis or fibroid phthisis, a disease which often terminated in death, or resulted in maladies over many years – loss of appetite, dyspepsia, gastro-intestinal catarrh, nausea, vomiting, metallic taste in the mouth, thirst, colic, constipation, headache and muscular pains.[64] Interestingly, brass-workers seemed to build up a tolerance during the week that was then lost over the weekend, and the symptoms of the ague, irregular fever, attacks of shivering, profuse sweating, nausea, thirst, headaches, and exhaustion, would reappear on Monday. Hence brass-founder's ague was popularly known as 'Monday fever'.[65] According to one study, French brass-workers often suffered from 'a particular form of delirium, with hallucinations of hearing and of touch, accompanied by excitement of the sexual organs', but this was unheard-of in England, and was dismissed by one authority as the product, not of industrial processes but of absinthe.[66]

Brass-founder's ague was something of an esoteric disease: not so mercury poisoning – 'mad as a hatter' was a common phrase, but others besides felt-hat makers worked with mercury and so ran the risk of brain disease – among them the silverers of mirrors, barometer and other instrument-makers, and furriers. By the time the 1878 Factory and Workshop Act prohibited young people from working on the silvering of mirrors where mercury was used, it was already a dying trade, and soon the electro-plating process replaced mercury in mirror-making. But mercury was still widely used among Jewish and Italian mirror-makers working in their homes.[67] Not until 1899 did mercury poisoning become a notifiable industrial disease. Excessive saliva, loosened teeth, nausea, vomiting, gastric pains and cramps, tremors, and general loss of strength were among the symptoms observed among those who handled mercury.[68]

The effects of various forms of employment upon health can be quickly grasped from the tables on pages 280–1 and 282, and perhaps the squeamish reader at this stage might want to turn directly to them. The description of industrial suffering we have so far given is far from complete however. Bleach-makers, for example, constantly exposed to chlorine gas, and working, as late as the 1850s, up to sixteen or eighteen hours a day in temperatures that reached 130°F, contracted consumption, conjunctivitis, bronchitis and asthma, and chrome-workers handled bichromatic of potash, which could lead to the perforation or even complete destruction of the navel septum and ulcers.[69] Those workers engaged in making the rubberized waterproof clothing, so popular in that era, breathed in naphtha vapours at work, and these caused giddiness, nausea, and loss of appetite. In a study conducted by the Royal Infirmary and the Victoria Hospital for Consumption in Edinburgh over an eight-year period, some 85 per cent of the rubber workers admitted as patients were suffering from respiratory ailments.[70] Nausea while working was also the common experience of house-painters and workers in paint factories. The paints used were generally lead-based, and to add to the dangers were inflammable, and their vapours not only led to a feeling of nausea, but to vomiting, loss of appetite, colic, and, in extreme cases, to bleeding in the ears and nose and 'temporary dementia'.[71] Among the many miseries endured by that sad and motley crew, the exploited house-painters in R. Tressell's *The Ragged Trousered Philanthropists*, was paint-poisoning. The feeling of nausea that was part and parcel of using quick-drying paints in closed rooms never left them. Either the painters had long lay-offs or were forced to work around the clock on a rushed job: they had their lunch 'on the floor beside them and ate and drank and worked at the same time – a paint-brushful of white-lead in one hand, and a piece of bread and margarine in the other.'[72]

Among the worst affected by industrial diseases was the vast army of textile workers – over 1,000,000 strong in 1891. Simon and his team at the Privy Council had drawn attention in the 1860s to the occupational hazards encountered in the overheated and ill-ventilated mills, but there were only minor improvements over the remainder of the century, and at the end of the century, J. T. Arlidge was still drawing attention to the same evils of fibre-laden air and a steamy, overheated atmosphere. Add to these, he wrote, the 'constrained positions of the body, and want of physical out-door exercise, and we cannot fail to recognize a series of hygiene conditions and surroundings which must sap the health, lower vitality, engender constitutional weakness, and deteriorate the race, besides being accountable for setting up active present disease, and thereby increasing in every direction the rate of mortality, and lessening the value of life.'[73] Arlidge presented quite a catalogue of the 'incidental causes of ill-health among cotton operatives:

> they are, dust from the cotton itself in the early processes of manufacture; heat with more or less watery vapour, combined in the weaving department with dust from the Cornish clay employed for sizing; long standing and a drooping posture in the spinning and doubling department; monotony of work; continuous strain upon the attention, and excessive noise with vibration of machinery. To these must be added vitiated air from excessive consumption of gas, from overcrowding, and general defects of ventilation. And it is no wonder that accidents abound, considering the extent of machinery, the velocity of movement, the proximity of machines to watch over, the loosely hanging gearing and the liability to the loosing and flying off of some parts of the machines.[74]

Quite specifically, though, it was the irritation by the cotton dust of the pharynx and larynx, manifested first in the morning cough, and developing into phthisis, bronchitis, and sometimes leading to pneumonia, that was the curse of the cotton worker. It is therefore hardly surprising that cotton workers had a death rate from respiratory diseases some two-and-a-half times higher than that for agricultural workers: the table on page 282 shows, however, that it was still far lower than that of workers in the Potteries.

Perhaps the most publicized of all working conditions were those in the coal mining industry. Not only did the drama of tragic mining accidents draw attention to the industry as a whole, but there was, quite understandably, something horrifying to the public imagination about an industry which required long hours of labour in narrow, low tunnels in total darkness. Legislation in the early- and mid-Victorian period was also concerned with the low moral standards and the nudity in the mines, and the underground employment of women and children was restricted. Less publicized, however, were the severe industrial diseases associated with coal mining. At the best, working a narrow seam could lead to serious skin lesions to the knees and elbows; at worst, mining meant death by emphysema or silicosis. In between were a variety of debilitating ailments. Coal-mining was not a concentrated industry but was scattered throughout England, Wales, and Scotland, and conditions varied enormously from area to area and pit to pit. Thus while deaths from respiratory diseases (excluding t.b.) among the Lancashire miners were 75 per cent higher than the national average, in the nation as a whole the death rate of miners from all diseases did not exceed the national average. Although the death rate (among males between 45 and 55 years of age) among miners in South Wales was 24.47 per thousand living, compared with the national average of 21.37, in the coal-fields of Durham and Northumberland it was only 16.35.[75] The mortality in this age-group for all miners in Britain was (as the table shows) below the national average and compared extremely favourably with that of tin-makers. The unhealthy work conditions were somewhat masked by the fact that miners were, by a self-selecting process, generally a strong and healthy group. Since death rates varied so enormously from area to area it was argued that domestic and other conditions, rather than working conditions, were the most important factors determining the miners' health. Arlidge, at the end of the century, was less than sympathetic to the newly-aroused interest in working conditions in the mines. The miners, he wrote,

> awaken public sympathy largely because of their work under ground; for aversion to darkness is engrained in human nature. Still, there are no decisive facts to prove that work in the dark, *per se*, is of distinct injury to human beings. The horses in pits, who remain for months, and even years, under ground, are fat and flourishing; and miners are seldom under ground above eight hours at a stretch, and not that every day in the week . . . Certainly, his physical surroundings are superior to those of mill hands and of most people occupied in trades.[76]

Nevertheless coal-miners (and there were still 1,127,000 of them in 1913) at the end of the century were forced to work 'in an atmosphere vitiated by coal dust, by foul air, and by excessively high temperatures'.[77] Thus 'black spit' continued to take its toll and even Arlidge admitted that conditions down the pit led to the 'peculiar loss of control over the muscular apparatus of the eye' – the characteristic miner's disease of nystagmus.[78] This disease was slow but certain in its course. One unfortunate miner who contracted the disease gave the following account:

Up to the last two years before I failed I had no trouble with my eyes and always earned good money. During the last two years my eyes got weak, but I struggled on, hoping things would mend. I lost days and days, and on times a week. At the end it was not safe for me to go to the face without the help of another man. I could not recognise anybody, and had to walk in with my lamp held behind my back. I could always tell by the sound if it was safe. My wages fell a pound a week, and the manager stopped me at last and told me that it was not safe to allow me to work any longer.

In 1912 it was said that 10,000 or so men and boys could not work due to nystagmus.[79] Nystagmus did not attract much attention, no public protest or appeal was mounted to end it; it failed to arouse the concern of the Privy Council or Local Government Board's medical departments; it remained untouched by legislation. And yet it affected the health and lives of thousands of miners. Typical of so many occupational diseases it resulted, not in death, so much as in debility, loss of status, and financial insecurity. And like so many other industrial and occupational diseases it simply cannot be ignored in any discussion of the quality of life in Victorian Britain and the health of the nation.

IV

It is dangerous to assume that death rates issued by the Registrar-General and other official sources for various occupations accurately reflect working conditions or the incidence of industrial disease, for a wide variety of influences were at work, among them domestic hygiene and housing conditions, public sewerage and water, diet, and general living standards. Further complicating the issue was the elimination of the weak from certain arduous trades. As Dr Ogle, at the Office of the Registrar-General, wrote, many industries 'are in fact carried on by a body of comparatively picked men; stronger in the beginning and maintained at a high level by the continual drafting out of those whose strength falls below the mark.'[80] Greenhow, Arlidge, and others interested in public health and occupational diseases were careful to point out how difficult it was to draw up any simple causal connection between certain hazards on one hand and the death rate among operatives on the other. It was argued, for example, that the high death rates prevailing among cutlery- and file-workers and the low rates among miners might in part be explained by the notoriously high incidence of drunkenness among the former and the general sobriety of the latter. The following tables, covering the years 1890–92, and compiled by Dr Ogle from some 500,000 returns, should be read then with due caution. The figures relate only to deaths of male workers between the ages of forty-five and fifty-five, the period in which, we may assume, the ravages of slow disease began to take their toll.

Death rates for males, between 45 and 55 years of age, per thousand living

Occupation	Death-rate
Inn-keepers	44.48
Pottery, Earthenware	42.97
Dock, Wharf labourers	40.71
File makers	40.06
Lead workers	37.62
Costermongers	37.08
Cutlery, Scissors	35.60
Tin miners	33.20
Glass	32.14
General labourers (London)	31.94
Chimney Sweeps	31.43
Carmen and Carriers	28.01
Brass	26.05
Musicians	26.01
Cotton (Lancashire)	25.11
Coal miners (S. Wales)	24.27
Butchers	22.65
Bricklayers	22.04
Tailors	21.98
National Average	21.37
Medical Men (Surgeons, G.Ps)	21.04
Blacksmiths	20.74
Wool (West Riding)	20.58
Fishmongers	20.13
Tin-plate	20.08
Coal miners (national average)	19.42
Paper	18.84
Fishermen	18.61
Barristers	17.72

Occupation	Death-rate
Railway porters	16.98
Coal miners	16.35
(Northumberland & Durham)	
Railway engine drivers	16.09
Domestic servants	15.85
Grocers	14.34
School-teachers	14.31
Farm labourers	13.56
Hosiery	12.15
Clergyman	10.52
Farmers	10.16
Artisans, Mechanics	8.83

[81]

Some brief word of explanation is needed for some of these figures. Inn-keepers at the head of the list as the most unhealthy occupational group might cause some bewilderment until it is realized that the Registrar-General included alcoholism and disease of the liver in his figures. Apparently many inn-keepers were their own best customers, for they had a death rate from alcoholism some seven times greater than the national average and some six times higher for both gout and liver diseases! Ten times as many London publicans died from alcoholism as the national average for all employed males. Pottery and earthenware workers suffered greatly from respiratory diseases affecting the heart and lungs, as did metal workers, and file-makers had a death rate almost double the national average for gout, phthisis, respiratory diseases, nervous diseases, and urinary infections. Lead-workers had a death rate almost three times higher than the national average for nervous diseases, two-and-a-half times higher for deaths from digestive diseases, and some four times higher for deaths from urinary diseases.[82] The high mortality of dock and wharf labourers should also be noted, indicating, perhaps, their general standards of living and the hazards of working in an undernourished state outdoors in London's climate: among the causes for their high mortality were consumption, pneumonia, and other respiratory diseases. Interestingly, as a group, general labourers, who, unlike factory workers, received no protection from general industrial sanitary and health codes, had a higher mortality rate at each age group than the factory operatives.[83]

That many industrial occupations were still hazardous at the end of the century is perhaps better illustrated by the following table, taken from the same comprehensive study conducted by the Office of the Registrar-General. The statistics are for male workers only: for comparative purposes a base figure of 100 is used for agricultural workers. Once again there is a danger of too simplistic a connection between the trade and the incidence of death; yet deaths from diseases of the respiratory system do suggest the degree of atmospheric purity of the workshop or factory:

Occupation	Deaths from Diseases of the Respiratory System
Agricultural workers	100
Coal Miners	133
Wool Manufacturers	202
Cotton Manufacturers	244
Lead Workers	247
Chimney Sweeps	249
Brass Workers	250
Zinc Workers	266
Copper Miners	307
Copper Workers	317
Lead Miners	319
File Makers	373
Tin Miners	400
Cutlery, Scissor Makers	407
Potters, Earthenware Workers	453

[84]

Appalling as is this wide range of mortality according to occupation, it tells only part of the story and does not convey the extent of the suffering brought on by slow, but not fatal illnesses, or the illnesses which other members of the family suffered as a result of privation when the principal bread-winners were forced from their jobs by occupational disease. Local authorities pointed out that the victims of industrial diseases and their families often dropped into the ranks of paupers. The observation (which we noted earlier in this chapter) of Dr White at the end of the century on the file-cutters of Sheffield applies with equal force to countless trades throughout the country. In industry after industry workers who had contracted some form of occupational disease did, indeed, 'too frequently become a burden on the community' or on their own families. Thus 'the canker of industrial diseases' must be numbered among the causes of pauperism and family destitution.[85]

In 1904, some three years after the various factory and workshop acts were consolidated, the Inter-Departmental Committee on Physical Deterioration maintained that the new act had been neglected in the Potteries, where it was most needed, and that there was still inadequate control over children in poor health entering workshops. Workshops were still largely beyond the arm of the factory laws, and in 1901 there were far more workshops than factories – 143,065 compared to 97,845.[86] In Leicester, when the small, old hosiery workshops gave way to factories in the 1870s there was a much more satisfactory control of working conditions, with a corresponding improvement in the health of the workers.[87] When, at the end of the century, a House of Lords Select Committee followed up the investigations of a decade of social reformers and went into the sweatshops and small workshops of East London, they were appalled at the lack of ventilation and the disregard for the health of the girls, and shocked at the ease with which the sanitary laws were circumvented. Inspectors could be spotted a mile off, workgirls were sent home (to avoid prosecution for overcrowding) and windows, normally shut tight, were hastily opened at the first sight of an inspector. Health regulations in the little sweatshops that were characteristic of the cheap clothing industry remained a farce throughout the late Victorian period. It was necessary for inspectors to prove that the labour performed in the home or workshop constituted 'the whole or principal means of living of the family' for the domestic setting to come under the provisions of the laws governing workshops. This requirement, combined with the reluctance of the authorities to invade what appeared on the surface to be a home, put sweatshops and much domestic industry beyond reach of the law. The 1891 Factory Act, following the Report of the House of Lords Select Committee on the Sweating System, permitted inspection of workshops without a writ or warrant and marked the beginnings of somewhat closer control of workshops.[88]

The Inter-Departmental Committee on Physical Deterioration discovered, much to its dismay, that the laws protecting young children were also often ignored. Although the new Factory Act of 1901 required the physical examination of all young persons applying for factory work, there was no such provision for youngsters in workshops, and although it did apply to mines, it was often ignored. 'It does not matter to the managers', one witness told the Committee, 'whether they [young miners] are scrofulous, rickety, phthisical, or anything else – they get them into the pit.'[89] In 1904 there were some 2,000 certifying surgeons to examine young workers entering the factories, but their main contribution lay in the future, and at the end of Victoria's reign there were still far too many young men and women who entered a life of factory work but whose physical condition was not up to the labour expected of them, or sufficiently sound to withstand the heat, humidity, overcrowding or contaminated air still encountered in many factories.[90] One must unfortunately conclude that, despite the many improvements in the final third of the century, the general observation of two early historians of the factory reform movement is pertinent for the control of industrial diseases and the provision of healthier working surroundings:

> We cannot adopt the enthusiastic tone of some who have written of the English Factory Acts as if the conditions of labour had thereby been completely transformed and humanised. On the contrary, closer study reveals the fact that an extraordinary timidity has beset all our efforts in the matter.[91]

Had Britain's industrial workers been able to leave the factories and workshops at the end of the day and return to healthy homes, perhaps their working conditions would not have exacted too heavy a toll upon their health. What these workers needed after a day's labour was rest and a modicum of domestic comfort. To sustain good health and to recuperate they required fresh air, good ventilation, sound sanitation, running water, and a basically sound diet. As we have seen, these last three requirements were all too often the exception rather than the rule, and certainly not widely available until the final quarter of the century. To what extent the working-class home was a setting for good health and a base for sound physical growth and regeneration the next chapter attempts to show.

11
'Home Sweet Home'

'Overcrowding was perhaps the most important of all causes contributing to the origin and spread of preventable disease.'
Sir Thomas Crawford, President of the Sanitary Institute, *Public Health*, III, 32 (December 1890), p. 143.

From its earliest stages the public health movement had focused on the connection between bad housing and bad health: and with obvious justification, for by bad housing was meant non-existent or faulty plumbing, irregular, insanitary, or inconvenient supplies of water, and rudimentary excrement removal, and, as we have seen, these were all regarded as causes of fever. But bad housing also came to mean poorly-constructed jerry-built houses, insanitary not only because they lacked certain amenities, but also because they were, by their very construction, unsound. Bad housing became synonymous with slums – dilapidated, overcrowded tenements, clustered together in the congested 'rookeries' and 'fever-nests' of the inner city. As the century progressed it became increasingly apparent that the growing structure of public health rested on *domestic* foundations and that the nation could not be healthy unless it housed its masses in healthy homes.

This chapter is not concerned with the underlying economic causes of overcrowding, regional housing variations, or the housing reform movement as an integral part of broader social policy, and for these as well as for housing standards measured in architectural terms and standards of comfort, the reader should consult the small body of literature which has, belatedly, appeared on these subjects.[1] In terms of public health the 'housing question' essentially boils down to two broad, and not always related problems – dwellings 'unfit for human habitation' and overcrowding.

Whatever the sanitary facilities, the very fact that the slum dwelling was foul-smelling, overcrowded, and unventilated was sufficient to condemn it in the eyes of men who associated stink and foetid, close, and stifling atmosphere with disease-ridden miasma. Fresh air and good through-ventilation were something of a national obsession. Since fresh air currents were held to be nature's way of dispersing dangerous effluvias, the ill-ventilated dwellings of the poor were cause for considerable alarm. The undernourished inhabitants of an un-heated flat had an understandable aversion to draughts, but the closed tenement window was as offensive to the middle-class reformer as was the closed carriage window to the typical railway traveller. One speaker before the Social Science Association in 1862 went so far as to observe that

> Inadequate dwelling-house ventilation was . . . the monster evil of civilization. In addition to the vast mass of disease of which it was the direct parent, it was indirectly responsible for much of that engendered by uncleanliness in person, habitation, and surroundings; for want of ventilation, by habituating the sense of smell to impure air, gradually blinded its delicacy, till, the safeguard of a healthful instinct which loathes fetidity being lost, man sank down into an abyss of filth to which no parallel could be found in the brute creation.[2]

To Charles Dickens, Coketown (an amalgam of Preston, Oldham, and Manchester) forced its inhabitants to dwell in 'an ugly citadel, where nature was as strongly bricked out as killing air and gases were bricked in', and to Dr Southwood Smith this lack of ventilation and pure air rendered the slum dwelling as potentially lethal as any disease-ridden tropical marsh:

> The room of a fever patient, in a small and heated apartment of London, with no perflation of fresh air, is perfectly analagous to a stagnant pool in Ethiopia full of the bodies of dead locusts. The poison generated in both cases is the same; the difference is merely in the degree of its potency. Nature with her burning sun, her stilted and pent-up wind, her stagnant and teeming marsh, manufactures plague on a large and fearful scale. Poverty in her hut, covered with her rags, surrounded by her filth, striving with all her might to keep out the pure air and to increase the heat, imitates Nature but too successfully; the process and the product are the same, the only difference is in the magnitude of the result. Penury and ignorance can thus, at any time and in any place, create a mortal plague.[3]

John Simon associated slum dwellings with a 'filthy atmosphere . . . spreading within it the taint of some contagious fever', and he defined and condemned overcrowding as a condition in which 'no obtainable quantity of ventilation will keep the air of a dwelling space free from hurtfully large accumulations of animal effluvium.'[4] To Dr Tidy, the MOH of Islington, 'congregation always rears degeneration', and to the President of the Association of MOH it was certain that 'over-crowding by itself will stunt the human race'.[5]

The concentration of dwellings within working-class districts and of people within dwellings was seen as a form of both physical and moral pollution. 'If human beings are crowded together', the Rev John Montgomery told the Social Science Association in 1860, 'moral corruption takes place, as certainly as fermentation or putrefaction in a heap of organic matter.'[6] His analogy, a linking of the 'residuum' with excrescence and decomposing matter, was a common one at the time, as was the analogy between human density on the one hand and swarming vermin and insects on the other. In Dickens's *Bleak House* they are practically interchangeable – the 'swarm of misery' in the slums 'bred a crowd of foul existence that crawls in and out of gaps in the walls and boards; and coils itself to sleep, in maggot numbers, where the rain drops in.' In a similar vein the *Nottingham Review* drew attention to a court which 'swarmed with population. Maggots in carrion flesh, or mites in cheese, could not be huddled more closely together . . .'[7]

As belief in fatal 'miasma' slowly gave way to an acceptance of the views that diseases either spread through infection by air or water-borne germs, or through contact, urban congestion continued to be seen as inimical to good health. Indeed, congested living as a prime cause of disease became an axiom which required no clear proof, so apparent was it to contemporaries. To Dr Duncan of Liverpool, the 'prevalence of fever in any street, court, or house, is generally proportioned to the density of population'; to Lord Shaftesbury who devoted his long life to housing reform, 'of all the agencies which disposed the human body to disease, none were so fatal as overcrowding in small dwellings.'[8] In 1842 a government commission of enquiry was told bluntly, as if the connection required no further medical explanation, that among the working classes in Ebbw Vale, 'fevers are very prevalent from the smallness of their houses and the number of persons residing in them'; some three decades later Edward Smith, whom we have encountered as one of John Simon's team at the Privy Council, declared that 'overcrowding has probably killed more than all other evil conditions whatever'.[9]

Although the clear connection between disease and overcrowding in insanitary dwellings could not be scientifically demonstrated until the epidemiologists could point to the transmission of germs by infection and contagion, Victorian health reformers were convinced that such a connection in fact existed. Well before the exact nature of the transference and spread of epidemic disease was understood it was clear that fever existed in its most virulent form in densely-packed dwellings.

Just as today there is a greater incidence of common colds and 'flu in winter, not because viruses are more powerful or prevalent in winter, but partly because people spend more time indoors, so, too, in the nineteenth century overcrowding increased the chances of contracting influenza, consumption, and the host of childhood diseases such as measles, scarlet fever, whooping cough, and any disease conveyed by droplets of saliva.[10] The risk of infection in overcrowded quarters was increased by the prevalence of one-roomed living and of the sharing of beds by the healthy, the sick, and the dying.[11]

That cramped quarters led to the sharing of beds was common knowledge to social investigators and (through countless reform tracts, novels, journalistic exposés, and government investigations) to the public at large.[12] In mid-century Darlington, to take just one case, six children, ranging in age from two to seventeen, shared a single room with their parents, an adult brother, and an uncle. What makes this particular example of urban crowding interesting, but yet not unrepresentative, is that all the children had contracted smallpox and that they slept, huddled together, on the floor.[13] Although the poverty, which in part produced the overcrowding, also explains the absence of beds which so appalled the health authorities (beds did, after all, offer some protection against rising damp and vermin and bugs), it was more generally the lack of space, rather than of money, which accounted for either the absence of, or, more often the sharing of beds.

Nineteenth-century health officials often drew up tables to illustrate the connection between population density and overcrowding on one hand and disease and death on the other. In his report for 1892 the MOH for London, for example, presented the following table:

Percentage of total Population overcrowded	Death rates, all causes
15	17.51
15–20	19.51
20–25	20.27
25–30	21.75
30–35	23.92
over 35	25.07

[14]

Similarly the death rates in Glasgow were linked to overcrowding and the following figures were given in 1901:

Type of Accommodation	Death rate per 1000
one room	32.7
two rooms	21.3
three rooms	13.7
four rooms	11.2

15

And in 1907 the Registrar-General's Office released figures which may stand as typical of numerous attempts to draw a direct correlation between high death rates and overcrowding:

Persons per square mile	Mean death rate
27 districts with an average density of 136	11.63
40 districts with an average density of 1303	18.53
18 districts with an average density of 4424	21.56
5 districts with an average density of 7480	26.54
4 districts with an average density of 55,563	34.82

16

Interesting and suggestive as these tables are, no such simple correlation can be drawn. For generally where overcrowding and high urban densities existed, there, too, casual labour, seasonal unemployment and year-round underemployment existed, and thus also poverty and its inevitable consequences, especially malnutrition, insanitary conditions, and poor medical services. It is, therefore, extremely difficult to apportion, among all these various conditions, responsibility for high death rates in congested areas and to isolate overcrowding from other equally pertinent factors. When Dr Niven, the MOH for Oldham, analyzed the dramatic decline in his town's general death rate (from 30 per thousand in 1872 to 20 per thousand in 1889) he mentioned the improvement in housing (especially the cessation of building back-to-backs in 1865 and the closing of all cellar dwellings in 1872), but he also included the replacements of cesspools by cans, the notification of infectious diseases in 1880, the provision of a fever hospital, and the improvement of the carding rooms in the cotton factories.[17]

That factors other than population density were involved in the high death rates prevailing in most working-class districts should by now be apparent from contemporary statistics. Although Liverpool with its density in 1881 of 106.3 persons per acre (the highest of any major city in the British Isles) also had the highest general death rates from all causes (26.7 per thousand) and from the principal zymotic diseases

(4.5 per thousand), it was not much more unhealthy than Cork (26.2 and 4.0, respectively), which had a population density of only 35.4 per acre. Dublin, with a population density of only 14.1 per acre had a higher general death rate than Liverpool, Glasgow, Manchester, Edinburgh, London, or Birmingham, which had population densities ranging from 84.9 (Glasgow) to 47.9 (Birmingham). Sheffield, with a population density of less than one-third that of Birmingham or Brighton, had a higher general death rate than either.[18]

But, for the reasons discussed, overcrowding attracted the attention of sanitary reformers. The causes of overcrowding are complex and belong more properly to the economic and social history of housing than to public health. What must be stressed here is that it would have been remarkable, given the rapid growth of the industrial towns, if there had been no overcrowding. Although a multitude of other forces were at work – among them land values, construction costs, the investment potential in working-class housing, rent levels, regularity of employment and wage-levels, effective demand and consumer preferences and expectations – it was above all the dynamic population growth of Britain's industrial cities which placed an immense burden on existing housing stock and on the ability of the building industries to provide low-cost dwellings when and where industrial workers wanted them. We have already noted in Chapter 1 how the major cities of Britain experienced population explosions of staggering proportions and intensity. To avoid overcrowding, Manchester which grew from 75,000 to 303,000 over the first half of the century would have had to build at least 2,500 rooms every year for fifty years to accommodate the increase – an enormous undertaking. In a single decade (1851–61) Barrow-in-Furness's population multiplied by 400 per cent and by another 278 per cent in the following decade; Middlesbrough, Cardiff, and other towns more than doubled their populations over a single decade.[19] It was basically this intensive localized population growth which produced or aggravated overcrowding.

In fact the efforts of the building industry to keep pace with demand were quite remarkable, and national figures show that person-to-house density fell from 5.5 to 5.1 between 1851 and 1911. But such figures are very misleading and mask the indisputable fact that in vast areas of most great industrial towns overcrowding had become the norm. Between 1801 and 1871, although the nation's housing stock grew from roughly 1,575,923 houses to 4,259, 117, the number of surplus families (excess of families over houses) had increased from 320,800 to almost 790,000.[20] Even the most efficiently organized large-scale building industry would have been hard pressed to keep up with population growth in the inner cities, and the British building industry, generally small-scale, subject to bankruptcies, and fluctuations in output, and primarily more concerned with satisfying the growing middle-class market, where risks were fewer and returns on investment higher, can hardly be termed efficient, at least from the viewpoint of the working classes.

The degree of domestic overcrowding which resulted is briefly examined later in this chapter. But even if overcrowding within houses had not existed, the intense concentration of the burgeoning population within towns – population density on the ground – would still have created in itself a severe health hazard, placing an enormous strain upon sewer and water facilities, saturating the sub-soil with its waste products, competing for air within the city, spreading the risk of infection and contagion. The rapid growth of the industrial towns produced staggering population densities. Liverpool had 138,224 people per square mile, Manchester approximately 100,000, Leeds roughly 87,000.[21] Most of us have a clearer idea of an acre (roughly 70 yards by 70 yards) than of a square mile – a substantial upper middle-class suburban house, with a fair-sized front and back garden might stand on a third of an acre. Yet in 1881 in Liverpool, taking the city as a whole, good areas with bad, some 106 people per acre was the average, in Manchester it was eighty, in Edinburgh fifty-five, and in London fifty-one.[22] Greenock's central parishes contained an average of 470 persons an acre, large sections of Liverpool had over 300 people an acre, as did parts of Leeds, sections of the City of London had 291 people to the acre and there were parts of central Glasgow where 1,000 people were packed to an acre of ground![23] Little wonder that when Dickens and others described the inner city they turned to the evocative analogy of the swarming world of insect life.

As the century progressed the pressure of population upon the central districts was partly relieved (at varying tempos according to the availability of land, the willingness to incorporate common and enclosed land, and the mobility of labour) by the development of working-class suburbs. Although health reformers and officials universally praised the suburbs for their healthier air and lower population densities, there was also some concern that the hasty, speculative building in the suburbs presented their own health problems. The suburbs were often beyond the jurisdiction of sanitary officials, surveyors and building inspectors, and the houses, cheaply constructed and speedily run up, were, partly as a consequence, jerry-built. Thus

George Godwin, the editor of *The Builder*, a district surveyor, and a keen housing reformer, condemned the way the working-class suburb was being constructed:

> See the mode in which thousands of houses in the suburbs of the Metropolis and elsewhere are commenced; without any excavation; the basement floor of thin, gaping boards placed within six inches of the damp ground; with slight walls of ill-burnt bricks and muddy mortar, sucking up the moisture and giving it out in the apartments; ill-made drains, untapped, pouring forth bad air; and you scarcely need more causes for a low state of health.

All too often the suburbs were 'embryo slums'.[24] But essentially it is the pressure of population within the built-up areas of the Victorian town which concerns us here, for it was that pressure which endangered the progress of public health. The response to the pressure – overbuilding, especially in closed courts, the development of back-to-back housing, the occupation of cellars, and overcrowding within houses ill-adapted to multi-occupancy – threatened to nullify or at least diminish, the great advances made in other areas of public health.

II

As the urban population increased so every available piece of land was pressed into use, courts, alleys, back yards, small parcels of empty lots, until dwellings pressed upon one another as closely as in any Italian hill-town or walled city. Dickens's favourite word for the teeming warrens of London which he knew so well was 'labyrinthine', and indeed, throughout London, in the West End, even in the mews off elegant Mayfair and Regent's Street, as in the East End and south of the Thames, working-class dwellings were packed so closely together that to the visitor they presented a bewildering, intricate and impenetrable maze. In many cities the topographical consequence of high density upon the ground was overbuilding within closed, or partially closed, courts or alleys and lanes. In fashionable mid-century Leamington Spa, as in other resorts, market, and cathedral towns, small houses, often of only two rooms some eight feet square were squeezed into tiny courts.[25] In Nottingham houses were run up in closed courts (that is without through-ventilation and virtually closed at both ends), which were approached through a tunnel often as narrow as thirty inches, and up to thirty feet long.[26] In Liverpool intensive building resulted in courts consisting of parallel rows of dwellings with as little as six feet of space between them. Until the building codes of the 1840s they rarely had as much as fifteen feet of air-space between them. Only five of the two hundred courts in Liverpool's Exchange Ward had openings at either end; in the town as a whole approximately one-third of the 1,982 courts were closed at both ends, and thousands of other inhabitants lived in what were virtually tightly-packed *cul de sacs* with small openings at the ends.[27]

In Glasgow only 542 of the more than 3,000 courts in the towns had entrances more than ten feet wide. In Greenock the tenements were so closely packed together that, accordingly to a local saying, 'the rain had no place to fall'.[28] But it was Liverpool which most startled contemporary reformers. When Dr George Buchanan visited the city in 1864 to investigate the typhus epidemic for the Privy Council he discovered that there were 18,610 houses crammed into over 3,000 small courts. According to the Borough Engineer of Liverpool:

> The houses are generally built back to back; one end of the court as a rule is closed either by houses or, which is worse, by the privies and ashpits; or a worse state of things still, the privies and ashpits are placed at the entrance of the court, and the only air supplied to the inhabitants must pass over their foul contents. But even this miserable state of things can be outdone. There are courts, which, by a perverted ingenuity, have been formed in the following manner: An ordinary street house has had its lobby converted into a common passage leading to the back yard. The passage is of course roofed over, and is, in fact, a tunnel from which the back room of the original house, now converted into a separate dwelling, has its entrance. The back yard has been filled with other houses in such manner as to have only the continuation of the tunnel for access, and from this little area of three feet wide the houses receive their supply of light and air. The passage is generally terminated by the privy and ashpit common to all the wretched dwellings.[29]

The courts of Liverpool were notorious but most large cities had their large areas of densely-concentrated houses – Edinburgh, for example, had its Wynds, Nottingham its 'Shambles', Manchester its 'Gibraltar' and London its Agar Town, Seven Dials, and Jacob's Island, districts so fantastic in their tumble-down congestion that they practically defied description. John Simon's literary powers were, however, equal to the task of evoking the labyrinthine courts and alleys of the City of London at mid-century:

> The inhabitants of open streets can hardly conceive the complicated turnings, the narrow inlets, the close parallels of houses, and high barriers to light and air, which are the common characteristics of our courts and alleys and which give an additional noxiousness even to their

cesspools and their filth . . . A man of ordinary dimensions almost hesitates, lest he should immovably wedge himself, with whomsoever he may meet, in the low and narrow crevice which is called the entrance to some such court or alley; and having passed that ordeal, he finds himself as in a well, with little light, with less ventilation, amid a dense population of human beings, with an atmosphere hardly respirable from its closeness and pollution. The stranger, during his visit, feels his breathing constrained, as though he were in a diving-bell; and experiences afterwards a sensible and immediate relief as he emerges again into the comparatively open street.

Simon added that there were 'many, very many, courts within the City, to which the above description accurately applies' and he forcefully argued that the houses within them were bound to be 'permanently unfit for habitation'.[30]

One form of overbuilding where land was expensive or scarce was to join houses together back-to-back, and in many northern towns this became the characteristic form of domestic architecture. The back-to-back had no through-ventilation, either from back-to-back, or, except the end houses of the terrace, from side-to-side. Probably this form of housing attracted criticism out of all proportion to its numbers, or indeed, to its seriousness as a health problem. But back-to-backs were a clearly identifiable violation of the concept of good ventilation and as such they became the object of reformers' attacks. The back-to-back or 'honeycomb' dwelling offered cheap, high-density, accommodation, and, unlike the multi-storey tenement, there was no working-class resistance to them and so they offered a fairly safe investment to builders.[31] In the mid-1880s over 70 per cent of Leeds' houses were back-to-backs (some 49,000); Sheffield had 38,000 in 1865 and Birmingham still had 42,000 in 1914.[32] Manchester, Bradford, Huddersfield, Shipley, Keighley, all had large concentrations of back-to-backs; their construction and acceptance in the North, especially in Yorkshire, appears to have little to do with special factors of site, costs, rents, or local conditions, and one historian has speculated that perhaps they were products of ' "cultural" factors of the sort that have produced local differentiation in the demand for fish-and-chips, Yorkshire pudding, Rugby League, and Lancashire hot-pot'.[33]

In no town were back-to-backs so prevalent as in Leeds: 'no other town continued to build them for so long nor fought so tenaciously to retain them.'[34] Between 1875 and 1887 two-thirds of the 16,070 new houses build in Leeds were back-to-backs, as were a quarter of the

2,000 houses built there between 1910 and 1914. Leeds continued to build back-to-backs until 1937, and in 1920 71 per cent of the town's housing stock consisted of back-to-backs – quite remarkably this was the same proportion as in 1801! Most of the houses were very small, some of them only one-up, one-down, and only five yards by five yards in total size – though cramped, they were at least well-suited to the size of available building lots in Leeds.[35]

To most health authorities, or at least to the reformers, back-to-backs were clearly insanitary due to the placement of their privies and to their lack of ventilation. At the end of the century the MOHs for Oldham and for Birkenhead considered the banning of back-to-backs a very significant contributing factor to the decline of the general death rates in their towns.[36] Dr Tattersall, the MOH for Oldham, told the Society of MOH in 1895 that both the infant and general death rates were far higher in the back-to-backs than in the town as a whole – 112.89 compared to 80.8 and 33.4 compared to 25.9, respectively.[37] A year earlier the Sanitary Institute of Great Britain had been told that deaths from tuberculosis ran some 50 per cent higher in back-to-backs than in houses with through-ventilation, and in 1910 a government inquiry concluded that even in the 'relatively good' examples, back-to-backs had a general death rate for their inhabitants some 15–20 per cent higher than in comparable dwellings with through-ventilation.[38] Although the same *caveat* made earlier about making any facile equation between poor housing standards and high death rates applies with equal force to back-to-backs, to most contemporaries they were so obviously undesirable that no careful analysis was required, and throughout the North local authorities tried to ban them. Manchester prohibited the construction of back-to-backs in 1844, Nottingham in 1845, in 1860 Bradford required open space to the rear and side of every new dwelling, Liverpool banned back-to-backs in 1861, Leeds in 1866, York in 1870 and Birmingham in 1876.[39] These by-laws were honoured more in the breach and back-to-backs not only continued to exist but continued also to be built down through the century. Finally in 1909 the Housing, Town Planning Act placed a general prohibition upon all future construction of back-to-backs – 'Notwithstanding anything in any local act or by-law in force in any borough or district, it shall not be lawful to erect any back-to-back houses intended to be used as dwellings for the working classes.' There was, however, a loophole in the Act, for it allowed future construction of back-to-backs in all cases where street plans had been approved before 1 May, 1909. Taking advantage of this escape clause, Leeds, as we have just seen, continued to permit extensive construction of back-to-backs.[40]

The reasons behind the local authorities' reluctance to enforce their own by-laws are clear – back-to-backs, whatever their disadvantages, did make efficient use of building plots, they were cheap to construct and hence to rent, and for all but the end-houses they at least guaranteed some measure of warmth. Thus, when in the 1840s a building act which would have placed a general prohibition on future back-to-backs was introduced into Parliament, it met with determined and organized opposition. The Leeds Town Clerk argued that alternative accommodation for the poor could cost up to 30 per cent more. Liverpool argued before the Health of Towns Committee (1840) that back-to-back construction not only 'renders the buildings warmer and drier and more fit for habitation', but also reduces building costs, 'thus bringing the rent within the limits of the Poor'. Similarly, the master builder, Thomas Cubitt, told the Royal Commission on the Sanitary State of Large Towns (1844) in no uncertain terms that the back-to-back was a form of low-cost construction and 'if we prevent it we prevent houses for the accommodation of poor people'. A year later Nottingham's Enclosure Act, which effectively banned back-to-backs, was opposed and then neglected on the grounds that its implementation would result only in higher rents for the working man. Thus back-to-backs continued as a characteristic feature of the growing northern industrial towns.[41]

To Victorian reformers no form of dwelling so clearly demonstrated the evil consequences of the pressure of population upon existing housing stock as the occupation of cellars. Today basement flats in fashionable mews and terrace houses are at a premium, but these are a far cry from the cellars which were occupied by the poorest classes in the nineteenth century. These cellars must be seen in the context of rudimentary street drainage and sewerage – they were thus often the unfortunate receptacles for the foetid matter which saturated much of the urban sub-strata and thus they became, so to speak, a form of residential sewer. Even where this wretched state of affairs did not exist they were still, for the most part, insanitary, dark, unventilated and overcrowded. In the eyes of respectable Victorians their occupants were inevitably regarded as a sub-species of cave-dwellers, scarcely human, a form of 'low-life', a tribe of 'troglodytes' and 'human moles'.[42]

It was not only the most impoverished immigrants or the Irish alone who were forced to make their homes in the cellars.[43] Thousands of families lived in cellars and were forced to dwell, eat, sleep, and breed in 'cellars [which] are the very picture of loathsomeness . . . disgusting receptacles of every species of vermin that can infest the human body'.[44] In Liverpool in the late eighteenth century roughly one-eighth of the population, it was estimated, lived in 'subterraneous and unhealthy habitations', and in 1841 these dwellings were attacked for their 'impure atmosphere' and 'defective ventilation'. They presented, it was said, 'in miniature a picture of the Black Hole of Calcutta'.[45] By that date the great influx of impoverished Irish was at full tide and Dr Duncan estimated that 'upwards of 8,000 inhabited cellars' now existed, containing about 38,000 people or some 22 per cent of the entire population of the town.[46] Many of these cellars were only 10′ by 12′, and in a survey conducted in 1841 it was discovered that many were 5′ or 6′ beneath the ground, that 3,000 of them were damp, and a further 140 thoroughly wet.[47] According to Duncan:

> there are of course few cellars entirely free from damp; many of those in low situations are literally inundated after a fall of rain. To remedy the evil the inhabitants frequently make little holes or wells at the foot of the cellar steps or in the floor itself; and notwithstanding these contrivances, it has been necessary in some cases to take the door off its hinges and lay it on the floor supported by bricks, in order to protect the inhabitants from the wet. Nor is this the full extent of the evil; the fluid matter of the court privies sometimes oozes through the adjoining cellars, rendering them uninhabitable by anyone whose olfactories retain the slightest sensibility. In one cellar in Lace-street I was told that the filthy water thus collected measured not less than two feet in depth; and in another cellar, a well, four feet deep, into which this stinking fluid was allowed to drain, was discovered below the bed where the family slept.[48]

Similar evidence was given before the Royal Commission on the Sanitary State of Large Towns and Populous Districts in 1845:

> Liverpool contains a multitude of inhabited cellars, close and damp, with no drain nor any convenience . . . Some time ago I visited a poor woman in distress, the wife of a labouring man; she had been confined only a few days, and herself and infant were lying on straw in a vault . . . with a clay floor impervious to water. There was no light or ventilation in [the cellar] and the air was dreadful. I had to walk on bricks across the floor to reach her bedside, as the floor itself was flooded with stagnant water. This is by no means an extraordinary case . . . [there are] hordes of poor creatures living in cellars which are almost as bad and offensive as charnel-houses.[49]

Though Liverpool was perhaps the worst city in Britain, it was by no means the only one with extensive cellar dwellings. In Manchester in the 1840s some 12 per cent of the population were cellar-dwellers, and there were few of the older industrial towns which did not have streets of cellar-dwellings; newer towns were better.[50] The cellars were the subject of reformers' invective and, more important, of local efforts at reform, in the first wave of sanitary reforms of the 1840s. Thus Liverpool cleared over 1,000 cellars of people between July 1844 and February 1845. By 1851 over 5000 cellars had been closed for human habitation, but at great human cost, for the 20,000 inhabitants who were ejected only increased overcrowding all around.[51] It is to the Corporation's credit that it took such energetic measures to eradicate the cellar dwellings for which it had gained some notoriety: given the town's housing stock and the general overcrowding which prevailed, the rise in domestic standards for the evicted was probably less certain than their rise to and above street level. But as the quotations on the previous page suggest, any surfacing would in itself be a healthy action. According to official statistics which were something of an underestimate, Manchester had over 18,000 cellar dwellers in 1843. Although the Building and Sanitary Regulations Committee began to alter and control cellar dwellings, beginning in 1845, and made sanitary improvements to dwellings occupied by more than 26,000 people, these efforts in the 1840s were largely nullified by the enormous influx of immigrants into the city.[52] A concerted and sustained attack on the problem had to wait until 1868, when the newly-formed Health Committee tackled the problem with such vigour that by 1872, 2,400 cellars were closed for occupation and by 1874 only 108 cellars remained, occupied mainly by old people. These remaining cellars were gradually shut down as the inhabitants died or moved and by 1882 there were 'only' 945 cellar dwellers left in Manchester.[53]

It is hardly necessary to dwell upon the insanitary nature of cellar dwellings – at the best damp, at the worst oozing with raw sewage and ill-ventilated, they were the perfect nexus for disease. For those suffering from pulmonary illnesses and for those who contracted typhus and other fevers they were often death-traps, to those suffering from arthritis or rheumatism the cellars were cells which aggravated and perpetuated their discomfort. Few precise analyses of the connection between cellar dwelling and mortality were taken in the nineteenth century – although George Buchanan argued from his survey of Liverpool undertaken in 1864 for the Privy Council that the general death rate in the cellars was some 35 per cent higher than among the working classes in general – and, given the pythogenic theory, no such analyses were necessary in the minds of reformers.[54] That the lower classes were often, in their habitations, literally lower, and that they were denied

298

the purifying and cleansing power of fresh air was in itself an affront to Victorian sensibilities. In the 1866 Sanitary Act all cellars were declared 'unfit for human habitation', and thus national legislation endorsed and reinforced legislation that had been passed on the local level. The continued existence of cellars for dwelling places down into the 1860s and after served to publicize the severity of the 'housing question' and forcefully demonstrated that the increasingly successful public health movement had to tackle the problem of insufficient housing – of overcrowding.

III

To Victorian sanitary reformers and to the governing classes as a whole overcrowding was for many reasons an intolerable evil. It bred drunkenness, crime, and sexual immorality; it destroyed the sanctity of the 'home', and of the family within it; it concentrated the masses in a politicially dangerous way; it disposed the mind to socialism or nihilism; it encouraged atheism; it helped to spread diseases. Overcrowding, in short, created the spectre of the moral and physical degeneration of the national stock.

But to the poor themselves overcrowding was a seemingly immutable condition, an inevitable portion of their lot. Although thousands of working-class families fled their overcrowded dwellings for the houses which the middle-classes deserted in their exodus to the suburbs, or moved into model dwellings or purpose-built houses, thus proving that a desire to improve their habitations was natural among the working, as among other classes, there were few organized attempts on the part of the working classes to improve housing conditions. There were some working-class building societies and housing associations, it is true, and various other self-help schemes, but these were never very extensive and there were few rent riots and, until very late in the century, almost no working-class participation in the housing reform movement.[55]

At the beginning of the era reformers and health officials commented on the dull acceptance of what, to more delicate minds, were unacceptable conditions. As the MOH for the West Derby Poor Law Union put it: 'Amidst the greatest destitution and want of domestic comfort, I have never heard, during the course of 12 years' practice, a complaint of inconvenient accommodation.' Late in the century, *Justice*, the organ of the Social Democratic Federation complained how difficult it was to interest the urban masses, the 'dumb-driven cattle', in housing reform, for, it asserted, 'the slum dweller in nine cases out of ten loves his slum'. Left-wing organizations bemoaned the fact that they could not get working men to support housing reformers at local elections; as the Workmen's National Housing Council admitted in 1901, 'whoever else takes the housing question seriously, the mass of those most seriously affected by it – the working people – have not done so.' Dr Southwood Smith, as we have noted, had an explanation:

> Now this want of complaint, under such circumstances, appears to me to constitute a very melancholy part of this condition; it shows that physical wretchedness has done its worst on the human sufferer, for it has destroyed his mind. The wretchedness being greater than humanity can bear, annihilates the mental faculties – the faculties distinctive of the human being.

Southwood Smith added, 'There is a kind of satisfaction in the thought, for it sets a limit to the capacity of suffering, which would otherwise be without bond.'[56]

Perhaps Southwood Smith was partially correct, but other reasons immediately suggest themselves: the poor were powerless, complaints about insanitary conditions often led to eviction, or, if and when the improvements were made, to higher rents; sanitary reforms and enactments against overcrowding – measures which reformers hoped the working man would support – only hurt him, leading in the first instance to higher rentals and in the latter to eviction. As we shall see when housing reform came to mean slum clearance it was seen by the poor as a destructive force, demolishing their homes without guarantee of rehousing. And while the casual labourer, crowded into a single room, might envy the more spacious flat of the artisan (and the concentrated nature of the city doubtless encouraged such comparison), he was no more capable of changing the rent structure or of influencing the supply of houses than is the average citizen today. He was, in short, the victim of the relative levels of rent and wages, and his 'passivity', if such it can be called, was merely a realistic knowledge of that fact.

Another reason might be offered. Many of the inhabitants of the great industrial towns were immigrants from the country where domestic conditions were often abysmal. Thus their level of expectation was very low. Their immediate past, as much as their exigencies and realities of the present, conditioned their expectations for the future. It is with this in mind that we should look briefly at rural housing conditions before turning to the urban housing problem which, until late in the century, was the primary focus of housing and health reformers.

To Cobbett, travelling throughout England in the 1820s, rural cottages were 'little better than pig-beds' and he was dismayed and disgusted at the 'hovels made of mud and straw'.[57] Mud cottages could be found throughout the British Isles down into the present century. In Wales, doctors visiting the homes of the rural poor described how they sank into the mud floors: to get some needed ventilation into the cabins they had to punch holes in the mud walls – it is not recorded how their patients reacted![58] Old cottages of thatch struck the Victorians as the perfect picture of rustic simplicity and bucolic delight, as they do us today, but the nineteenth-century reality was that most of them were hopelessly old, with oozing floors, porous walls and roofs that leaked. Cottages near Aylesbury in Buckinghamshire were representative examples of outworn, decrepit housing stock, typical in their state of dilapidation and disrepair:

> The vegetable substances, mixed with the mud to make it bind, rapidly decompose, leaving the walls porous. The earth of the floor is full of vegetable matter, and from there being nothing to cut off its contact with the surrounding mould, it is peculiarly liable to damp! The floor is frequently charged with animal matter thrown upon it by the inmates, and this rapidly decomposes by the alternate action of heat and moisture. Thatch placed in contact with such walls speedily decays, yielding a gas of the most deleterious quality.[59]

These mud or clay and straw cottages – stud and mud in the South, wattle and daub in the Home Counties, post and plaster in the North – at least generally had thick walls, but once they absorbed dampness they retained it. In Ayrshire, 'floors are frequently depressed a few inches below the street, and composed of clay full of inequalities so they are constantly dirty and generally wet; indeed, floors which neither admit of washing nor scrubbing cannot be otherwise.'[60] In Dorset, a local doctor claimed that he had 'often seen the springs bursting through the mud floors of some of the cottages, and little channels cut from the centre under the doorways to carry off the water.'[61]

The presence of dung and animals in the cottages, the 'deadly lassitude' of the inhabitants and their 'hopeless surrendering up to filth' struck the Privy Council inspectors as animalistic.[62] Dr Hunter could scarcely believe the condition of some of the dwellings he encountered in his investigation of rural conditions. In Bedfordshire, one cottage had 'plaster walls which leaned and bulged very like a

lady's dress in curtsey. One gable end was convex, the other concave
... A long stick served as prop to prevent the chimney from falling.
The doorway and window were rhomboidal.'[63] Although the Irish
were held to be the worst offenders in sharing their accommodation
with their livestock, they were, in fact, by no means unique, and
throughout the British Isles the habitations of the rural labourers were
often indistinguishable from barns and stables. As late as 1892 *Public
Health* contained a description of a typical crofter's cottage in Harris
in the Western Isles (famous, of course, for its cloth):

> The House is divided into three compartments, with only one door of
> entrance. The first compartment is used for housing the cattle, and the
> manure and liquid filth are allowed to accumulate for twelve months
> before the place is cleaned out. Immediately adjoining is the second
> compartment or kitchen usually divided by a rudely constructed
> wooden partition from the cattle – in some instance there is no partition
> at all; the third or innermost compartment is the bedroom, containing
> two, four or five beds.[64]

One could argue that however badly constructed and insanitary
rural cottages at their worst might be, at least with rural depopulation
and the great flow to the towns they were uncrowded. But this was not
the case. In the first half of the century not a single rural county had an
absolute population decrease, and many experienced increases up to
the national average.[65] Low rural wages and hence the inability to pay
rents which would make building an attractive investment, the greater
profitability of urban construction, the decline in the old practice of
boarding agricultural workers with the farmer's family, enclosures
and other rural 'improvements' which encouraged the demolition of
old housing stock, all combined to create a serious rural housing
shortage. In 1864 Dr Hunter surveyed 821 parishes and rural town-
ships in all forty counties for the Privy Council (in all, some 5,373
dwellings occupied by 24,770 people). He discovered that between
1851 and 1861, although there had been a net increase of 16,497
people, there had occurred a net *decrease* of some 3,118 cottages.
Only five per cent of the thousands of cottages Hunter investigated
had more than two bedrooms, and 40 per cent had only one.[66] In
Bedfordshire some 62 per cent of the cottages Hunter visited were
one-roomed affairs, and in both that county and in Lincolnshire
Hunter found innumerable cases of nine or more occupants in the
single room.[67] Commenting on this state of affairs, which he called a
'reproach to the civilisation of England', Simon wrote that the ordinary laws of supply and demand hardly pertained in the countryside:

'Even the base principle of *caveat emptor* is inapplicable, where prime necessaries of life are concerned, and no alternative purchase can be made.'[68]

Rather ironically, it was only considerably later in the century, after generations of migration from the countryside made the remaining labourers more valuable, that housing conditions improved.[69] Yet an official survey just before the First World War revealed that slightly over half the rural parishes of England suffered from a housing shortage and that an estimated 120,000 new cottages were necessary.[70] Despite improvements in rural sanitary administration later in the century and the availability of government loans to rural authorities for housing purposes, the general standard of rural housing remained pitifully low. When Queen Victoria died the general situation had improved little from that described in the report of a Labour Commission some seven years earlier:

> The accommodation provided in respect of the number, size and comfort of the rooms, the sanitary condition and the water supply are lamentably deficient generally, and require amendment ... rent has generally no relation to the size of the cottage, its condition as regards repair or sanitary arrangements, or to the earnings of the occupant. . .[71]

The compressed picture we have given of rural housing conditions cannot do justice to their enormous variety. Cottages of course could vary in standards of comfort, construction, and sanitary arrangements, even within a small village let alone within the British Isles as a whole. There were many improving landlords who took a keen interest in the dwellings of their tenants – the Earls of Winchester and Leicester and the Dukes of Rutland, Northumberland, and Newcastle, for example – and there can be little doubt that taking the country as a whole, there was a rising standard of accommodation.[72] Yet one must sadly agree with John Burnett that,

> The truth behind the Victorian's sentimental image of the countryman was that agricultural labourers existed at the lowest standard of life of any fully-employed section of the community, and that they were, in general, miserably rewarded for long and arduous work, that they were ill-fed, ill-clothed, and ill-housed and, until late in the century, uneducated, unenfranchised, unorganized and unrepresented.[73]

We have seen earlier in this study that country and town were linked closely together in several aspects affecting public health – the transportation of cattle on the hoof into towns for example, or the sale of town manure to the countryside. It is tempting to speculate that standards of urban housing were also affected by conditions prevailing in the countryside. Rural labourers migrating to the towns – and it should be remembered that all large Victorian towns were immigrant towns – brought with them their customary low sanitary standards and perhaps the psychology of low expectations. They were leaving districts in which, as late as mid-century, a rent of 1s 6d a week was standard, and thus they doubtless had difficulty adjusting to the considerably higher rents (in London the space available for 1s 6d in the countryside could cost 4s 6d or more) of the towns. Bombarded with a bewildering and seductively novel range of consumer attractions in the town, music halls, new foodstuffs, workmen's clubs, insurance schemes, to name just a few, the temptation must have been great to settle for the one- or two-roomed living they were accustomed to, and to put their higher (yet often irregular) wages to other uses. Sanitary reformers continually railed against this, but inertia, accustomed standards and a psychological resistance to higher rents encouraged overcrowding even when regular employment might have provided better dwellings. Similarly it is perhaps not far-fetched to suggest that whatever the attractions of their new urban environment and the network of community and companionship which the immigrants quickly established there, the uprooting from their old villages may have produced a disorientation which, exacerbated by the industrial conditions we have studied, encouraged the hard drinking which so exasperated and frustrated those reformers who tirelessly pointed out that the working man often sacrificed healthy accommodation for harmful alcohol. In turn it could be argued, as in fact Shaftesbury, Kingsley, Dickens and others did argue, that the hellishness of the urban slum not only stimulated hard drinking but practically made it a psychological necessity – the quickest road out of Manchester was, as the saying went, drunken oblivion.[74]

Some observers hoped that overcrowding might be just a temporary condition of the great urban population explosion and that it would disappear once the towns settled down to a more normal growth rate. Liverpool, for example, saw the arrival of 300,000 Irishmen in a six-month period, and with 1,342 families out of the 4,814 families surveyed in the Vauxhall ward having no form of support and the average family income there at only 9s 3d a week, overcrowding was an inevitable accompaniment of the growth. Dr Duncan discovered in 1846 that some of the more unfortunate were 'sleeping in privies and even in the open streets' and one family 'had taken up their residence in an old boiler'.[75] Similarly, Bradford was a town which, according to the Privy Council, was 'making a slow and steady progress in town reform' when it was

> burst in upon by many thousands of immigrants, who are stowed away in cellars and garrets, while authorities and employers are at issue whether more importance should be attached to the quantity or to the quality of proposed new buildings

The Privy Council noted that, with towns expanding so rapidly, very 'slight industrial and other local changes could rapidly and irresistably develop a high degree of overcrowding.'[76]

But in fact overcrowding was not a temporary condition, a transitory phase in the development of the nineteenth-century town. Late Victorian statistics show only too well the ineluctable nature of the problem. In 1891 11.2 per cent of the entire population of England and Wales, or some 3,500,000 people were, according to official statistics which tended to underestimate things, overcrowded.[77] And these national figures (just like national general death rates), mask the seriousness of things at the local level. Thus while the 1901 figure for overcrowding in the nation as a whole was 8.2 per cent, the figure for Gateshead was 31.2, for Berwick 33.8, for Newcastle 28.6, for Tynemouth 30.9 and for London 18.6.[78] And although the national figure had been reduced to 7.8 per cent in 1911, the continued high degree of overcrowding in the major cities was appalling, as the following table indicates:

Tenement dwellers overcrowded in 1911 %	Total number of people overcrowded
Glasgow	55.9	421,739
Dundee	48.2	77,391
Aberdeen	37.9	59,879
Edinburgh	32.7	99,842
Newcastle	31.6	81.140
London	17.8	758,786
Leeds	11.0	48.057
Swansea	10.6	11,658
Birmingham	10.1	51,447
Liverpool	10.1	71,184
Sheffield	8.4	37,375
Manchester	7.2	49,797

[79]

Even these statistics fail to convey the degree of overcrowding within working-class neighbourhoods, for they are for the entire town and for all classes and as the towns grew geographically so they absorbed far less densely-packed areas. The amount of overcrowding within the older districts was much higher. Thus, while in Edinburgh as a whole, 'only' 32.7 per cent of the population was overcrowded, the figure for the North Canongate district was 76 per cent! Similarly, behind the 1901 census figure for London of 18.6 per cent overcrowded, lies the darker reality of overcrowding within the older central districts – Whitechapel had 48.3 per cent of its population in overcrowded dwellings, Holborn 29.8 per cent, Shoreditch 27.3 per cent, Bethnal Green 26.9 per cent, and Stepney 25.6 per cent.[80] The domestic reality behind the widely-known but cold statistics was often conveyed by the journalists and in the more sensational anthropological forays into the slums which did much to make the 'housing question' a burning social question by the last quarter of the century. Typical of the contemporary reaction was *The Working Man*, which wrote in 1866 that, wherever overcrowding existed,

> there can be no delicacy, no refinement, no purity of feeling. . . . Decency of thought and act is impossible. The very instinct of decency is destroyed. Nor does the calamity of manners end here. Irritability is produced, not only by bad air, which affects the nerves, but by ceaseless contact of persons and tongues, which engenders ill-will, hatred, quarrels without end, offences which are never fogotten and never forgiven. Domestic estrangements grow up amongst those most nearly allied by blood and who should be attached by unchanging affection. People who seldom meet seldom quarrel.

In an unintentionally ironic analysis of the family, *The Working Man* argued that if the working-class family were less a unit bonded together in mutual love and respect than the upper- or middle-class family, it was mainly because members of the latter classes could choose when and where to see one another. But in the working-class dwelling, 'where dirt, din, and discomfort constantly reign, where escape is out of the question and privacy impossible', it was impossible to expect to find 'kind feelings, respectful manners, and the fine charm of deference, which lies at the bottom of all true politeness. . . .'[81] Simon and a host of medical officers throughout the country stressed the effects of overcrowding (and especially one-roomed living) upon health, but the public at large was much more concerned with its effect upon domestic, and hence civic, virtues. It was a concern which many health reformers were not above exploiting in the cause of sanitary progress.[82]

Concern for better housing was an integral part of the early public health movement and was synonymous with it. Robert Baker's house-to-house survey, undertaken for the Statistical Committee of the Leeds Corporation in 1837–9 and his subsequent sanitary map of the city, published in 1842, the reports of the 1838–9 Poor Law Commission, of the 1840 Health of Towns Committee, and of Chadwick and the Royal Commission on the Sanitary State of Large Towns and Populous Districts, together with the surveys of the Statistical Society of London and the Health of Towns Association, all made the connection between bad housing and 'fever'. Although the main emphasis of all this exploratory work was upon sewers and general sanitary matters, the investigations could hardly stop at the threshold of the dwellings, and the deleterious effects of overcrowding upon the health of the inhabitants were clearly perceived. Indeed, the Royal Commission of 1842 exhibited considerable curiosity about the domestic arrangements and degree of overcrowding to be found in the homes of the poor. But the primary concern – and, it must be said, the primary *need* – of the day was sewerage and drainage, not the construction of houses or the prevention of overcrowding within them.

Nevertheless the early public health movement not only drew attention to housing conditions but encouraged the first tentative steps towards reform. The Health of Towns Committee of 1840, for example, had called for a building code, and a ban on all back-to-backs, windowless cellars, and closed courts. As the Committee pointed out there was 'no building act to enforce the dwellings of these workmen being properly constructed; no drainage act to enforce their being properly drained; no general or local regulations to enforce the commonest provisions for cleanliness and comfort.'[83] Although no immediate legislation resulted from the Select Committee, it had drawn, in a clear manner, the need for building codes, and, following Chadwick's great *Report on the Sanitary Condition of the Labouring Population*, this need became even more apparent. Chadwick's *Report*, it is true, stressed more the need for sanitary engineering than for better housing, but one impact of his strenuous and, indeed, biased editing of the scores of investigations carried out by poor law and other doctors, was to associate bad health with bad housing.[84] Master of both publicity and pressure politics that he was, Chadwick, first by his use of the Poor Law Commission to investigate the causes of fever in London, and then with his detailed study of sanitary conditions throughout the land, propelled housing reform into the centre of the political arena.

But the official response was to call yet another commission of inquiry – the Royal Commission on the Sanitary State of Large Towns and Populous Districts (1844). Although historians have seen this Commission as largely Chadwickian, it did, in fact, represent an important departure, for it spent considerable time examining domestic conditions which created illness and it put greater stress, than had Chadwick, upon overcrowding. It deplored the extent of overcrowding and called for a central inspector of housing. It drew attention to the connection between overcrowding and unemployment caused by illness; it examined the possibility of large block dwellings, and it recommended that the local authorities should be able to demand that landlords of dwellings dangerous to public health clean or repair them at their own expense. The Report of the Commission contained the germ of much of the housing legislation which followed over the next two decades.

The Royal Commission's reports were supplemented by the continued exposés of the Statistical Society of London and the energetic work of publicity undertaken by the specially-formed pressure group, the Health of Towns Association (see Chapter 6). This early agitation for healthier towns quickly produced legislative results, although it could be argued that it was fear of cholera and not the mass of information which had been gathered, which prompted Parliament to act. At any rate, the first of several Nuisances Removal Acts was passed in 1846, followed by the creation of the Metropolitan Commission of Sewers and the Public Health Act of 1848. The 1846 Nuisances Removal and Diseases Prevention Act, as its title indicates, made the connection between 'nuisances' and disease explicit, and, included in the broad definition of a nuisance, was any dwelling in an unwholesome state. It empowered local boards of guardians to enforce sanitary improvements. The 1848 Public Health Act helped local authorities to inspect and regulate insanitary dwellings by creating Provisional Orders under which they could act quickly and inexpensively.

In view of all the publicity over the previous decade the legislative results up to 1850 were disappointing. The governments of the day were feeling their way slowly and were very conscious of the extent of the feeling against central government controls. That bad housing existed was now beyond doubt, but that the central government was the proper body to effect change was still questioned. Thus one housing reformer, writing in 1851, was typical of the age when he declared that the 'deep seated ulcer' of the slums affected 'the very vitals of the state and spreads its paralysing effect through every part of our social system,' and yet added, 'that as regards the well-being of the poor themselves nothing is so hurtful as too much interference, whether on the part of states or individuals.'[85]

Given the political philosophies of the age and the nature of the housing question it would have been quite remarkable if the central government had taken the initiative. Though the investigations had shown that housing conditions affected the nation's health they also demonstrated that those conditions varied enormously, both in severity and in nature, from locality to locality; and the legislation which was passed in this period was designed to encourage local authorities to address the problem. That these authorities were prepared to do so is indicated by the number of towns which, under the influence of the wide publicity created by the early public health movement, passed local acts or by-laws to regulate housing: Leeds and Liverpool in 1842, Birkenhead in 1843, London in 1844, Manchester in 1844 and 1845, Nottingham and St Helens in 1845, Newcastle and Burnley in 1846, the City of London in 1851 and so on. Some of these local acts were 'improvement' acts and their main purpose was to redevelop the urban centres, but most also contained some form of building code, regulating width of streets and courts, opening up courts, thus providing for some ventilation, establishing building standards for walls and windows, regulating cellars, and calling for the provision of privies.[86]

These Acts, both national and local, may be said to mark the first phase of the Victorian attempt to improve public health by improving houses. It was a phase characterized by building codes to improve future housing stock and 'nuisances' acts to improve existing houses. It was a good and necessary beginning, with the central state establishing broad guide-lines for local authorities to follow. It was also a legislative phase which indicated that the early Victorian governments were by no means bound to the doctrine of *laissez-faire* or reluctant to interfere in the rights of property. Even in this first phase of housing reform, the interests of public health took precedence over those of private property.

At the local level the various improvement acts and by-laws asserted the principle that property had its duties as well as its rights. At the national level the legislation passed at mid-century indicated that the government was prepared to extend the broad concepts of public health to housing. Three examples show this clearly. The Towns Improvement Clauses Act of 1847 (section 75) enabled authorities to demolish residences which were considered to be dangerous to neighbours. The Shaftesbury Act of 1851 (Labouring Classes Lodging Houses Act) enabled local authorities to purchase land for the purpose of erecting working-class dwellings and to borrow on the security of rates to do so. Though shrouded in ambiguity and unused (Shaftesbury sadly acknowledged in 1884 that it had remained a dead-letter; only Huddersfield used it to convert a large warehouse to model dwellings), it marked, quite remarkably, the acceptance of the principle of municipal socialism in housing. Although the only explanation for the rapid passage of an Act which broke so radically from cherished concepts of free-market competition in the supply of housing seems to lie both in Parliament's confusion that the Act applied to doss-houses rather than to permanent residences, and to a certain absent-mindedness on the part of Parliament, *The Times*, for one, did not miss the greater significance of its passage. The 'proper housing of the labouring population', it commented, 'seeing that it is not and cannot be left to the laws of free competition', was as legitimate an object of municipal enterprise as street improvements and the supply of water.[87] The third Act was the Nuisances Removal and Diseases Prevention Act of 1855. It enabled Poor Law guardians to enter and control overcrowding in private residences wherever they suspected epidemics, which, given the endemic nature of 'fever', should have resulted in continuous inspection. It also focused upon overcrowding as a 'nuisance' injurious to health and stipulated that, 'When a medical officer or two medical practitioners shall certify that a house is so overcrowded as to become dangerous to the health of the inhabitants, and the inhabitants shall consist of more than one family', the local authority shall 'cause proceedings to be taken before the justices to abate such overcrowding and the person permitting it shall be fined.' Though permissive, difficult to enforce (a later ruling in Queen's Bench decided that 'a nuisance is not a nuisance unless it can be proved to be injurious to health' – an almost impossible requirement before scientific epidemiology), and limited to multi-family dwellings, taken together with the Metropolis Local Management Act of the same year, which made the appointment of MOH compulsory throughout London, it marked a most significant step towards local inspection of domestic dwellings.

Just a few years earlier such inspection was unthinkable even to many dedicated housing and sanitary reformers, and most local administrators equated house-to-house visitations with an inquisitorial form of government that was better suited to Prussia than to the free society of England. Charles Kingsley, for example, as part of his 'muscular Christianity' which placed so great an emphasis upon bodily vigour and purity, had acknowledged how vital house-inspection was for public health: 'I am struck more and more with the amount of disease and death which no sanitary legislation whatsoever could touch', he wrote, 'unless you had a complete house-to-house inspection of a Government officer with powers to enter the house, to drain, and to ventilate it.' But such powers, Kingsley immediately cautioned, would be 'absurd and impossible, and would also be most harmful morally'.[88] Yet within a few years, far from being either 'absurd' or 'impossible', such inspection was routinely being carried out in Liverpool, Leicester, London, and elsewhere, and although it was not until after the Public Health Act of 1872, which required the appointment of MOH by local authorities, that house-to-house visitations became a regular feature of local public health administration, a bold new social policy had begun.

But it *was* only a beginning, and when in the mid-1860s Simon turned his attention to the problem of overcrowding the Privy Council quickly discovered that it existed on a disturbingly large scale throughout the nation. The Privy Council investigations, supported and supplemented by the efforts of the Social Science Association, marked the second stage of the application of state and municipal preventive medicine to the field of housing.

It is both interesting and significant that while the investigation of rural housing which Hunter carried out in 1864 for the Privy Council was simply entitled 'Inquiry on the State of Dwellings of Rural Labourers', his report on urban housing the following year was entitled 'Report . . . on the Housing of the Poorer Parts of the Population in Towns, particularly as regards the Existence of Dangerous Degrees of Overcrowding and the Use of Dwellings Unfit for Human Habitation'. While concern over general sanitary conditions and methods of construction still existed there was a tacit acknowledgement that if public health was to keep pace with the realities of urban growth it had to come to grips with the problem of overcrowding. Overcrowding was still seen as an integral part of general sanitary reform, as a 'nuisance' similar in effect to other nuisances such as bad drains and capable of remedy by the same measures (prohibitions and prosecutions), but it did mark a new awareness, and it was an awareness that bore immediate, if hardly effective, legislative results.

Hunter concluded that the Nuisances Removal Acts, which were left to the discretion of local magistrates, had proved incapable of dealing with the growing problem of overcrowding.[89] Building his case upon Hunter's evidence, Simon, in his Eighth Annual Report to the Privy Council, stressed the importance of housing for the health of the nation:

> Large as the inquiry was and copious as are the resulting details of information, the broad results may be told in these very few words – that, neither against degrees of overcrowding which conduce immensely to the multiplication of disease, as well as to obvious moral evils, nor against the use of dwellings which are permanently unfit for human habitation, can local authorities in towns, except to a certain extent in some privileged places, exercise any effectual control . . . When first, seventeen years ago, it devolved upon me (then officer of health for the City of London) to draw attention to the sanitary circumstances of great masses of metropolitan population, I showed, in regard of my then sphere of observation, that those evils were sufficient in their gigantic magnitude to neutralise whatever in other respects was being attempted for the improvement of health. And now . . . I affirm generally what was then but of partial application, and say that to provide for the public health in important centres of population must of necessity be a hopeless task, unless the administering authority be armed with ample powers to render impossible those conditions of lodgment which are of so deadly effect upon the poor.

Simon called for the extension of the system of registration, which had already been applied to common lodging houses of the 1d a night variety, to private dwellings, for the stricter control of cellar dwellings, and, most important, for a control of overcrowding based upon available air space, and, unlike the Nuisances Removal Act, applicable even when overcrowding occurred in a single family dwelling.[90] In calling for a new approach to housing, Simon was aware that the Nuisances Removal Acts had failed in their purpose. Simon was perhaps fortunate in his timing, for that old friend of sanitary reformers – cholera – reappeared, and although less devastating than in past epidemics, it was still sufficiently frightening to create an atmosphere favourable to reform.

The Sanitary Act of 1866 reflected Simon's recommendations. It enforced the connection of all houses to the main sewers, regulated cellar dwellings, and enabled the central government to *force* local authorities to conduct inquiries and make improvements to abate nuisances. Local sanitary authorities could now place all houses (private as well as common lodging houses) upon a register, and overcrowding was now made illegal both under a clear quantifiable definition, according to air-space (clause 35) and in terms of a general nuisance (clause 19 allowed local authorities to include as a 'nuisance' any 'house or part of a house' so overcrowded as to be dangerous or prejudicial to the health of inmates'). But these important clauses were, unfortunately, adoptive, not compulsory, and were applied in the most desultory fashion. Nevertheless, by defining overcrowding in terms of space as well as a nuisance, the Act tended to shift housing slightly away from sanitation and concepts of *quality* and placed it within the context of availability and *quantity*. Although the *Daily News* found the Act inquisitorial and 'almost despotic', Simon and the Metropolitan MOH soon had reservations of a different nature and almost immediately the Social Science Association began to agitate for an extension of the compulsory principle.[91]

The new phase in housing policy which the Sanitary Act indicated was about to begin was marked by an effort, sponsored by the central government, and conducted by local authorities, to improve public health by eradicating the slum. 'Improvements' in the period from the mid-1860s to the mid-1880s came to mean slum clearance and demolition. Although many varied forces were at work, including the desire to strengthen the tax base by increasing the rateable value of the newly-refurbished central districts and to effect a saving in poor relief by eliminating the unemployment and ill-health which medical officers traced to poor domestic conditions, the emphasis was on the demolition of slums both to effect the 'beautification' of the towns and to eradicate, in bold strokes, fever-nests which were a source of increasing embarrassment and concern to civic officials. It was a nationwide movement characterized by confidence, energy, determination, and, ultimately, frustration and increased awareness of the complexities of the 'housing question'.

Slum clearance was carried out under the Torrens Act (1868) and the Cross Act (1875) and their amendments, and under local improvement acts. The Torrens and Cross Acts, and their weaknesses, especially the costly legal procedures and high compensation given to owners of the slum property condemned for demolition, have been analyzed in several recent works and it is not necessary here to go into them in any great detail.[92] It is interesting to note, however, that in introducing his original bill in 1866, Torrens had stressed the connection betwen *overcrowding* and ill-health, while the much-emasculated and amended Act put the stress, in a much more traditional manner, upon *insanitary* housing. Similarly, Torrens's original bill would have given the local authorities rehousing powers, and, even more significantly, would have empowered the Home Secretary to compel the authorities to use them. Although Torrens vigorously defended his novel concept that authorities should be compelled to rehouse those evicted by local demolition schemes, he met with great opposition. The prevailing philosophy was that while it was a legitimate function of local government to demolish insanitary dwellings it was totally illegitimate for it to interfere in the free market to build houses. As one irate MP cried, the very idea of municipal housing was quite 'monstrous'. 'If such a principle were admitted he did not know where it could stop. The next demand made upon them [Parliament] might be to provide clothing if not carriages and horses for the poor'.[93] As passed, the Torrens Act enabled local authorities to demolish small groups of insanitary dwellings but left all rehousing to the vagaries of the housing market. Cross's Act, introduced in 1875, after considerable pressure from the Charity Organisation Society, the Social Science Association, and, most significantly in the context of the present work, the Royal College of Physicians, was designed not only to make possible slum clearance on a grander scale, but to tackle what had come to be recognized as an inseparable consequence of demolition, overcrowding in adjoining areas. The Royal College of Physicians, in its petition to the Prime Minister in 1874, had echoed a growing awareness that

> private enterprise is powerless to provide the fresh and improved accommodation which is required for those who have been expelled from their former habitations in addition to that which is called for by the constant increase of the population by reason of the impossibility of securing suitable sites for building.[94]

Cross's Act was Torrens's writ large, with rehousing clauses, and it marked an important step forward. Disraeli's famous 'Sanitas Sanitatum, Omnia Sanitas' electioneering speech had associated national health with national greatness and this housing act of his Home Secretary marked the first comprehensive housing legislation to be initiated by the Government. Cross had introduced his measure in highly emotional terms, calling the slums of England 'haunts of sickness and of death . . . where all is dark . . . a darkness of mind, body, and soul' and had called upon Parliament to 'assist in carrying out one of God's best and earliest laws – "let there be light" '.[95] He was determined that his bill should not suffer the same fate as Torrens's and he emphasized that the major intent of the Act was to guarantee that when local authorities cleaned 'out the rookeries for the benefit of the whole community, the persons driven from these rookeries should not be damaged by it'.[96]

The Cross Act (Artizans' and Labourers' Dwellings Improvement Act), according to the *Law Times* was 'altogether divergent from the *laissez-faire* doctrine, which for so long a period was held to be the guiding principle of English politics.'[97] But it was a permissive, not a compulsory act, and its compensation clauses so favoured propertied interests that it stifled action by local authorities. Whatever powers of building were allowed to local authorities were strictly for rehousing purposes only, although it is significant that these authorities were permitted to rehouse more people than they had evicted in their slum clearance schemes. Yet the wording of the Act hardly encouraged rebuilding by the local authorities, for it clearly stated that while it could sell or lease land cleared of slums to any 'body of trustees, society or societies, person or persons' to carry out the rehousing provisions of the Act, 'the local authority shall not themselves, without the express approval of the confirming authority [the central government] undertake the rebuilding of the houses.' Not only were the local authorities therefore expected to be the rehousing agency only in the last resort, but they were compelled, under the Act, to sell any dwellings they erected within ten years of completion. Cautiously worded, and tentative in form, the Cross Act nevertheless made extensive slum demolition possible not only for 'houses unfit for human habitation', but wherever 'diseases indicating a generally low condition of health' prevailed, and it recognized that rehousing must be an integral part of urban renewal and public health.[98]

Whatever their inadequacies, and they were many, the Torrens and Cross Acts helped to publicize the need for slum clearance and to legitimize it as a fit and proper function of municipal administration. But even before their passage, several towns had begun under local acts to tear down their most insanitary houses. The scale of the clearance schemes can be conveyed by a quick survey of the work of Liverpool, Glasgow, Edinburgh, Birmingham, and Manchester. Between 1858 and 1883 Liverpool, acting under local improvement acts, demolished much insanitary property. But the cost of the work – nearly £3,000,000 – served to reinforce fears of increased local taxes and so between 1871 and 1884 only one more clearance scheme was undertaken. Not until the late 1890s did the Corporation again turn its attention to clearing the vast areas of central blight.[99] Glasgow, whose 'structural arrangements' and 'condition of the population' had been described by Chadwick in 1842 as 'the worst of any we had seen in any part of Great Britain', had acted under the City of Glasgow Improvement Act (1866) to establish a municipal housing trust to demolish insanitary property, and it quickly set about improving eighty-eight acres of insanitary houses within the city. By 1876 it had displaced some 25,375 people. Yet it had erected only 1,646 new dwellings by 1902. Like so many other towns, Glasgow's efforts at slum clearance resulted in even greater pressure upon available housing. In 1902 a sanitary inspector discovered people sleeping in cupboards, under beds, and even on the rooftops![100] Glasgow also tackled the problem of insanitary dwellings under the Police Act of 1862. Under this Act dwellings of three rooms and under, with a total footage of under 2,000 cubic feet, were 'ticketed' – that is a metal ticket was placed on the outside of the dwelling indicating the number of occupants allowed by law (300 cubic feet for each person over eight years of age). By 1881 some 75,000 people, roughly one-seventh of the total population, were living in ticketed dwellings. Yet only one-half of the one-roomed dwellings were ticketed and the fines for overcrowding were absurdly low. Rather like the attempt in London to bring houses under a regular system of inspection by placing them on the registers of the local authorities, the system of ticketing in Glasgow did little to get at the problem of overcrowding.[101]

In Birmingham, under its dynamic mayor, Chamberlain, the Corporation had embarked upon what became the most-publicized central slum clearance scheme in England until the London County Council demolished the notorious 'Jago' in its Boundary Street Scheme towards the end of the century. Operating under a loan of £1,500,00, the Corporation purchased factories as well as private dwellings. By relocating the factories in the suburbs it not only set the tone for much urban redevelopment in the twentieth century, but it also, much to its own benefit, obviated the necessity to rehouse all those evicted, for it agreed, with reason, that the workforce could now find work and accommodation (provided by speculative builders) in the suburbs. It was, in some respects, more of a city beautification than a slum demolition and rehousing scheme, and factors peculiar to Birmingham (a high percentage of skilled and regularly employed labour, and factories sited in the central slum districts) made it an experiment difficult to follow elsewhere.[102] By 1875 Birmingham had completed its great central clearance scheme (amounting to some ninety-three acres); after that it undertook only one other scheme, completed in 1901.[103]

Manchester, operating under a local Borough Police Act (1844) between 1845 and 1847 had ordered sanitary improvements in dwellings occupied by over 26,000 people. Yet it embarked upon no great clearance schemes in the nineteenth century, partly because like so many towns it was deterred by the expenses that London and other towns were experiencing under the Cross Acts, partly because it hoped, against all the available evidence, 'that commercial development would help do the job for it'.[104] Certainly the fear of the additional burden to the rates was justified, but the do-nothing policy was advocated at a time when parts of central Manchester had five hundred people to the acre and when Liverpool's schemes were about to help bring its death rate down from above Manchester's to below it. Eventually, in 1891, the town did introduce its first improvement scheme.[105]

Edinburgh moved remarkably quickly after its MOH, Dr Little-john, had drawn attention to the city's slums in his *Report on the Sanitary Condition of Edinburgh*, in 1865. Within three months a £500,000 improvement scheme had been initiated. But it took twenty-two years to finish, and while 2,721 houses were demolished, only 340 were provided. In 1885 the Town Council commenced Open Court proceedings, in which owners of insanitary houses had to show cause why their dwellings should not be closed. These proceedings led to 1,606 houses being closed as unfit for human habitation between 1885 and 1890. Another 818 dwellings were demolished in the 1893 Improvement Scheme.[106]

By and large these various improvement schemes and those conducted under the Cross Act failed to accomplish the improvement in the nation's inner-city housing which housing reformers hoped for. Indeed, in the first decade after the passage of the Cross Act, only twelve towns outside London asked for permission to employ it (Birmingham, Derby, Devonport, Liverpool, Newcastle, Norwich, Nottingham, Swansea, Walsall, Wolverhampton, Greenock, and Leith); only Birmingham engaged in large-scale clearance, and in only four towns was there any concerted effort to rehouse those evicted.[107] At the root of the problem was the realization that if no buyers emerged for the cleared land the towns would suffer considerably – thus slum clearance remained, in the words of one historian, 'economically unorthodox, politically embarrassing, and of little direct electoral appeal'.[108]

Much of the concern over the slums in this period had focused upon London, partly because in the central districts the old housing stock and the degree of overcrowding were appalling, an embarrassment to all who looked to London, as the nation's largest town and the centre of an empire, for leadership and direction. Increasingly as the century progressed, London, and especially its East End, became the symbol for urban abuse, and a warning of the social, moral and political dangers of failing to include housing as an integral part of a broader public health policy. I have examined in detail elsewhere the efforts of London to clear away the acres of insanitary dwellings concentrated throughout its considerable area.[109] It is necessary here only to point out that despite all the hesitations and difficulties involved, and the various disagreements between the local vestries and the Metropolitan Board of Works (the agency for the Cross Acts in London) concerning their respective obligations under the Torrens and Cross Acts, significant improvements were effected. Indeed, before its dissolution in 1888 the Metropolitan Board of Works had undertaken twenty-two separate schemes, and had demolished some 7,400 insanitary dwellings inhabited by 29,000 people. In clearing a total of forty acres of congested slums in every central district of London except Bermondsey, Shoreditch and Bethnal Green, the Board appears to have been guided as much by the general death rate of the area, and its lack of ventilation, as by the actual physical or sanitary condition of the houses scheduled for demolition. In its first clearance scheme, begun in Whitechapel and Limehouse in 1876, the death rate for the area was over twice that of Whitechapel or London as a whole. Although London did not have many back-to-backs, they did exist in four of the areas which the Board cleared (Southwark, Westminster, Holborn, and Marylebone); the Board also cleared away some old wooden houses. In some of the areas scheduled for demolition the courtways were so narrow that the walls on either side could be touched with the elbows when walking through.[110] It is interesting to note that the Board had started three-quarters of all its demolition work within two years of the passage of the Cross Act and that it eased up considerably in its later years, partly because of the high costs and consequent burden on the rates. Although the Board was able to sell the land to various housing trusts and companies, (and these eventually housed 27,000 people), it was never able to recoup by sale the purchase price of the land and the cost of demolition, and by selling land at under its free market price it was virtually subsidizing the efforts of the various philanthropic groups engaged in the rehousing.[111] The London County Council, which replaced the Metropolitan Board of Works in 1889, continued its work of slum clearance: in all it cleared away some fifty-eight acres scattered throughout London. In the schemes it inherited from the Board, the London County Council received permission from the Local Government Board to rehouse only half the total number evicted (6,000 people), but in the schemes it commenced itself it rehoused almost as many people as it displaced.[112]

There can be little question that the slum clearance schemes, by destroying acres of fever-ridden, hopelessly unhealthy property, supplemented the advances made in other areas of public health. But there can also be no doubt that it was all accomplished at the cost of much human suffering. The earlier Nuisances Removal Acts and Torrens Acts, which also resulted in demolitions, had not been used to the full because the MOH, who could initiate proceedings, were reluctant to recommend demolition when there was no provision for the immediate rehousing of the evicted. All those most intimately connected with slum clearance and demolition were agreed that considerable human suffering resulted from 'indiscriminate ejectment'.[113] Thus one witness to the early attempts in Liverpool to get at cellar dwellings cautioned that the closing had been achieved at the expense 'of physical inconvenience and of moral injury'. The evicted, he added, had simply been driven into 'other inferior and ill-conditioned dwellings and have suffered great inconvenience from the change without deriving any sanatary [sic] benefits'.[114] Of the fifty or so street improvement schemes undertaken by the Metropolitan Board of Works in London only sixteen (beginning in 1879) provided for any rehousing at all, and the dispossessed had to compete with the evicted from dock building, railway termini construction and other commercial ventures for available space. George Godwin, the editor of the *Builder*, bitterly attacked the 'new street-makers [who] when they are asked where the displaced occupants of the garrets and cellars are to go, shout without a thought: "go to? – Anywhere".'[115] Actually the hope was that they would go to the suburbs, but this was clearly impossible for the casually-employed and all those whose jobs depended on being on the spot for the daily hiring. Indeed, as late as 1913, 40 per cent of the working-class residents of Westminster said they had to live close to their work.[116] In the graphic words of one casually-employed workman, 'I might as well go to America as go to the suburbs.'[117] One poor woman told an East End clergyman an all-too familiar tale of woe: 'I came to London twenty-five years ago and I have never lived in any room more than two years yet.'[118] Between 1902 and 1913 over 45,000 working-class rooms in central London and some 70,000 working-class rooms in London as a whole were pulled down for various 'improvements': of these only 15,073 were demolished to make way for new working-class dwellings.[119] Demolition and improvement schemes were thus a mixed blessing.

Similarly, legislation regulating overcrowding under the Nuisances, or Sanitary Acts, or local by-laws (the Local Government Board set model by-laws of 300 cubic feet per adult and half that for children under ten) was rarely implemented by the MOH for these men, compassionate and well-informed, knew that it would only create immediate overcrowding in adjoining districts. In the opinion of the MOH for St Marylebone; 'sanitary improvement is a very car of juggernaut, pretty to look at, but which crushes them [the poor]', and he added, echoing the attitude of his fellow MOH, that, if the Torrens and Cross Acts had been vigorously enforced, 'an appalling amount of misery, of overcrowding, and of poverty would have been the result.'[120] To the MOH for Lambeth it was supremely ironic that 'insanitary areas may be in this way [slum clearance and enforcing legislation against overcrowding] manufactured by sanitary authorities.'[121] Even the Charity Organisation Society, which was often very blithe in its attitudes towards urban 'improvements', finally realized that 'all social changes must tell first and most heavily, on the poorer classes.' As one London MOH declared, 'Until tenements are built in proportion to those demolished at low rents, it is not humane to press on with large schemes.'[122]

Torrens had argued that, without the essential rehousing clauses, it 'would have been stupid, reckless, and cruel' of the local authorities to use his Act.[123] Yet although an amendment to his Act (passed in 1879) and the Cross Act did have rehousing clauses, they cannot be said to have been of direct benefit to the displaced. Writing in 1883, the MOH for St Marylebone noted that 'The present tendency of the Artizans Dwellings Acts . . . is to give a better and increased accommodation for the fairly paid artisan, but to decrease the living room of the labourer, of the needlewoman, and of the class generally denominated as poor.'[124] Behind this statement lay the realization that the dwellings built to rehouse the evicted were generally too expensive for the class whose dwellings were demolished by slum clearance schemes.

This is not the place to discuss in detail the model dwelling movement, which, inspired by a mixture of evangelical concern and practical reform motives, married philanthropy and capitalism (generally the model dwelling companies aimed at a five per cent profit margin) in an attempt to add to the housing stock.[125] The movement received a great fillip from the Cross Acts, which made centrally-located land available to them at below market cost, and the model dwelling companies were, in that sense, the first subsidized housing offered on a large scale. At first glance the numbers housed by the various model dwelling companies might seem considerable. Up to 1910 the major agencies in London (the most famous of which was the Peabody Trust) had built over 100,000 rooms.[126] Though never on the same scale, the model dwelling movement also made an impact in several provincial towns.[127] Condemned for being cheerless piles and 'barracky' 'Bastilles', criticized for charging rents which only the artisan class could afford, and attacked for their stern regimentation of the occupants, the model dwellings nevertheless had some influence upon the health of the nation.[128] They helped to focus attention upon the need to build in the central districts, and although no direct and conclusive proof is possible, it may also be hazarded that they helped to raise the standard of expectation of the working classes. According to the Agent for the Grosvenor and Northampton estates in London, model dwellings set 'a good example of cleanliness and decent behaviour in the whole neighbourhood', and to the MOH for the St Saviour's Board of Works model dwellings were 'small plots of civilization cultivated in the midst of a wide waste of barbarism'.[129] In areas like Whitechapel, where in 1900 there were over 15,000 people living in model dwellings, and in Shoreditch where 8,450 people lived in model dwellings in 1914, the model blocks stood as advertisements, in brick and stone, for cleanliness and sanitary housing.[130] Though often segregated from the slum streets around them by formidable railings and great gates, their underlying philosophy of healthy accommodation may have filtered down through the neighbourhood.

Certainly their rules reinforced the sanitary idea. Thus, in the Peabody blocks, among the long lists of rules we find:

> No applicants for rooms will be entertained unless every member of the applicant's family has been vaccinated or agrees to comply with the Vaccination Act, and further agrees to have every case of infectious disease removed to the proper hospital . . . The passages, steps, closets, and lavatory windows must be washed every Saturday and swept every morning before 10 o'clock. This must be done by the tenants in turn. Washing must be done only in the laundry . . . Refuse must not be thrown out of the windows . . . Tenants are required to report to the superintendent any births, deaths, or infectious diseases occurring in their rooms. Any tenant not complying with this rule will receive notice to quit.[131]

The *Pall Mall Gazette* wryly observed that the Peabody blocks 'do not answer to an Englishman's idea of home', and while this observation was no doubt correct, they did answer to the sanitarians' concept of what a healthy dwelling should be.[132] Thus while *The Times* could be critical of their outward and interior appearance, it had nothing but praise for the sanitary and domestic provisions found in the Peabody dwellings:

Drainage and ventilation have been insured with the utmost possible care; the instant removal of dust and refuse is effected by the means of shafts . . . the passages are kept clean and lighted with gas without any cost to the tenants; water from cisterns in the roof is distributed by pipes into every tenement and there are baths free for all who desire to use them. Laundries with ringing machines and drying lofts are at the service of every inmate, who is thus relieved from the inconvenience of damp vapours in his apartments and the consequent damage to his furniture and bedding. Every living room or kitchen is abundantly provided with cupboards, shelving, and other conveniences, and each fire place includes a boiler and oven.[133]

Formidable and unfriendly, not inexpensive to construct or rent, insufficient in number to solve the problem of overcrowding, the model blocks at their best did demonstrate the possibility of bringing sanitary living and advanced sanitary engineering and conveniences down to the poor. They also indicated that, with adequate sanitary provisions, density was not itself a lethal force. Thus in one of the buildings of the Metropolitan Association for Improving the Dwelling of the Industrious Classes, the density reached 1,625 people per acre: but the death rate in the Association's dwellings was only fourteen per thousand compared to twenty-four per thousand in London as a whole.[134]

The model dwelling movement helped to pave the way for the third stage of housing reform in Victorian England – the stage of municipal endeavour. Like the model dwelling movement, the achievements of municipal housing were not considerable in terms of numbers housed, and the Victorian era marks an uncertain beginning rather than a full-scale movement. But, again like model dwellings, the council flats which were erected in Liverpool, Glasgow, London, Manchester, and other major cities, mark an acknowledgement of the need for new housing stock of a high sanitary standard, and the recognition that with proper sanitary design high-density living could be healthy. For better or worse they helped promote the idea of block dwellings: by 1911 3.4 per cent of the total housing stock in England and Wales was in the form of block dwellings; South Shields had 72 per cent of its housing in blocks, Newcastle 55.6 per cent, and London 17.8 per cent (in Holborn the figure was over 60 per cent).[135] Liverpool had pioneered municipal dwellings with its St Martin's Cottages, completed in 1869 on land it had cleared of slums; but it was not until much later in the century under the Housing Acts of 1885 and 1890 that local authorities embarked upon housing schemes of any magnitude. By 1901 the Glasgow City Improvement Trust had erected

1,697 houses; Dublin, which erected its first dwellings in 1888, had built twelve blocks before the war; Edinburgh by 1890 had provided some 237 houses; Sheffield by 1919 had constructed 617 houses; Liverpool before the First World War had almost 10,000 people living in nearly 3,000 municipal dwellings; Manchester had 2,140 people; Glasgow had 3,639 people in municipal dwellings; and in London almost 17,000 rooms had been provided by the London County Council for rehousing purposes and almost 13,000 rooms were added as fresh housing. Another 8,000 rooms were added by local boroughs and district councils in Greater London and adjoining areas.[136] Taken as percentages of total housing stock they are clearly just a beginning: Liverpool had the highest percentage of its population living in municipal dwellings, but the figure was only 1.31 per cent; in London the figure was 0.76, in Manchester 0.34, Sheffield, 0.34; Swansea, 0.93; Glasgow 0.47; Edinburgh 0.61.[137] In 1914 the Local Government Board praised the efforts of the local authorities but added that 'we cannot profess to be satisfied with the progress which has been made in the direction of the provision of new housing by local authorities.'[138] For the most part built to a high standard and cost, they were rarely occupied by the evicted of municipal slum clearance schemes, and the unwillingness of the authorities to come to the Government for the low-interest loans that were available suggests that housing was never fully accepted, even in London or Liverpool, as an essential component of an integrated public health programme.[139]

Following a decade of sensational exposés in the press and often fervent agitation by a newly-awakened Christian conscience, the 1885 Housing Act restated the power of municipalities to clear land, rehouse the evicted, and to build new dwellings. Under pressure from such groups as the Workmen's National Housing Council, a Housing Act was passed in 1900 which made municipal ownership of dwellings easier (it enabled local authorities to purchase land for housing purposes outside their own boundaries). Finally in 1903 the 'imperative tone' came to housing legislation when the Housing Act of that year enabled the Local Government Board to force local authorities to implement the Torrens and Cross Acts. The central government continued to offer incentives in the form of low-cost long-term loans for housing purposes but it would have been too great a departure from the accepted philosophy of government for the State to *insist* that municipalities enter the housing market on a large scale.

The Edwardian era did, however, see a marked departure from that philosophy. The Housing, Town Planning Act of 1909 did for new housing stock what the 1903 Act did for rehousing – it enabled the Local Government Board to force local authorities to act. Upon the petition of four resident householders the Board could, after a public enquiry, declare the local authority in default, and order it to carry out the work: the Board could also force the local authorities to revoke their by-laws if, in its opinion, they 'unreasonably impeded' the erection of working-class dwellings. Understandably, doubts were raised about the central government's new powers to involve the local ratepayers in considerable expenditure for housing the poor. Once the central government had the powers to coerce local authorities to build, the demand for direct government grants – that is, subsidized State housing – was bound to be raised. Indeed the Housing of the Working Classes (Ireland) Act of 1908 established a housing fund of £180,000 to be used as grants-in-aid to assist local housing schemes: an Act passed in 1914 established a fund of £4,000,000 for housing for government employees in rural areas in England and Wales, and marked, in a dramatically new way, the direct entry of the State in the provision of working-class dwellings.[140] Although direct government grants had been attacked in Parliament in 1912 as a wild proposal, combining 'the maximum of officious interference with everybody, the apotheosis of centralization and bureaucracy, finance that is thoroughly unsound, and political economy that would be condemned in a girl's high school', by the outbreak of the First World War the central government had, somewhat reluctantly, become directly involved in adding to the nation's housing stock.[141]

It was the conclusion of a period which began with the unauthorized use by Chadwick of the Poor Law Commission to investigate the connection between fever, poverty and housing conditions. Over the next seventy years or so it became increasingly clear that housing was, at root, a problem of poverty. Indeed, perhaps of all manifestations of poverty the teeming slum was the most obvious, just as it was the most ineluctable. To all those familiar with the costs of construction and central land costs on one hand and the uncertain employment, low wages and the exigencies of the family budget on the other, healthy, uncrowded accommodation for the urban masses raised, in the words of the Chairman of the London County Council's Housing Committee, 'the vexed question of the relation between rent and wages, which easily slides into that of capital and labour.'[142] As John Burns said, slums were 'created primarily by poverty of pocket. Wherever casual labour was endemic poverty was epidemic, and squalour must prevail.'[143] *The Times*, as was often the case, put it most succinctly, when in 1883, at the height of a national agitation over slum conditions, it sadly reflected that 'the housing of the great mass of workers . . . is a question, we say, of wages.'[144] To those involved in public health the awareness of the economic foundations of the 'housing question' provoked a sense of despair and helplessness.

Throughout the nineteenth century the poor were accused of mismanaging their budgets and they were often indicted for spending far too much on drink and far too little on rent. But if the public health movement, especially the daily experience of evangelicals and others in the slums, proved anything, it was that while it was easy to point to 'vice' and poor budgeting as a cause of slum living, in the case of thousands of 'respectable' families the accusation was blatantly unjustified. The emphasis of the great reform exposés of the 1880s and of the accumulated evidence of the Royal Commission on the Housing of the Working Classes was to show convincingly that there were throughout the country thousands of working-class families who followed all the cherished precepts of Smilesian self-help and bourgeois respectability, who did not drink, or gamble, or spend their wages frivolously, who managed to stay in regular employment, and yet who still could not afford adequate or healthy dwellings, however carefully they nurtured and juggled their budgets. To say, as so many did, that the poor ought to spend a higher proportion of their wages on rent was to display a pitiful ignorance of the uncertain nature of their employment, their fear of sudden unemployment, and the marginal quantity and quality of their diet. As early as 1851 Hector Gavin concluded his survey of *The Habitations of the Industrial Classes* by declaring that 'the poor pay in rent a very large proportion of their earnings, and that the sum they thus pay is greatly disproportioned to the accommodation provided for them.'[145] Over half a century later, in early twentieth-century Glasgow, many of the working classes were paying only 11 or 12 per cent of their wages in return for sub-standard housing; but, as one historian of Glasgow's working-class housing points out, it is difficult to see how they could afford any more, given their low wages and the uncertainty of employment – 'It was not the low percentage of income allocated to rent . . . which was the cause of their poor living conditions', he concludes, 'it was that the income level of labourers in a wide range of Glasgow's industries was too low to allow a man to keep his wife and children in decent accommodation.'[146]

At the end of this long career, when he wrote his *English Sanitary Institutions* (1890), Simon stressed that the housing question could not be separated 'from various other questions regarding poverty' and that it 'more and more compelled thought on poverty in general.' His realization that overcrowding and slum conditions were hardly to be improved by sanitary legislation alone, since their improvement ultimately depended upon 'how far poverty can be turned into non-poverty, how far the poor can be made less poor', revealed a sense of frustration that was common to all the MOH whose work took them daily into the slums of Victorian Britain. 'Overcrowding', wrote one MOH, 'is a poverty problem, nothing more nor less', while another, giving vent to his sense of inadequacy, declared that 'poverty and high rents' were the basic cause of overcrowding and he had no control over these.[147] John Foot, the hard-working MOH for Bethnal Green, maintained in 1905 that 'poverty and the inability to pay the rent is the cause of 98 per cent of all the cases [of overcrowding] that come under our notice.' Foot and his staff found it distressing and unproductive to apply the legislation against those who were overcrowded 'because of their inability to pay rents impossible to their straitened circumstances'. With wages averaging 21s a week in his neighbourhood, and with average rents of 7s a week for the two rooms which most medium-sized families would require to stay on the side of the law, it is little wonder that in Bethnal Green overcrowding was 'a good hardy annual flourishing all the year round' and 'an economic question right through'. Like so many other health authorities Foot sadly concluded that 'until the conditions of life producing it [overcrowding] are entirely remodelled, no permanent improvement can in the main be hoped for.'[148]

If, as the *Medical Times* declared in 1884, 'overcrowding was . . . merely a question of the relationship between wages and rents', it was quite clear that there was not very much health authorities could do about it. 'What are the main causes of overcrowding?', asked the MOH for Kensington: 'Poverty and high rents', he answered, and 'over these conditions the Local Authority has no power.'[149]

IV

There can be little doubt that in terms of sanitary standards and public health the nineteenth century made remarkable progress in slum clearance. The utterly fantastic, labyrinthine slums of the past, with their tumbledown, old housing stock, subterranean dwellings, narrow courtways, and densely-packed tenements were swept away, and street and other 'improvements', commercial construction, railways, and other forces of urban development transformed the topography of the major British cities. So marked were the changes that even the popular novelist, playwright and housing reformer, George Sims, a man who well knew the human cost of slum clearance, could hardly refrain from striking a congratulatory note in his *In London's Heart* (1900):

> To a man who has long been absent from the mother of cities, the first walk must be exceedingly interesting. Change has been in every direction. During his absence narrow streets have yielded to broad, handsome thoroughfares; whole areas that were once little better than slums have been cleared, and vast hotels and splendid shops stand where, only a few years back, the thieves and ruffians of London herded.[150]

But behind the new thoroughfares slums still existed, somewhat more out of sight and, because of improvements in sewerage and water supply, and all the other advances in preventive medicine we have discussed, somewhat out of the public mind since they no longer constituted a major threat to the health of the nation. Despite the housing provided by the speculative builder in the working-class suburb, the model dwelling movement, and late-Victorian and Edwardian municipal enterprise, the official figures for overcrowding in 1911 stood at 3,000,000. This was an underestimate, like most official figures on overcrowding: probably 6,000,000 people, roughly one-fifth of the entire population, was overcrowded.[151] Just after the First World War it was estimated that at least 805,000 houses were needed to relieve overcrowding.[152] In the Black Country between one-third and one-fifth of the entire urban population was overcrowded at the end of the century; along the Tyne it was one-third.[153]

Healthy housing was one of the cornerstones of the sanitary reformers' philosophy and programme. It was to so many of them the very heart of the matter, the reform without which all other reforms would be weakened. 'When a man is emancipated from this physical degradation' of overcrowded living, wrote one reformer at mid-century, 'and exposed to air and light, his feelings are elevated, his health improves, his whole nature expands, and then, if there be the seeds of goodness in him, they swell, burst, grow, flower, and bear fruit.'[154] It was a noble programme and indicates the missionary zeal and proselytizing fervor of much of the Victorian public health movement. Unfortunately, for most of the labouring classes, it was unrealized. In the final analysis, the public health movement which achieved so much in the public sphere in the nineteenth century, was only partially successful when it tackled the thorny problem of the slum. So long as public health depended on private wage levels and general economic conditions the fullest aspirations of health reformers would remain only hopes and dreams.

12

'A Nation of Good Animals'?

'The first requisite of life is to be a good animal, and to be a nation of good animals is the first condition of national prosperity.'

Herbert Spencer, quoted in John F. Sykes, *Public Health Problems* (1892), p. 28.

As the Victorian era drew to a close there was much for public health officials and social reformers to reflect upon with satisfaction. Wherever one turned there was evidence that the Victorian achievement was considerable – better water supplies, better excrement removal and street cleaning, a better working environment, better personal hygiene and (although, as we have seen, improvements came late), better diet, milk supplies and isolation facilities. All these, when combined with the growing science of epidemiology and immunology resulted in better national health. The death rate (corrected for both age and sex) declined from 20.5 (1861) to 16.9 (1901).[1] Dramatic improvements in health were recorded in every age group except that for babies from birth to a year old. Between the decades 1841–50 and 1891–1900 the death rate declined by over 12% in the 0–4 year-old age group, by over 50% in the 5–24 year-old group, by almost 38% in the 25–34 group and by almost 19% in the 35–44 age group.[2] Life expectancy increased at birth from 40.2 (1841) to 51.5 (1911) for England and Wales as a whole, and by 1911 Londoners could expect to live to almost 50 rather than only 35, as in 1841. The improvements in the quality of city life resulted in a reduction in the ratio of urban to rural deaths from 124:100 (1851–61) to 114:100 (1891–1901).[3] Quite clearly the self-congratulatory tone of *Public Health* in the Diamond Jubilee year of 1897, which was quoted at the beginning of this book, was justified – the Victorian achievement in the field of public health was, indeed, 'worthy'.[4]

Even Charles Masterman, who felt that 'an amount remains to be done which may well tax the energies of philanthropists and statesmen for years to come', and who, as we shall see, wrote despairingly of urban conditions, allowed that there had been great progress over the past century. 'Public bodies, the London County Council and similar authorities in the great provincial cities', he wrote in his introductory essay, 'Realities at Home', for the collection of essays, *The Heart of Empire* (1901)

> have been pushing their activities into the dark places of the earth; slum areas are broken up, sanitary regulations enforced, the policeman and the inspector at every corner. A series of factory acts, building acts, public health acts, have continually assailed the worst of these evils . . . the forces of progress are against these older social diseases, which eventually must disappear before the machinery which is brought against them.[5]

Yet alongside the sense of accomplishment was a feeling of failure, or at least of urgency. At the end of the century there was certainly no complacency or weakening of the reform impulse. This was partly due to the self-generating reform impetus which had built up steadily over the past decades and to the machinery (especially the growing power of the MOH) to which it had given rise, and partly to the stimulus of the shocking exposés into slum conditions and the statistical work of Rowntree and Booth. But there were also new forces which modified the sense of achievement and served as a spur for future reform.

In an earlier chapter I quoted Simon's conviction that the mere absence of fatal diseases did not necessarily imply good health.[6] To Masterman this was the essential point, one which to a great degree nullified much of the progress of the past century. For a new 'type' of Englishman had emerged, one who did not necessarily succumb to the epidemic diseases which had ravaged England earlier in the nineteenth century, but who, nevertheless, could hardly be considered healthy. 'The death-rate, indeed, steadily falls', Masterman wrote, 'but this appears due far more to improved sanitation and increased medicinal skill than to improved vitality.' There was now 'a perpetual presence of a multitude of minor disorders, irritability, digestive disorganisations, producing a sum total of preventable suffering . . .'[7] It was a vision of a lethargic, sickly people which was shared by many others at the time, including H. G. Wells, who in his novels *Tono-Bungay* and *The New Machiavelli* described a population dependent on stimulants and relishes to awaken dead palates and on patent medicines and nostrums (of which 'Tono-Bungay' was one) to help relieve the many ailments and debilities from which they suffered: '. . . there seem to be more boards by the railway every time I pass', Wells wrote of the South London suburb of 'Bromstead', 'advertising pills and pickles, tonics and condiments, and suchlike solicitudes of a people with no natural health or appetite left in them. . . .'[8] For Wells, Masterman, and indeed for many MOH and scores of journalists and politicians, the greatest challenge, as the new century dawned, lay in the new, sickly urban 'type' which, thanks to sanitary science, now survived to perpetuate and so, it was argued, weaken the national stock. As Masterman put it, 'more of the unfit now drag out a stunted existence, and transmit the bloodless, ineffective type to succeeding generations.'[9] Public health thus became caught up in an emotional debate over national physical degeneration.

Concern for possible race deterioration antedates Darwin and was especially strong around the time of the Crimean War when Charles Kingsley and others argued, somewhat calculatingly, that sanitary reforms were the basis for future military strength. Hector Gavin, for example, wrote that over 42% of town-bred recruits and over 17% of rural, had been rejected as unfit by the army – figures which he used to indicate both the comparative unhealthiness of towns and the relationship between good health and national security, a relationship which in an urbanizing nation like England was especially critical.[10] Kingsley bluntly stated that 'unless the physical deterioration of the lower classes is stopped by bold sanitary reform . . . we shall soon have rifles but no men to shoulder them', and Farr cautioned that England was 'on the verge of a great calamity', for 'if degeneration should extend and large numbers of the English race be divested of its noblest characteristics, their reclamation would be an arduous if not impracticable undertaking . . . How few genuine instances are there', he asked, 'of the regeneration of a fallen man, class, or nation?' Farr maintained that 'to a nation of good and noble men Death is a less evil than Degradation of Race' and he predicted that, 'out of the existing seed, to raise races of men to a divine perfection' would be 'the final problem of Public Medicine'.[11] In 1857 the *City Press*, in an article entitled, and linking, 'Wars Abroad and Reforms at Home', wrote that it was good that the Crimean War had served to cast light on 'the physical condition of the masses, whence our soldiers and sailors must be obtained', for 'it is at times like this that the necessity of providing for the people healthy, out of door recreations, healthy habitations, and means of cleanliness and instruction becomes apparent'. Two years later the Social Science Association was told that 'the British soldier has never crossed bayonets with his equal', but 'the crowding of the population in large towns without sanitary provisions' was enfeebling the nation. Hence the 'State has a direct interest in guarding against a deterioration of our race.'[12]

The great agitation over physical degeneration which swept England during the Boer War was in several respects similar to the discussion a half-century earlier. Like it, it was intimately related to military strength and was fuelled by statistics of rejected recruits and by military set-backs in a major war. It, too, was linked to a realization that England was a nation primarily of town dwellers and that, since urban conditions bred a weakened race, deterioration of the national stock would probably ensue.[13] But there were crucial differences also. The earlier talk of race deterioration had stemmed from a small circle of health reformers and was rarely heard beyond that circle. Now the agitation was taken up in the daily, periodical, and specialized medical press and resulted in an official government inquiry, the Inter-Departmental Committee on Physical Deterioration (appointed in September 1903). A more important difference, however, is that whereas previously the cry of race deterioration had been raised to stress the *need* for social reform some now raised it to warn of the *dangers* of such reforms. The new cry, as we shall shortly see, was that the environmental and sanitary improvements of the past were actually weakening the national stock.

Although other evidence was cited (including an increase in the number of female babies born and a decline in the birth rate), the prime 'proof' of possible national physical deterioration was the appallingly high percentage of rejections of volunteers for the army. No careful *comparative* analysis was undertaken of the rejection rate at the end of the century and earlier, but the *total* numbers rejected clearly indicated to many contemporaries that the English were now so hopelessly puny and enfeebled that some deterioration must have occurred.[14] According to official army statistics, of 679,703 men medically examined for enlistment between 1893 and 1902, 234,914 were rejected as medically unfit, or 34.6% of the total. Of those accepted, some 5,849 'broke down within three months of enlistment', and another 14,259 were discharged as invalids within two years. As if these figures were not bad enough it was pointed out that they were for those volunteers only who were passed on by the recruiters to army medical officers; an 'appallingly large' number had already been rejected by the recruiters themselves for being under-weight, under-height, or unfit.[15] Again, according to army figures, almost half the volunteers in Manchester in 1902 were rejected for 'reasons of physical incapacity' (and during the Boer War less than 10% of the volunteers were considered fit enough to send abroad to fight!); at Hounslow recruiting station the rejection rate was 39.5%, in Liverpool and Newcastle over 38%, and in Belfast over 37%. In York,

Leeds and Sheffield almost 27% of the recruits between 1897 and 1901 were rejected as completely unfit and another 29% were accepted only provisionally. Rowntree concluded from these statistics that only half of the manpower of the nation, roughly, was sufficiently fit for military service.[16] In 1845 only 10.5% of the men in the army were under 5' 6"; in 1900 the figure was 56.5% and the percentage of men weighing under 8st 8lbs increased from 15.9 (1871) to 26.9 (1898) and 30.1 (1900).[17] Under pressure during the Boer War the army began to enlist men down to a minimum height of 5'.[18] The dangers inherent in these statistics hardly needed elaboration: as Lord Rosebery so cogently put it, 'it is of no use having an Empire without an Imperial Race.'[19]

The acute problems of recruitment were given a national airing when Major-General Sir John Frederick Maurice published two articles, full of statistics, urgent pleading and dire warnings ('Where to Get Men' and 'National Health: a Soldier's Study') in the *Contemporary Review* in 1902 and 1903.[20] The shocking revelations of physical decline, or at least of stunted growth, received the full glare of national publicity at a time when the public had already become acquainted with the spectre of race degeneration and national decline through the propaganda of the 'restrictionists' who wanted strong immigration laws to exclude 'undesirable' aliens (i.e. East European Jews), who, it was argued, were flooding England with an inferior stock which was capable of living at incredibly low standards, 'which to the more highly developed Englishman and Englishwoman', wrote the Secretary of the Association for Preventing the Immigration of Destitute Aliens, 'mean disease and death.'[21]

The debate was also conducted in the pages of *Lancet*, the *British Medical Journal*, and *Public Health*, and although there was some support for the notion of physical deterioration, most of the medical men writing on the subject agreed with the Royal College of Surgeons and the Royal College of Physicians that there was little evidence to sustain the pessimists' views.[22] Arthur Newsholme, the MOH for Brighton, like many others argued that it was unscientific and misleading to judge an entire nation by the quality of its recruits who were drawn mainly from the 'outcast' and unemployed ranks, and Henry Armstrong, the MOH for Newcastle, cited as evidence the fact that hats and gloves were now made in bigger sizes and that England had done extremely well against Australia, a nation of ranchers, at cricket. Armstrong wrote with some acerbity that 'the overweening desire to make out that our nation is going to wreck and our population

deteriorating which certain persons encourage, may itself be an indication of degeneracy on their part.'[23]

To MOH and sanitary reformers the most alarming feature of the
whole issue was that, ironically, sanitary and other improvements,
despite the evidence of declining death rates, were actually held
responsible for national physical deterioration. For example, in his
article, 'The Deterioration in the National Physique', which appeared
in the *Nineteenth Century*, George Shee wrote that 'sanitary science
and hygiene have made prodigious strides . . . The result has been a
great reduction in the death-rate', but only 'superficial observers' saw
in the declining death rate 'a sign of improvement in national health
and vigour.'[24] More explicitly, Dr J. B. Haycroft argued in his Milray
Lectures that 'I do not see how we can shirk the fact that preventive
medicine and civilisation between them have already deteriorated in a
marked degree the healthy vigour of our race . . . Preventive medicine
is trying a unique experiment, and the effect is already discernible –
race-decay.'[25] To the Social Darwinians of the day the achievements of
the public health movement thus ran directly counter to the laws of
nature, in which the weak died, and from which Man, even in society,
could not divorce himself.[26]

Two developments of Social Darwinism were the eugenics movement and an organized attempt to slow down all social legislation,
especially that relating to public health. It is significant that the first
issue of the *Eugenics Review* (April 1909) emphasized that the social
legislation of the day was 'penalizing the fit for the sake of the unfit',
while one of the Eugenics Laboratory lecturers complained that 'practically all social legislation has been based on the [false] assumption
that better environment meant race progress.' The *Eugenics Review*
heartily agreed with a correspondent to *The Times* who wrote that

> all recent social legislation . . . has actually penalized the fitter classes of
> society in the interests of the less fit . . . We take the human rubbish . . .
> and give it compulsory education, Housing Acts, inspection of all sorts
> and at all seasons, at the expense of the fitter class, and imagine that
> better results will ensue than if we left the whole business alone. Are we
> right? or are the horse breeders right?[27]

While organized groups, like the Liberty and Property Defence
League, condemned social legislation for being 'socialistic' and called
for 'self-help versus state help', the Social Darwinians regarded such
legislation as counter-productive and 'unnatural', the fruit of a mis-
guided and 'maudlin sentiment'.[28] To L. T. Hobhouse they had
brought the unfeeling and cruel law of the jungle into society:

Were the losers in the struggle [for survival] left to welter in dire poverty? They would the sooner die out. Were housing conditions a disgrace to civilization? They were the natural environment of an unfit class and the means whereby such a class prepared the way for its own extinction. Was infant mortality excessive? It weeded out the sickly and the weaklings. Was there pestilence or famine? So many of the unfit would perish. Did tuberculosis claim a heavy toll? The tubercular germs are great selectors, skilled at probing the weak spots of living tissue.

In short, 'if natural selection is the foundation of all progress, it follows that mutual aid is the persistent enemy of progress.'[29]

Though potentially very dangerous to the continuing development of the public health movement, this strain of Social Darwinian thought was not powerful enough to stem, still less to turn back, the flow of legislation. In fact the debate over physical degeneration on balance definitely acted as a stimulus to reform. The MOH in general, of course, opposed the notion that public health had created a weakened national stock: on the contrary, vigorously administered, it served to elevate the race. As John Sykes argued, although there was undoubtedly 'a strong tendency to degeneration ever present in crowded communities', the 'power and exercise, from the cradle to the grave, of the knowledge possessed of the laws of health, must not only have a preventive effect, but also a regenerative result upon communities enfeebled by the unhealthy conditions of great towns and cities.'[30] The claim that preventive medicine enabled the feeble to struggle on and undermine the national stock was attractive to many, but even more compelling was the counter-argument that what was now needed was a new round of legislation which would address the problem of physical weakness and debility. If infectious diseases had been tackled and an industrial and domestic environment hazardous to health improved to the point where the unhealthy now survived in large numbers then surely, it was argued, it was up to the next generation to build on that achievement and devise a new programme that would raise the general level of health. Rather than lament the fact that the frail and feeble now survived, the purpose of society should be to elevate their physical standard – to accomplish what Simon had so desperately called for, the elimination of everything which stood in the way of really good health and bodily vigour.

One result of the debate over physical deterioration was that attention was now focused even more critically than before on the relationship between the social consequences of urbanization and good national health. To Masterman the overwhelming force working to counteract all the public health improvements of the past, great as these were, was the evolution of a 'New Town Type':

> in the past twenty-five years a force has been operating in the raw materials of which the city is composed. The texture has been transformed as by some subtle alchemy. The second generation of the immigrants [from country to town] has been reared in the courts and crowded ways of the great metropolis, with cramped physical accessories, not, fretful life, and long hours of sedentary and unhealthful toil. the problem of the coming years is just the problem of this New Town type: on their race development and action depend the future progress of the Anglo-Saxon race, and for the next half-century at least the policy of the British Empire in the world.[31]

Masterman unrealistically saw country living in terms of 'the spacious places of the old, silent life of England; close to the ground, vibrating to the lengthy, unhurried processes of Nature.' In contrast, high-density city living had produced 'a characteristic *physical* type of town dweller: stunted, narrow-chested, easily wearied; yet voluble, excitable, with little ballast, stamina, or endurance – seeking stimulus in drink, in betting, in any unaccustomed conflicts at home and abroad.'[32]

To some the solution lay in counteracting these pernicious urban influences by encouraging games and physical fitness in the schools and to 'countrify' the town by creating more parks and moving industry, as far as possible, back into the country.[33] Arthur Newsholme was just one of many suggesting that 'life in the country should be encouraged, and the urbanization of the population discouraged in every possible way.'[34] One way to accomplish this was to create new, totally planned communities, which combined the best features of town and country – an idea which had occupied the early socialists, Owen, St Simon, and Fourier. The planned, healthy community was an essential component of national health in Benjamin Ward Richardson's *Hygeia*, which was first published as a Presidential Address to the Health Section of the Social Science Association in 1875. 'Hygeia' was a city of spotless cleanliness and hygiene – 'in our model city', wrote Richardson, 'certain forms of disease would find no possible home, or, at worst, a home so transient as not to affect the mortality in any serious degree'. It was limited in population to 100,000 residents and had a maximum density of 25 persons per acre.[35] The creation of model towns by the industrialists Lever (Port Sunlight, outside Liverpool, commenced in 1888), Cadbury (Bournville, outside Birmingham, begun in 1880, but with the main development in 1893), and

Rowntree (New Earswick, outside York, begun in 1901), and the creation of Letchworth, as the first garden city in 1903 and Hampstead Garden Suburb in 1905, all had for their inspiration much broader impulses than the improvement in the standard of public health, but they must be seen, at least in part, as one response to the heightened concern for national health and strength at the end of Victoria's reign.[36] The objectives of the model and garden cities were well expressed by Ebenezer Howard, one of the most influential men in the new movement: 'to raise the standard of health and comfort of all true workers of whatever grade – the means by which these objects are to be achieved being a healthy, rational and economic combination of town and country life, and this on land owned by the municipality.'[37] When at the height of the national debate on physical degeneration the *British Medical Journal* argued that the way 'to prevent deterioration . . . and raise the standard of national physique' was to 'get the children of the poor . . . out of the gutters and slums', it did not advocate the accepted policy of slum clearance and re-housing, but, rather, asked its readers to support the work of the Garden City Association and the new concept of town planning.[38]

This concept received legislative support from the Liberals in the Housing, Town Planning Act of 1909, which permitted and encouraged local authorities to embark on planning schemes. What is significant about the Act was that it wove urban planning into public health and placed it under the direction of the Local Government Board which could order local authorities to prepare and submit a town planning scheme when a public inquiry decided one was necessary. Other sections of the Act made it obligatory for County Councils to appoint full-time, tenured MOH and for local authorities to establish public health and housing committees. As we saw in the last chapter, it also forced them, at the discretion of the Local Government Board, to embark on new working-class housing schemes. Little wonder that *The Times*, which had for so long been a staunch supporter of mandatory slum clearance and a general supervision by the central government over local public health bodies, felt that things had now gone too far. It bitterly condemned the 'dictatorial supremacy of the Local Government Board' and 'the passion of the government for compulsion, for the suppression of freedom, and for irresponsible bureaucratic control, for everything opposed to true Liberalism.' The paper passionately argued that 'the ideal of collective socialism is an all-embracing bureaucracy which shall wrap its tentacles around everything and everybody and squeeze all the individual life out of them. The Town Planning Bill in an innocent guise was a step, and no inconsiderable one, in that direction.'[39] But despite *The Times*' hysteria, the improvement in the nation's health by the creation of totally planned, semi-rural urban communities was, in the Edwardian period, just a dream for the future.[39]

If urban planning was one possible approach, another more immediately fruitful one was to concentrate less on the bricks and mortar, the *physical* aspects of the city, and more closely on its occupants, the *flesh and blood* of the city, and especially on the children who were born and bred there. To eugenicists it was essential that attention to the individual took precedence over attention to the environment:

> the first thing is good stock, and the second thing is good stock, and the third thing is good stock, and when you have paid attention to these three things, fit environment will keep your material in good condition. No environmental or educational grindstone is of service, unless the tool to be ground is of genuine steel – of tough race and tempered stock.[40]

This new approach, with its primacy of the individual's general physique and well-being over environmental factors, can be seen in the labours and report of the Inter-Departmental Committee on Physical Deterioration which, though it showed concern over slum housing conditions and so hardly ignored the urban environment, spent far more time on the effects of urban poverty upon the health and stamina of the masses.[41] The Committee did not discover any clear evidence of physical deterioration, but it did accumulate detailed and new evidence of the depressingly low standard of health and physique of the working classes and especially of the children and infants. Its *Report* called for a programme which placed more emphasis on the mitigation of the consequences of poverty than upon the control of specific diseases, and it went well beyond what might have been expected of it (a strongly worded demand for the strict enforcement of existing health codes) to demand what might be called a charter of physical rights for children – the teaching of child-care, cooking, and domestic science to schoolchildren, the encouragement in schools and outside of physical exercise and sports (including gymnastics and swimming for girls and boys), and the better medical examination and feeding of schoolchildren, together with the better regulation of day nurseries.[42]

What this amounted to was the acknowledgement that the standard of national health now depended on raising the nutritional standards and physical fitness of the next generation. As early as 1905 the Local Government Board issued a circular to all Boards of Guardians instructing them to pay for the food of all needy schoolchildren, and in 1906 the Education (Provision of Meals) Act was passed. Together with the new concern for physical fitness and an outdoor life for youngsters (seen in the work of the National League for Physical Education and Improvement and the formation in 1907 of the Boy Scouts and in 1909 of the Girl Guides), the establishment of municipal crèches and milk depots, and a growing awareness of the importance of maternal health, the Act marked a new approach to the needs of the individual, one which equated good health with physical strength and bodily stamina as much as with absence of illness. As one doctor put it in a discussion on the Report of the Inter-Departmental Committee on Physical Deterioration:

> He thought they were just at the beginning of a great advance movement in public health. Up to the present they had been occupied in environment, with the improvement of the environment of the individual. They had made great progress in that direction, and now they were beginning to attack the individual himself.[43]

The rest of the Liberal legislative programme, especially the Education (Administrative Provisions) Act, 1907 (which required educational authorities to conduct medical inspections of school-children), the provision of old age pensions and labour exchanges, and the 1911 National Health Insurance Act (which provided sick pay, free medicine, limited unemployment benefits and public medical care, including maternity, disablement, and sanatorium benefits), indicated that at last the thorny problem of the physical consequences of poverty was being tackled in earnest.[44] As we have noted, concern over poverty and the realization that it lay at the root of many of the problems of public health presented a challenge to the MOH. 'Poverty', wrote Edward Smith in his *Manual for MOH* (1873), 'is a very complex social problem, and a fruitful source of disease.' For Simon it was a major underlying cause of disease and ill-health and he returned to it again and again through his long career. In 1864, in his Sixth Annual Report as MOH to the Privy Council, he insisted that 'the masses will scarcely be healthy unless, to their very base, they be at least moderately prosperous', and in his Thirteenth Report (for 1870) he lamented the fact that preventable illness fell mainly

> upon the most helpless classes of the community: upon the poor, the ignorant, the subordinate, the immature: upon classes, which in great part through want of knowledge, and in great part because of their dependent position, cannot effectually remonstrate for themselves against the miseries thus brought upon them . . .[45]

Simon, was however, a realist, and he knew that while there was nothing he could do about poverty, beyond bringing it to the attention of his superiors, there *was* a lot he could do about the pressing problems of death and disease. If really good health depended upon the eradication of poverty then it unfortunately lay beyond his reach: much of the mortality and morbidity of the age, on the other hand, was preventable, and Simon brought to the task all his energies and reformist zeal. The focus of the public health reformers can hardly be considered to be narrow. It was eminently practical, for they were, after all, practitioners of *preventive* medicine and their appointed task was to prevent the preventable, that is, to confine themselves to the realm of the possible. For the most part their social and political philosophy did not permit them to question, still less to challenge, the underlying fabric of society. Had they done so they would certainly have run the risk of jeopardizing their position and so undermining the machinery of public health. Hence, while aware of the deeper, underlying causes of much mortality and morbidity, they plodded on with the essential work of effecting environmental and sanitary improvements.

As the nineteenth century drew to its close, however, it became a matter of common knowledge that the poor had not shared equally in the sanitary improvements and advances in public health and that, whatever the fears of the social Darwinians, their hold on life was still far more precarious than that of the more comfortable classes. In 1889 the Rev Samuel Barnet, who had spent much of his life administering to the East End poor and who was a leading force behind the settlement house movement, considered that the very poor were still outcasts in terms of health and hygiene:

> The mother among the poor, in her joy that a son is born into the world, cannot look forward to his life. What is it to her that science has proved stronger than disease? The rich man's family may grow up unbroken around the hearth. . . . The children of the poor must die, and the family circle is broken by death which carries off the weakly . . . What is it to the poor that it has been proved how cleanliness is the secret of health? They cannot have the latest sanitary appliances. They cannot take baths . . . or have constant change of clothing; they cannot secure that the streets shall be swept, or, as the inhabitants of Belgrave Square, protect themselves from the neighbourhood of a tallow-factory.

Barnett went on to mention the occupational hazards the poor faced and concluded that 'the poor, by bad air, by dirt, by accident, cannot live out half their days. The good news about health which science preaches to the rich is not preached to them.'[46] As we have seen, the statistics gathered by Rowntree indicated that almost one half of the residents of York did not earn enough money to keep themselves, as Rowntree put it, 'in a state of bare physical efficiency' and at the outbreak of the First World War probably one-third of all wage-earners in England and Wales were below Rowntree's poverty line. These figures simply underscored how far England had yet to go before she became 'a nation of good animals'.[47]

The awareness of poverty and its significance for the nation's health and strength served as a warning against complacency and a spur for future efforts. That life, despite the rapid growth of towns and the population as a whole, was no worse and in several respects considerably better than at any time in the nineteenth century, or that it was a healthier, more comfortable life than that for workers in the other industrialized countries of Europe, hardly alters the basic facts. Nor did it make them any more palatable to the reformers of the age. Fortunately men and women of compassion and sensitivity do not accept an undesirable *status quo* merely because prior conditions or conditions in other countries are worse. Private philanthropy, state, municipal, and local government action, the economy itself in the form of a higher standard of living, had all achieved much. So much, in fact, that the expectation in 1900 was that both the general and infant death rates would decline and that the general health standards of the poorest, as well as of other members of the community, would rise. It was to translating that expectation, via state and municipal policy, into reality, that the generation which followed the Victorians, a generation cruelly interrupted by war, dedicated themselves.

Notes

Unless otherwise stated, place of publication is London

Chapter One. 'The Setting'

1 Information on the Royal Family is from E. Longford, *Queen Victoria. Born to Succeed* (N.Y., 1964). For the state of the Thames, see *PP.XXXIII* (1867), 'First Report, RCRP (Thames)', p. 19. For pollution from the cement factory see *PP.XXV* (1920), 'Interim Report of the Committee on Smoke and Noxious Vapours Abatement', p.3.

2 For two excellent recent books see F. B. Smith, *The People's Health, 1830–1910* (1979) and B. Haley, *The Healthy Body and Victorian Culture* (Cambridge, Mass., 1978).

3 Rev C. Girdlestone, *Letters on the Unhealthy Condition of the Lower Classes of Dwellings, especially in Large Towns* (1845), pp. 4, 63.

4 J. Burnett, *A Social History of Housing, 1815–1970* (Newton Abbot, 1978), pp. 6–7, 139.

5 R. W. Breach and R. M. Hartwell, *British Economy and Society, 1870–1970* (1972). Table V, p. 378.

6 B. R. Mitchell and P. Deane, *Abstract of British Historical Statistics* (Cambridge, 1962), pp. 24–26.

7 C. Lock and J. Stephenson, eds., *Longman's Atlas of Modern British History* (1978), pp. 94–95.

8 *Ibid.*, p. 95.

9 F. Engels, *The Condition of the Working Classes in England* (1842), trans. W. O. Henderson and W. H. Chaloner (Oxford, 1958), pp. 105–106.

10 H. Gavin, *The Unhealthiness of London and the Necessity of Remedial Measures* (1847), p. 20. Gavin was Lecturer in Forensic Medicine at Charing Cross Hospital.

11 *Lancet*, 5 August 1843, p. 661.

12 The bias and preoccupations of the statisticians have been superbly analyzed by M. J. Cullen, *The Statistical Movement in Early Victorian Britain* (Brighton, 1975). See also J. M. Eyler, *Victorian Social Medicine. The Ideas and Methods of William Farr* (Baltimore, 1979) and J. M Eyler, 'Mortality Statistics and Victorian Health Policy: Program and Criticism', *Bulletin of the History of Medicine*, 50, 3

343

(Fall, 1976), for a much more sympathetic treatment of Farr's methods; see for example *Victorian Social Medicine*, pp. 193–4.

13 *Public Health*, VII, 86 (June, 1895), p. 321

14 K. J. Fielding, ed., *The Speeches of Charles Dickens* (1960), p. 128. This was in a speech commemorating the first anniversary of the Metropolitan Sanitary Association, 10 May 1851.

15 *Transactions of the Sanitary Institute of Great Britain* (1874), p. 274.

16 C. Kingsley, 'Great Cities and their Influence for Good and Evil', *Miscellanies*, II (1860), pp. 321, 328.

17 Lord Shaftesbury, *The Labourers' Friend*, July 1853, p. 100, quoted in N. Pope, *Dickens and Charity* (New York, 1978), p. 200.

18 R. Bickersteth, quoted in *ibid.*, p. 212.

19 What, he asked, were a few hours in some ragged school compared with the 'noxious, constant, ever-renewed lesson' of life in the slums. C. Dickens, 10 May 1851, in Fielding, *The Speeches of Charles Dickens*, p. 129.

20 Gavin, *The Unhealthiness of London*, pp. 65–66.

21 *Ibid.*, p. 34. My italics. Eyler, in his *Victorian Social Medicine*, stresses the passion and cautious optimism of William Farr at the Registrar-General's Office and regards him in this respect, as in others, as the epitome of 'Victorian socio-medical liberalism', p. 201.

22 *Public Health*, IX, 10 (January 1897), p. 286.

Chapter Two. 'The Massacre of the Innocents'

1 Throughout the book the phrases 'infant death rate' and 'infant mortality rate' refer to deaths in the 0–12 month age group, and are expressed in deaths per thousand live births.

2 An analysis of the infant death rate can 'be of great help in determining the significance of social causes (such as inadequate housing, food, and health services) in the evolution of ill-health', S. Leff, *Social Medicine* (1953), p. 82.

3 PP. XIV (1904), 'Sixty-fifth Annual Report of the Registrar-General, Pt. 1, 1904', p. xxxiv.

4 In the last quarter of the century the general death rate fell by eight per cent but the infant death rate declined by only one per cent, see G. Newman, *Infant Mortality. A Social Problem* (1906), pp. 2–3. *Public Health*, VI, 66 (October 1893), p. 18.

5 PP. XXXII (1904), 'Inter-Departmental Committee on Physical Deterioration. I. Report', p. xxxiv.

6 W. P. D. Logan, 'Mortality in England and Wales from 1848 to 1947', *Population Studies*, IV (1950–1), p. 169.

7 PP. XVII (1864) 'Twenty-fifth Annual Report of the Registrar-General, Supplement 1864', p. 11. Smith, *The People's Health*, p. 66.

In 1892 Preston's infant death rate was 227, Leicester's was 214, Blackburn's was 204. Prussia at that time had an infant death rate of 220, France of 216: see *Public Health*, VI, 66 (October 1893), p. 2, *ibid.*, III, 40 (August 1891), p. 500; *Annual Report of the MOH to the London County Council*, 1892, p. 10 and *PP*. XXXII (1913), 'Forty-second ARLGB, Supplement "In Continuation of the Report of the MOH . . . ." ' Dublin in 1898 had an infant death rate of 245.8, *PP*. XXXVII (1902), 'Supplement to the Twenty-ninth Annual Report of the Local Government Board for Ireland, 1900–1901, "Reports on the Sanitary Circumstances and Administration of Cities and Towns in Ireland" ', p. 5. As late as 1931–5 both Bombay and Calcutta had an infant death rate of over 250, see G. Z. Johnson, 'Health Conditions in Rural and Urban Areas of Developing Countries', *Population Studies*, XVII, Pt. 3 (March 1964), p. 295.

8 Smith, *The People's Health*, p. 67; *PP*. VII (1871), 'Select Committee on the Protection of Infant Life. Report', p. 170; J. D. J. Havard, *The Detection of Secret Homicide* (1960), pp. 64, 75; G. F. McCleary, *The Early History of the Infant Welfare Movement* (1933), p. 89.

9 Smith, *The People's Health*, p. 69. The infant death rate for illegitimate babies could approach 90 per cent or more: in Sheffield in the mid-1870s it was 582 compared to 162 for legitimate babies, *ibid.*, p. 70.

10 *Public Health*, VI, 66 (October, 1893), p. 20, and Newman, *Infant Mortality*, p. 6.

11 The devastating effect of an unhealthy environment was clearly revealed in the Registrar-General's figures. In the first month of life the infant death rate in Liverpool was roughly 45 per cent lower in a selected group of 'healthy districts' than for the town as a whole. By the eleventh month it was 400 per cent lower. *Ibid.*, pp. 39, 181.

12 R. Roberts, *The Classic Slum. Salford Life in the First Quarter of the Century* (1971), p. 109. See also D. J. Oddy, 'A Nutritional Analysis of Historical Evidence: the Working-Class Diet, 1800–1914', in D. J. Oddy and D. Miller, eds., *The Making of the Modern British Diet* (1976), p. 220. The effects of nutrition upon health in general are examined in the next chapter.

13 For rickets see the next chapter. For Maryland see H. Birch and J. Gussow, *Disadvantaged Children* (New York, 1970), p. 149.

14 Smith, *The People's Health*, p. 177. It was claimed in 1910 that children raised in a single-roomed flat were, at age fourteen some 21.3″ and 4.7lbs below the national average for height and weight, *ibid.*, pp. 75, 118, 178. The World Health Organization has found that babies born to mothers suffering from malnutrition may be partially deficient in iron, calcium, iodine, and many vitamins, see World Health Organization, *Technical Report Series* (1967), no. 377, 'Joint FAO/WHO Expert Committee on Nutrition', p. 20.

15 Birch and Gussow, *Disadvantaged Children*, pp. 95–7, 118. See also J. Boget, G. Briggs, and D. Calloway, *Nutrition and Physical Fitness*

(Philadelphia, 1973), p. 38. World Health Organization, *Technical Report Series* (1970), no. 457, 'The Prevention of Perinatal Mortality and Morbidity', p. 15.

16 *PP.* XXI (1843) 'Fifth Annual Report of the Registrar-General (1843), appendix' p. 185. See also *PP.* XVII (1864) 'Twenty-fifth Annual Report of the Registrar-General, supplement 1864, p. 190; Smith, *The People's Health*, p. 13. The maternal death rate was six per thousand births in 1847, 4.9 in 1871 and 4.03 in 1903, *ibid.*

17 J. Donnison, 'The Development of the Profession on Midwife in England, from 1750 to 1902', London University, Ph.D thesis (1974), p. 21.

18 For childbirth practices see *ibid.*, and J. Miller, ' "Temple and Sewer": Childbirth, Prudery and Victoria Regina', in A. S. Wohl, ed., *The Victorian Family: Structure and Stresses* (1978), and Smith, *The People's Health*, chapter 1. Despite Queen Victoria's use of chloroform (it was called chloroform *à la reine*), there were many doctors who continued to agree with Sir Anthony Carlisle that 'it is always mischievous to tamper with pregnant women, under the pretence of hastening, easing, or retarding the most portentous and delicate work of the creation', *Lancet*, 5 May 1827, p. 146.

19 *PP.* XX (1873) 'Thirty-fourth Annual Report of the Registrar-General (Abstracts of 1871), supplement, "Report of the Infant Mortality Committee of the Obstetrical Society of London, 1870" ', pp. 225–6. Donnison, 'The Development of the Profession of Midwife, p. 108. J. M. Kerr, R. W. Johnstone and M. H. Phillips, *Historical Review of British Obstetrics and Gynaecology* (Edinburgh, 1954), p. 6; P. Horn, *The Victorian Country Child* (Kineton, 1974), p. 1.

20 Donnison, 'The Development of the Profession of Midwife', pp. 136–7; T. Forbes, 'The Regulation of English Midwives in the Eighteenth and Nineteenth Centuries, *Medical History*, XV (October 1971), p. 358.

21 *PP.* XX (1873) 'Thirty-fourth Annual Report of the Registrar-General, supplement, "Report of the Infant Mortality Committee" ', pp. 226, 407.

22 Quoted in Forbes, *Medical History*, XV (October, 1971), p. 355.

23 Mrs Layton, 'Memories of Seventy Years', in M. L. Davies, ed., *Life as We have Known it, by Co-operative Working Women* (New York, 1975), pp. 43ff. See *ibid.*, p. 45 for an excellent account of the nerve-wracking examination for the midwives' certificate.

24 *PP.* XXXIX (1914), 'Forty-third ARLGB, Supplement, "Infant Mortality in Lancashire" ', p. 88.

25 *PP.* XXV (1914–16), 'Forty-fourth ARLGB Supplement, "Report on Maternal Mortality in Connection with Childbearing and its relation to Infant Mortality" ', *passim*.

26 Although the Local Government Board suspected that rural perinatal deaths were due partly to the low standard of rural midwifery, it

realized that the government preferred to leave the organization and regulation of most aspects of the medical profession to the doctors themselves.

27 For the incompetence of doctors and conditions in lying-in hospitals see Smith, *The People's Health*, chapter 1.

28 For a splendid analysis of the coroners see Havard, *The Detection of Secret Homicide*. In 1903 Newman stated that prematurity and congenital diseases accounted between them for over 19 per cent of all infant deaths, Newman, *Infant Mortality*, p. 46.

29 G. F. Gibberd, *A Short Textbook of Midwifery* (1960), p. 563.

30 Smith, *The People's Health*, p. 67. See also J. M. Tanner, *Growth at Adolescence* (Oxford, 1955), p. 131.

31 J. Fredrick and A. Anderson, 'Factors Associated with Spontaneous Pre-term Birth', *British Journal of Obstetrics and Gynaecology*, 83 (May, 1976), pp. 342ff.

32 *Ibid.*, pp. 344–5. During the siege of Leningrad in the Second World War 40 per cent of all births were premature and the rate of still-births increased by 56 per cent, see Boget, Briggs and Calloway, *Nutrition and Physical Fitness*, p. 444.

33 Newman, *Infant Mortality*, p. 220. See also Eyler, *Victorian Social Medicine*, p. 157.

34 Mrs B. Drake, 'A Study of Infant Life in Westminster', *Journal of the Statistical Society of London*, LXXI (1908), quoted in Smith, *The People's Health*, p. 125.

35 W. Radcliffe, *Milestones in Midwifery* (Bristol, 1967), p. 96. Hence, for example, small or deformed pelvises were detected too late.

36 *PP.* XX (1873) 'Thirty-fourth Annual Report of the Registrar-General supplement (Abstracts of 1871), "Report of the Infant Mortality Committee" ', p. 228.

37 Quoted in H. Siebert, 'The Progress of Ideas Regarding the Causation and Control of Infant Mortality', *Bulletin of the History of Medicine*, VIII, 4 (April 1940), p. 552.

38 Newsholme, *Public Health*, III, 29 (September 1890), p. 135; *ibid.*, III, 40 (August 1891), p. 508.

39 A. F. Harris [MOH, Sunderland], *Transactions of the Sanitary Institute of Great Britain*, IV (1882–3), p. 122.

40 Horn, *The Victoruan Country Child*, p. 171.

41 *Transactions of the Sanitary Institute of Great Britain*, XIX (1898), p. 437.

42 Smith, *The People's Health*, p. 109.

43 *Transactions of the Sanitary Institute of Great Britain*, IV (1882–3), p. 123.

44 *Ibid*, I (1879), p. 283.

45 *Public Health*, VI, 66 (October 1893), p. 19.

46 Newman, *Infant Mortality*, table, p. 46.

47 Child Poverty Action Group, *Must These Babies Die of Cold?* (1976).

48 Birch and Gussow, *Disadvantaged Children*, p. 179.

49 World Health Organization, *Technical Report Series* (1970), no 457, 'The Prevention of Perinatal Mortality and Morbidity', pp. 8, 9. See also A. Burgess and R. F. A. Dean, eds., *Malnutrition and Food Habits* (1962), p. 3: 'the chief cause [of infant mortality] is the combination of disease and malnutrition, the one precipitating and perpetuating the other'. See also Oddy in Oddy and Miller, eds., *The Making of the Modern British Diet*, p. 229.

50 For commercial baby food see *PP*. XXXII (1913), 'Forty-second ARLGB, Supplement, "Second Report on Infant and Child Mortality" ', p. 87.

51 *PP*. XXVII. 2 (1862), 'Fourth ARMOHPC, for 1861, appendix five, "Report by Dr E. Greenhow on the Circumstances under which there is an Excessive Mortality of Young Children among certain Manufacturing Populations" ', p. 194. Smith, *The People's Health*, p. 83, and see pp. 83ff., for a splendid discussion of feeding practices.

52 *PP*. XXVIII (1864), 'Sixth ARMOHPC, for 1863, appendix fourteen, "Excessive Mortality of Infants" ', p. 458.

53 *PP*. XXXII (1904), 'Inter-Departmental Committee on Physical Deterioration. I. Report', p. 57; Smith, *The People's Health*, p. 83.

54 *PP*. XXXIX (1914), 'Forty-third ARLGB, for 1913–14', pp. 20ff.; Smith, *The People's Health*, pp. 84–85.

55 R. M. Goldblum, *et al*, 'Antibody-forming cells in human colostrum after oral immunization', *Nature*, 257, 5529 (30 October 1975), p. 797.

56 *PP*. XXXVII (1878), 'Seventh ARLGB, for 1877–8', p. xliv; *PP*. XXVIII (1883), 'Twelfth ARLGB, for 1882–3', p. cvi; *PP*. XXXVII (1899), 'Twenty-eighth ARLGB, for 1898', p. cxxxiii (the figure was 9.9 per cent). See also Smith, *The People's Health*, p. 214.

57 In Newcastle, for example, about one-third of all the milk in 1895 came from the town's seventy-three cowsheds, see J. C. Drummond and A. Wilbraham, *The Englishman's Food* (1950), p. 300.

58 *PP*. XXXII (1904), 'Inter-Departmental Committee on Physical Deterioration. I. Report', p. 52; see also *Public Health*, XIII, 12 (September 1901), pp. 82ff.

59 Smith, *The People's Health*, pp. 212, 214.

60 *PP*. XXXII (1904), 'Inter-Departmental Committee on Physical Deterioration. I. Report', p. 53; Smith, *The People's Health*, p. 214, Public Health, XIII, 12 (September 1901), pp. 820, 826ff.

61 Smith, *The People's Health*, p. 114; Drummond and Wilbraham, *The Englishman's Food*, pp. 377, 379.

62 Smith, *The People's Health*, pp. 88, 374. Even india-rubber teats were difficult to clean, see *PP*. XXXII (1904), 'Inter-Departmental Committee on Physical Deterioration. I. Report', p. 53.

63 H. Ashby, 'Infant Feeding in Relation of Infant Mortality', Manchester and Salford Sanitary Association, *Health Lectures for the People*, V (1881–2), pp. 79, 86.

64 *PP*. XXV (1889), 'Supplement in Continuation of the Report of the Medical Officer [of the Local Government Board], for 1877. . . .'

65 Newman, *Infant Mortality*, p. 19. G. F. McCleary, *The Early History of the Infant Welfare Movement* (1933), p. 24.

66 Or 13.9 per cent of all deaths of infants. First was prematurity and congenital diseases accounting for 19.1 per cent or over 23,000 deaths, see Newman, *Infant Mortality*, p. 46. The diarrhoeal death rate is probably an underestimate as the category did not include deaths from 'atrophy' and 'debility' after diarrhoea, see Smith, *The People's Health*, p. 87.

67 M. W. Beaver, 'Population, Infant Mortality and Milk', *Population Studies*, XXVII, Pt. 2 (July 1973), p. 251.

68 For contemporary medical views on breast and bottle feeding see Smith, *The People's Health*, pp. 90–95. Charles Creighton in his *A History of Epidemics in Britain*, II (1894), p. 767, was much more cautious than most, for while he saw the dangers of bottle feeding, he argued that many of the babies who succumbed to infantile diarrhoea were in a generally weak condition and if they had survived it would have been as weak and rickety children.

69 Newman, *Infant Mortality*, pp. 238, 242.

70 *Public Health*, XII, 9 (June 1900), p. 679.

71 For Preston see *ibid*., VII, 82 (February 1895), p. 172; for Birmingham, *ibid*., VI, 66 (October 1893), p. 19; for Liverpool, *ibid*., XI, 6 (March 1899), p. 435; for Brighton, Newman, *Infant Mortality*, p. 251; for Leeds, Smith, *The People's Health*, p. 100. See also *PP*. XXXII (1904), 'Inter-Departmental Committee on Physical Deterioration. I. Report', p. 50.

72 *PP*. XXXIX (1914), 'Forty-third ARLGB, Supplement, "In Continuation of a Report by the MOH of the Board for 1913–14, containing a Third Report on Infant Mortality. . ." ', pp. 9, 124, 134. See also *PP*. XXXII (1913), 'Forty-second ARLGB, "Supplement to the Report of the MOH of the Board, 1912–13, containing a Second Report on Infant and Child Mortality" ', pp. 59, 82ff.

73 Newman, *Infant Mortality*, p. 247.

74 *Public Health*, VII, 79 (November 1894), p. 163. See also *Transactions of the Sanitary Institute of Great Britain*, (1897), p. 85.

75 *PP*. XXVIII (1864), 'Sixth ARMOHPC, for 1863, appendix fourteen, "Excessive Mortality of Infants" ', p. 458.

76 World Health Organization, *Technical Report Series*, 1965, no. 314, 'Nutrition and Infection', and *ibid*., 1967, no. 377 'Joint FAO/WHO Expert Committee on Nutrition'.

77 *PP*. XXIX (1860), 'Second ARMOHPC', for 1859', p. 64; *PP*. XXVII (1862), 'Fourth ARMOHPC, for 1861", p. 33; J. Simon, *English Sanitary Institution* (1890), p. 298.

78 For awareness of the complexities of the issue, see *PP*. XXXIX (1914), 'Forty-third ARLGB, for 1913–14, Supplement ". . . infant mortality" '.

79 *Public Health*, III, 40 (August 1891), p. 500; *PP.* XXXIII (1864), 'Eighth ARMOHPC, for 1867', p. 179.

80 *Lancet*, 6 November 1875, p. 680, my italics. See also *ibid.*, 23 October 1875.

81 *PP.* XXXII (1913), 'Forty-second ARLGB, Supplement ". . . Child Mortality" ', p. 89.

82 *PP.* XXXII (1904), 'Inter-Departmental Committee on Physical Deterioration. I. Report', p. 29.

83 Manchester and Salford Sanitary Association, *Health of the People* (1875–76), I, p. 158. For Lord Shaftesbury, see M. Hewitt, *Wives and Mothers in Victorian Industry* (1958), p. 10, and for Mrs Ranyard, see W. C. Dowling, 'The Ladies' Sanitary Association and the Origins of the Health Visiting Service', London University, MA thesis (1963), pp. 84ff.

84 Dr Reid, 'Infant Mortality and Female Labour', Liverpool Congress of the Royal Sanitary Institute, 1893. Reid offered the generalization that where married women worked the infant death rate was some 28 per cent higher, see also Smith, *The People's Health*, p. 95.

85 *Public Health*, X, 124 (August 1898), p. 377.

86 *PP.* XXXII (1913), 'Forty-second ARLGB, Supplement, "Second Report . . . Infant and Child Mortality" ', p. 73. This survey followed one conducted in 1910 which covered rural counties.

87 *Ibid.*, p. 57.

88 *Ibid.*, p. 65. Low summer temperatures were important in keeping down summer diarrhoea.

89 Leicester, for example, at the end of the century had 6,700 pails, 11,000 ashpits, 17,000 ash-bins, and only 13,000 w.cs, *Public Health*, VII, 85 (May 1895) p. 281.; see also *PP.* XXXIX (1914), 'Forty-third ARLGB, for 1913–14, Supplement, "Third Report . . . Infant Mortality" ', pp. 12ff.

90 *Ibid.*, p. 20. Another study at the end of the century of 124 Preston cotton mill female workers revealed that two went back within a month; thirty-eight within one to two months, forty-two within two to three months, and thirty-four between six and twelve months. Two did not return, see Newman, *Infant Mortality*, p. 124.

91 *PP.* XXXIX (1914), 'Forty-third ARLGB, for 1913–14, Supplement, "Third Report . . . Infant Mortality" ', pp. 12ff. There were considerable regional differences: in Dundee and Preston, two towns with high infant mortality rates, the jute, hemp, and cotton mill girls worked longer into their pregnancies – 14 per cent up to one week before delivery – than the better-paid textile workers of Paisley, *ibid*.

92 *PP.* XXV (1914–16), 'Forty-fourth ARLGB, for 1914–16, Supplement, "Report on Maternal Mortality in connection with Childbearing and its relation to Infant Mortality" ', p. 56. See also Mrs Wrigley, 'A Plate-Layer's Wife', in Davies, ed., *Life as We Have Known It*, p. 61. For a rare comment on the effect of hard work upon pregnancy see H.

Jones, *Journal of the Statistical Society of London*, 54 (March 1894), p. 4, 'premature birth [is] associated it would seem with the employment of young married women in industrial occupations.'

93 *Transactions of the Sanitary Institute of Great Britain*, IV (1882–3), p. 128.

94 Hewitt, *Working Wives*, p. 135. *PP*. XXV (1863), 'Fifth ARMOHPC, appendix five "Dr Buchanan, Report Relating to the Sanitary Condition of the Cotton Towns of Lancashire and Cheshire" ', p. 304. *PP*. XXXIX (1914), 'Forty-third ARLGB, for 1913–14, Supplement, ". . . Infant Mortality" ', p. 128.

95 Hewitt, *Working Wives*, pp. 171ff.

96 As early as 1862 John Simon had seen the economic aspects of the problem – 'at the root of the evil [of working mothers] is an influence with which English law has never professed to deal. Money is on one side; penury on the other. Domestic obligation is outbidden in the labour market.' His solution was to establish factory nurseries. *PP*. XXVII (1862), 'Fourth ARMOHPC, for 1861', p. 35.

97 *Transactions of the Sanitary Institute of Great Britain*, XV (1894), p. 507.

98 *PP*. VII (1871), 'Select Committee on Infant Life. II. Minutes of Evidence', p. 153. Manchester and Salford Sanitary Association, *Health Lectures for the People*, III, (1879–80) p. 137. In this respect France was far more advanced than England.

99 Quoted in A. Redford, *The History of Local Government in Manchester* (1939), III, p. 136.

100 *Transactions of the National Association for the Promotion of Social Science*, 1874, pp. 574, 577, W. Cooke Taylor. Miss Todd, *ibid.*, p. 589.

101 *Transactions of the Sanitary Institute of Great Britain*, XV (1894), p. 500; *PP*. XXXII (1904), 'Inter-Departmental Committee on Physical Deterioration. II. Minutes of Evidence, p. 147.

102 D. E. Forsythe, 'The Evolution of Child Welfare Services in England and Wales', *Journal of the Royal Institute of Public Health and Hygiene*, 29 (January-December 1966), p. 161. For Dufour's clinic and Pierre Budin's work at the Charité Hospital, and for American milk depots, see McCleary, *The Early History of the Infant Welfare Movement*, pp. 70ff. See also B. D. White, *A History of the Corporation of Liverpool, 1835–1914* (Liverpool, 1951), p. 124.

103 At Battersea the cost of milk was 3d a day for infants under six months, and 4d a day for infants between six and twelve months; *Lancet*, 2 August 1902, McCleary, *The Early History of the Infant Welfare Movement*, p. 126.

104 Smith, *The People's Health*, p. 114.

105 *PP*. XXVII (1864), 'Sixth ARMOHPC, for 1863 appendix fourteen, "Dr Hunter . . . Excessive Mortality of Infants" ', p. 457. The best account is in Havard, *The Detection of Secret Homicide*. See also *PP*., XXVII. 2 (1862), 'Fourth ARMOHPC, for 1861, appendix five, "Report by Dr E. Greenhow . . ." '.

106 Havard. *The Detection of Secret Homicide*, p. 52.

107 Quoted in *ibid*., p. 61. *Lancet*, 14 September 1861, p. 256.

108 *Public Health*, VII, 82 (February 1895), p. 164.

109 *Ibid*.

110 *Transactions of the Sanitary Institute of Great Britain*, IV (1882–3), p. 126; *ibid*., XXI (1900), p. 177, Horn, *The Victorian Country Child*, p. 169; *Public Health*, VI, 77 (September 1894), p. 425. Newman, *Infant Mortality*, pp. 210–211. *British Medical Journal*, 5 December 1903, p. 1471.

111 *Ibid. Public Health*, VI, 77 (September, 1894), p. 429. The Children Act, 1908, made a drunken parent who slept with a child under three, who subsequently died of suffocation, liable for its death.

112 Sudden Infant Death Syndrome is still a mystery, although recently the bacterium clostridium botulinum has been identified as having some possible connection. For an interesting analysis see T. L. Savitt, 'Smothering and Overlaying of Virginia Slave Children: a Suggested Explanation', *Bulletin of the History of Medicine*, 49, 3 (Fall 1975).

113 Havard, *The Detection of Secret Homicide*, pp. 55ff.; *PP*. VII (1871), 'Select Committee on Infant Life', p. 102.

114 *PP*. XXVII. 2 (1862), 'Fourth ARMOHPC, for 1861, appendix five "Report by Dr E. Greenhow. . . ." ', p. 195. In Coventry twelve druggists sold over ten gallons of Godfrey's Cordial weekly, *ibid*. See also Smith, *The People's Health*, p. 97.

115 E. Lomax, 'The Uses and Abuses of Opiates in Nineteenth-Century England', *Bulletin of the History of Medicine*, XLVII, I (January-February 1973), p. 169.

116 *PP*. XXVIII (1864), 'Sixth ARMOHPC, for 1863', p. 81. Norfolk and Lincolnshire between them consumed half of the opium imported into the country in 1867, Horn, *The Victorian Country Child*, p. 169.

117 *PP*. XXVIII (1864), 'Sixth ARMOHPC, for 1863, appendix fourteen "Dr Hunter, Excessive Mortality of Infants" ', pp. 459–460.

118 Lomax, *Bulletin of the History of Medicine*, XLVII, I (January-February 1973), p. 168. See also Smith, *The People's Health*, p. 96. Mrs Beeton felt that 'unprincipled nurses' gave 'deadly narcotics' to their charges to ensure for themselves 'a night of many unbroken hours', I. Beeton, *The Book of Household Management* (1861, facsimile ed. 1968), pp. 1032–1033.

119 *PP*. XXVII. 2 (1862) 'Fourth ARMOHPC, for 1861, appendix five, "Report by Dr Greenhow. . . ." ', p. 195.

120 Havard, *The Detection of Secret Homicide*, p. 53.

121 *PP*. XXVII. 2 (1862), 'Fourth ARMOHPC, for 1861, appendix five, "Report by Dr Greenhow. . . ." ', p. 195.

122 Lomax, *Bulletin of the History of Medicine*, XLVII, I (January-February 1973), p. 171. *PP*. XXVIII (1864), 'Sixth ARMOHPC, for 1863, appendix fourteen, "Dr Hunter, Excessive Mortaility of Infants" ', p. 460.

123 Lomax, *Bulletin of the History of Medicine*, XLVII, I (January-February 1973), p. 174.

124 The medical profession was divided on the issue of the dangers of opium; the lucrative opium import trade stood to lose by controls, and the Pharmaceutical Society was reluctant to see its equally lucrative retail distribution of opium affected by the reclassification of the drug, *ibid.*, pp. 173ff.

125 Roberts, *The Classic Slum*, p. 126.

126 Smith, *The People's Health*, p. 98.

127 Lomax, *Bulletin of the History of Medicine*, XLVII, I (January-February 1973), p. 169.

128 *Transactions of the National Association for the Promotion of Social Science*, 1866, p. 583.

129 Dowling, 'The Ladies' Sanitary Association', pp. 84ff.

130 Ladies' Sanitary Association, *Tracts*, (n.d.) 'The Sick Child's Cry and Other Household Verses on Health, Happiness and Ventilation'.

131 Dowling, 'The Ladies' Sanitary Association', *passim. Transactions of the Sanitary Institute of Great Britain*, XIX, 1898, p. 435. The obstetrician was Thomas Turner.

132 The officers of the National Society for the Prevention of Cruelty to Children were, for example, generally well received. For conflicting evidence see Smith, *The People's Health*, pp. 116–117.

133 See the next chapter, pp. 67–9.

134 In 1907 the City of Westminster Health Society made over 10,000 visits and inspected over 2,000 children, see Smith, *The People's Health*, p. 115.

135 *Transactions of the Sanitary Institute of Great Britain*, XIX (1898), pp. 567–8; *ibid.* XX (1899), p. 238, and *Public Health*, III, 29 (September 1890), p. 135.

136 F. Petty, *The Pudding Lady* (1910), p. 20.

137 Dowling, 'The Ladies' Sanitary Association', p. 84.

138 *PP.* XXXII (1913), 'Forty-second ARLGB, for 1912–13', pp. iii–iv.

139 *Ibid*, 'Supplement, "Second Report on Infant and Child Mortality" ', p. 56. The MOH for Stoke-on-Trent and Blackburn thought that the loss of earnings would be detrimental to the health of the children, *Transactions of the Sanitary Institute of Great Britain* (1894), pp. 565–6. See Eyler, *Victorian Social Medicine*, pp. 152–3 for the connection, which Farr recognized, between a low birth rate and a low death rate.

140 Scotland's infant death rate was 126, Ireland's 103, Newman, *Infant Mortality*, appendix, p. 328.

141 *Ibid.*

142 Ballard, quoted in *ibid.*, p. 16.

143 *PP.* XXXII (1913), 'Forty-second ARLGB, for 1912–13, supplement, "Second Report on Infant and Child Mortality" ', p. 73. Newman, *Infant Mortality*, p. 177.

144 Even today there is a considerable difference in infant death rates between the classes, see Leff, *Social Medicine*, p. 89, and M. Lerner, 'Social Differences in Physical Health', in J. Kosa and I. Zola, eds., *Poverty and Health* (Cambridge, Mass., 1975), table III, p. 108. The map is taken from *PP*. XXXII (1913), 'Forty-second ARLGB, for 1912–13, supplement, "Second Report on Infant and Child Mortality" ', p. 18. See also Smith, *The People's Health*, p. 69.

145 *PP*. XXVII. 2 (1862), 'Fourth ARMOHPC, for 1861, appendix five, "Report by Dr Greenhow. . . ." ', p. 192. Simon, quoted in Newman, *Infant Mortality*, p. 96.

146 A. James and N. Hill, eds., *Mrs John Brown, 1847–1935* (1937), pp. 52–3.

147 A. S. Jasper, *A Hoxton Childhood* (1969), p. 14.

148 S. Reynolds, *A Poor Man's House* (1908, reprinted 1980), pp. 71, 74. For the similar grief of a working-class mother and her determination to give her baby a proper funeral, see [T. Wright], 'The Riverside Visitor', *The Pinch of Poverty. Sufferings and Heroism of the London Poor* (1892), pp. 269ff.

Chapter Three.. 'Tolerable Human Types'

1 P. Deane and W. A. Cole, *British Economic Growth, 1688–1959* (Cambridge, 1962), pp. 27–8. Using a base figure of 100 for 1850, real wages, adjusted for unemployment were: 132 (1877–1880), 142 (1883–1886), and 184 (1900), *ibid.*, table 7, p. 25.

2 G. Barnsby, 'The Standard of Living in the Black Country during the Nineteenth Century', *Economic History Review*, 2nd Series, XXIV, 2 (1971), p. 223. For an interesting criticism see C. Griffen, 'The Standard of Living in the Black Country in the Nineteenth Century: a comment', *ibid.*, XXVI, 3 (1973). See also D. Blythell, 'The History of the Poor', *English Historical Review*, 89 (April 1974), p. 372.

3 T. L. Richardson, 'The Agricultural Labourer's Standard of Living in Kent, 1790–1840', in Oddy and Miller, eds., *The Making of the Modern British Diet*, pp. 108–11.

4 R. Newton, *Victorian Exeter, 1837–1914* (Leicester, 1968), pp. 149–50.

5 A. T. McCabe, 'The Standard of Living on Merseyside, 1850–1875', in S. P. Bell, ed., *Victorian Lancashire* (Newton Abbot, 1974), pp. 141–7. Using a base figure of 100 for real wages in 1850, McCabe argues that throughout much of the period he studied real wages did not rise above the upper 70s.

6 These estimates are drawn from Charles Booth, see A. S. Wohl, *The Eternal Slum. Housing and Social Policy in Victorian London* (1977), pp. 312, 315.

7 *PP*. LXXXI (1887), 'Tabulations of Statements made by men living in Certain Selected Districts of London in March, 1887', p. 34. For casual labour see G. Stedman Jones, *Outcast London. A Study of the Relationship Between Classes in Victorian Society* (1971).

8 B. S. Rowntree, *Poverty. A Study of Town Life* (1901), pp. 133, 135, quoted in Oddy and Miller, eds., *The Making of the Modern British Diet*, pp. 215–16.

9 *PP*. CVIII (1912–13), 'Report of an Enquiry by the Board of Trade into the Earnings and Hours of Labour of Workpeople of the United Kingdom', p. 28, quoted in *ibid.*, p. 215.

10 *Lancet*, 10 March 1832, p. 827. For an interesting general discussion of the various factors involved in poverty and their connection with disease, see B. Luckin, 'Death and Survival in the City: approaches to the history of disease', *Urban History Yearbook*, 1980 (Leicester, 1980).

11 A. Ciocco and D. Perrott, 'Statistics on Sickness as a Cause of Poverty. An Historical Review of U.S. and English Data', *Journal of the History of Medicine and Allied Sciences*, XII (January 1957), pp. 45–6.

12 Quoted in *ibid.*, pp. 57–8; For York, *ibid.*, p. 53.

13 This is dealt with at some length in R. Hodgkinson, *The Origins of the National Health Service*, (1967).

14 For this awareness in Scotland see especially, G. Bell, *Day and Night in the Wynds of Edinburgh and Blackfriars Wynd Analyzed* (1849–50, reprinted Wakefield, 1973), J. H. F. Brotherston, *Observations on the Early Public Health Movement in Scotland* (1952), and F. McKichan, 'Stirling, 1780–1880: the Response of Burgh government to the Problems of Urban Growth', University of Glasgow, M. Litt thesis. (1972).

15 Quoted in Brotherston, *Observations on the Early Public Health Movement*, p. 59.

16 *Lancet*, 1 April 1843, p. 9.

17 *Transactions of the Sanitary Institute of Great Britain*, VI (1884–5), p. 154.

18 *Ibid.*, pp. 79–80.

19 Fear of revolution as a stimulus to social reform is very important in the housing reform movement, see Wohl, *The Eternal Slum*, especially pp. 64, 65, 74, 205, 218, and 230.

20 In this, as in other things, the MOH were far more aware than either politicians or the general public.

21 J. Hollingshead, *Ragged London in 1861* (1861), pp. 282, 287.

22 *Public Health*, II, 21 (January 1890), p. 269.

23 Petty, *The Pudding Lady, passim*.

24 *PP*. XXXII (1904), 'Inter-Departmental Committee on Physical Deterioration. I. Report', p. 33.

25 Areas like Crediton in Devon, where each cottage had its own pigstye, erected at the landlord's expense, or where tenants were given grass-

land to keep a cow, such as on the estates of the Dukes of Devonshire and Derbyshire, were the exception, Horn, *The Victorian Country Child*, p. 10.

26 *PP*. XXVIII (1864), 'Sixth ARMOHPC, for 1863, appendix six, "Report by Dr Edward Smith, FRS. on the Food of the Poorer Labouring Classes in England" ', p. 248. Much of the meat was bacon, which 'may be cut up easily into small portions and fried, producing drippings for children to be eaten with dry bread . . . or making a rapid dish with greens or potatoes . . .' It also kept well, *ibid*.

27 J. Burnett, *Plenty and Want. A Social History of Diet in England from 1815 to the Present Day* (1966), p. 3.

28 Quoted in *ibid*., p. 20.

29 Quoted in *ibid*., p. 25.

30 J. Burnett, 'Country Diet', in C. E. Mingay, ed., *The Victorian Countryside*, 2 (1981), p. 561. *PP*. XXVIII (1864), 'Sixth ARMOHPC for 1863, appendix six "Report by Dr Edward Smith FRS on the Food . . ." ', p. 246.

31 G. E. Evans, *Where Beards Wag All. The Relevance of the Oral Tradition* (1970), pp. 214, 215.

32 R. Salaman, *The History and Social Influence of the Potato* (Cambridge, 1949), pp. 528, 613. The 1860s were, Burnett concludes, the last decade of 'widespread bad feeding', but 'If sheer hunger had diminished by 1900, many labourers and their families [in the country] were still undernourished, especially in the protein foods, in calcium and in several vitamins', Burnett in Mingay, ed., *The Victorian Countryside*, 2, pp. 561, 565.

33 Burnett, *Plenty and Want*, p. 96. This may seem to contradict Burnett's earlier observation, but the diet of the urban labourer was more varied.

34 Roberts, *The Classic Slum*, p. 115.

35 E. Wallace, *People. A Short Autobiography* (1926), p. 18.

36 *PP*. XXVIII (1864), 'Sixth ARMOHPC, for 1863, appendix six "Report by Dr Edward Smith FRS on the Food . . ." ', pp. 220, 232–3, 241.

37 *PP*. XXVI (1865), 'Seventh ARMOHPC, for 1864, appendix eight, "Report by Dr Buchanan upon an Epidemic of Typhus . . . Liverpool" ', p. 481.

38 Burnett, *Plenty and Want*, p. 98.

39 *Ibid*., *passim*. Oddy in Oddy and Miller, eds., *The Making of the Modern British Diet*, and Oddy, 'Food in Nineteenth Century England: Nutrition in the First Urban Society', *Proceedings of the Nutrition Society*, 29 (1970), p. 7.

40 *Ibid*., and Oddy in Oddy and Miller, eds., *The Making of the Modern British Diet*, pp. 214ff.

41 *PP*. XXXII (1904), 'Inter-Departmental Committee on Physical Deterioration. I. Report', p. 66, and *ibid*., 'II. Minutes of Evidence', p. 25. For the three surveys in London see D. Rubinstein, *School*

Attendance in London, 1870–1904: A Social History (University of Hull Occasional Papers in Economic and Social History, No. I, Hull, 1969), p. 82. In 1871 the London School Board was told that the children 'fell off the form fainting through hunger', quoted in *ibid.*, p. 81. The London School Board in 1889 estimated that one of eight children was underfed. *Ibid.*, p. 82.

42 Oddy in Oddy and Miller, eds., *The Making of the Modern British Diet*, p. 216.

43 *Ibid.*, pp. 242–3.

44 Boget, Briggs, and Calloway, *Nutrition and Physical Fitness*, pp. 34, 38.

45 *PP.* XXVIII (1864), 'Sixth ARMOHPC, for 1863, appendix six, "Report by Dr Edward Smith FRS on the Food. . . ." ', p. 249.

46 Roberts, *The Classic Slum*, p. 104. For a feminist historian's use of this material see L. Oren, 'The Welfare of Women in Labouring Families in England, 1860–1950', *Feminist Studies*, I, 3–4 (Winter-Spring, 1973), pp. 108ff.

47 Burnett, *Plenty and Want*, p. 89. For bread reform societies see Ladies' Sanitary Association, *Twenty-third Annual Report* (1881), p. 28, and Dr J. Bell, 'Food Adulteration and Analysis', *International Health Exhibition* (1884), p. 17. For the terribly unhygienic conditions in the bakehouses see Smith, *The People's Health*, pp. 208–209.

48 Burnett, *Plenty and Want*, p. 89; Smith, *The People's Health*, pp. 210–211, and Drummond and Wilbraham, *The Englishman's Food*, pp. 390, 392.

49 *PP.* XXXVII. 1 (1878), 'Seventh ARLGB. for 1877–78', *passim.*

50 See the previous chapter, pp. 21–2.

51 London County Council, *Annual Report of the MOH, for 1898*, appendix 1, 'Preparation and Sale of Food in London', pp. 6, 9.

52 *PP.* XXV (1863), 'Fifth ARMOHPC, for 1862', p. 22.

53 *Lancet*, 9 July 1831, p. 449.

54 Hassall's analyses of adulterated food had first appeared in the *Lancet* between 1851 and 1855.

55 *PP.* XXXVI (1877), 'Sixth ARLGB, for 1876–7', p. lxxix; *PP.* XXVIII (1883), 'Twelvth ARLGB, for 1882', p. civ; *PP.* XXXVII (1899) 'Twenty-eighth ARLGB, for 1898', p. cxxxiii.

56 Smith, *The People's Health*, p. 213. Street vendors did not have to be licensed until 1912 and they, of course, provided much of the food for the poorer classes, *ibid.*, p. 204.

57 See especially the World Health Organization's reports cited in the previous chapter.

58 Salaman, *The History and Social Influence of the Potato*, p. 304. In 1848, when conditions improved, typhus deaths declined to under 46,000. By 1850 the corresponding figure was 23,545, *ibid.*

59 G. Rosen, 'Disease, Debility, and Death', in H. J. Dyos and M. Wolff, eds., *The Victorian City. Images and Realities* (1973), II, p. 655. Rosen believes that Gee underestimated the incidence of rickets.

60 *Lancet*, 19 January 1889, pp. 114–15.
61 See for example, *PP*. XVIII (1864) 'Sixth ARMOHPC, for 1863, appendix six, "Report by Dr Edward Smith on the Food ..." ', pp. 251, 274, 280, 285.
62 Boget, Briggs, and Calloway, *Nutrition and Physical Fitness*, p. 200.
63 *Ibid.*, pp. 202–3.
64 Major Greenwood, *Epidemics and Crowd Diseases. An Introduction to the Study of Epidemiology* (1935), pp. 110ff.
65 Mrs Pember Reeves, *Family Life on a Pound a Week* (1912), pp. 6–7.
66 Rowntree, *Poverty*, pp. 211–212.
67 *PP*. XXXII (1904), 'Inter-Departmental Committee on Physical Deterioration. I. Report', p. 3.
68 City of Edinburgh Charity Organisation Society, *Report on the Physical Condition of Fourteen Hundred School Children in the City, together with some Account of their Homes and Surroundings* (1906), pp. 24–6.
69 C. Booth, *Life and Labour of the People of London* (1902–3), III. *Poverty*, p. 207, quoted in W. D. Smith, *Stretching their Bodies. The History of Physical Education* (Newton Abbot, 1974), p. 96.
70 *PP*. XVII (1840), 'Second Annual Report of the Registrar-General, appendix, "Letter to the Registrar-General from William Farr" ', pp. 6–7. See also B. Harrison, *Drink and the Victorians. The Temperance Question in England, 1815–1872* (1971), p. 33.
71 National Temperance League, Annual Report for 1869–70, quoted in J. H. Warner, 'Physiological Theory and Therapeutic Explanation in the 1860s: the British Debate on the Medical Use of Alcohol', *Bulletin of the History of Medicine*, 54, 2 (Summer, 1980), p. 239. For Richard Todd, the British Medical Temperance Association, and the *Temperance Lancet* see N. Longmate, *The Waterdrinkers. A History of Temperance* (1968), p. 172. One doctor prescribed 6 pints of brandy over a 72 hour period! See B. Harrison, *Drink and the Victorians*, p. 307.
72 Longmate, *The Waterdrinkers*, pp. 180–1. See also R. M. MacLeod, 'The Edge of Hope: Social Policy and Chronic Alcoholism, 1870–1900', *Journal of the History of Medicine and Allied Sciences*, XXII (July 1967).
73 In 1875 1.3 gallons of spirits and in 1876 34.4 gallons of beer were consumed *per capita* annually; at the end of the century the figures were 1.1 and 32.5, respectively, P. Mathias, 'The British Tea Trade in the Nineteenth Century', in Oddy and Miller, eds., *The Making of the Modern British Diet*, p. 98. For other figures of consumption see Harrison, *Drink and the Victorians*, pp. 61, 67, 68.
74 A. E. Dingle, 'Drink and Working-Class Living Standards in Britain, 1870–1914', in Oddy and Miller, eds., *The Making of the Modern British Diet*, p. 120.
75 The working man would be encouraged to underestimate his consumption of alcohol by an awareness of teetotal propaganda and his realiza-

tion that he must present a picture of sobriety in order to qualify for charity. Charles Booth was surprised that 'so much should have been admitted', but he also thought that much had been held back, quoted in *ibid.*, p. 122.

76   *Ibid.*, pp. 128ff. Both Booth and Rowntree thought that alcohol was a major source of secondary poverty, *ibid.*, p. 117.

77   In Glasgow alone in the late Victorian period there were some 10,000 yearly commitments for drunkenness and of 781 families selected by the Edinburgh Charity Organization Society as representative of the working classes of the city, 425 were considered 'drunken'. Scottish cities were no worse than the English in this respect. MacLeod, *Journal of the History of Medicine and Allied Sciences*, XXII (July 1967), p. 232. City of Edinburgh Charity Organisation Society, *Report on the Physical Condition*, p. 17.

78   MacLeod, *Journal of the History of Medicine and Allied Sciences*, XXII (July 1967), p. 217. Yet we should note that according to Brian Harrison 11 of the leaders of the teetotal movement also campaigned for sanitary reform, *Drink and the Victorians*, p. 175. Teetotalers of course did stress that barley was far healthier when used in puddings, soup, or bread rather than alcohol and that alcohol was not nutritious, *ibid*, pp. 121, 122.

79   Quoted in Longmate, *The Waterdrinkers*, p. 131.

80   Quoted in Newman, *Infant Mortality*, p. 196.

81   *The Labourers' Friend Magazine*, CXII (July 1840), p. 104.

82   In 1847 over 27,000 houses in Edinburgh had no piped-in water, Smith, *The People's Health*, p. 216. For Birmingham and Newcastle see W. Robson, 'The Public Utility Services', in H. J. Laski, W. Ivor Jennings, and W. A. Robson, eds., *A Century of Municipal Progress, 1835–1935* (1935), pp. 312–313.

83   F. Sheppard, *London, 1808–1870. The Great Wen* (1971), p. 262.

84   For Wolverhampton see G. A. Barnsby, 'Social Conditions in the Black Country in the Nineteenth Century', University of Birmingham, Ph.D. thesis (1969); for Hanley, W. E. Townley, 'Urban Administration and Health: A Case Study of Hanley in the Mid-Nineteenth Century', University of Keele, M.A. thesis (1969), p. 298; for London, W. A. Robson, *The Government and Misgovernment of London* (1939), p. 107; for Bristol, L. Wright, *Clean and Decent. The Fascinating History of the Bathroom and Water Closet* (1926), p. 149.

85   N. Sunderland, *A History of Darlington* (Manchester, 1972), p. 90.

86   H. Macdonald, 'Public Health Legislation and Problems in Victorian Edinburgh, with Special Reference to the Work of Dr Littlejohn as Medical Officer of Health', University of Edinburgh Ph.D thesis (1971), p. 182. Barnsby, 'Social Conditions in the Black Country', p. 110.

87   Robson, in Laski, Jennings and Robson, eds., *A Century of Municipal Progress*, pp. 316–317.

88 *PP.* LXI (1878–9), 'Return of a House of Commons Order', pp. 55–6.

89 Redford, *The History of Local Government in Manchester*, III, p. 128.

90 Smith, *The People's Health*, p. 222.

91 A. J. Archer, 'A Study of Local Administration (1830–1875)', University of Wales, Bangor, M.A. thesis (1967), p. 91. The people of Lincoln were charged 2d a day for well water, S. F. Hill, *Victorian Lincoln* (Cambridge, 1974), p. 161. In Sheerness the poor tenants of cottages let at 2s a week were paying 10d a week for water by the bucket, *PP.* XXIX (1860), 'ARMOHPC, for 1859', pp. 37, 42.

92 Leff, *Social Medicine*, p. 79.

93 Roberts, *The Classic Slum*, p. 34, T. Willis, *Whatever Happened to Tom Mix?*, (1970), pp. 6–7.

94 W. Chaloner, *The Social and Economic Development of Crewe* (Manchester, 1950), quoted p. 206.

95 E. Hall, ed., *Canary Girls and Stockpots* (Luton, 1977), p. 27.

96 Quoted in M. W. Flinn, ed., *Report on the Sanitary State of the Labouring Population of Great Britain, by Edwin Chadwick* (Edinburgh, 1965), p. 136.

97 E. H. Gibson, 'Baths and Wash-houses in the English Public Health Agitation, 1839–48', *Journal of the History of Medicine and Allied Sciences* , IX, 4 (October, 1954), p. 398.

98 L. C. Parkes, *Hygiene and Public Health* (1889), p. 200; *Transactions of the Sanitary Institute of Great Britain*, XX (1899), p. 33.

99 D. Scannell, *Mother Knew Best* (1974), p. 9.

100 See for example, Hollingshead, *Ragged London in 1861*, p. 287.

101 E. Flint, *Hot Bread and Chips* (1963), p. 17. To Ted Willis's mother constant scrubbing was a means of preserving and displaying respectability – 'it was her way of flying a flag at the masthead, her signal to the world that whatever else we lacked, our self-respect was still with us.' Her refrain was 'elbow-grease costs nothing'. Willis, *Whatever Happened to Tom Mix?*, pp. 13, 15.

102 Roberts, *The Classic Slum*, p. 37. F. M. Jones in his 'The Aesthetic of the Nineteenth Century Industrial Town', in H. J. Dyos, ed., *The Study of Urban History* (1968), p. 179, speculates that the drive for cleanliness filled a 'keenly felt aesthetic defence against the general dirt and dullness'.

103 Quoted in Horn, *The Victorian Country Child*, p. 9.

104 Roberts, *The Classic Slum*, pp. 78–9.

105 *PP.* VII (1871), 'Select Committee on the Protection of Infant Life. II. Minutes of Evidence', p. 157.

106 Edinburgh Charity Organisation Society, *Report on the Physical Condition*, p. 41. In the Stroud Union in 1904 16.9% of the urban children and 29.4% of the rural, had verminous heads. No wonder schoolteachers wore sulphur bags in the hems of their skirts. See J. S. Hurt, *Elementary Schooling and the Working Classes, 1860–1918* (1979),

p. 102. In London, 23,573 children were verminous, of 50,694 inspected, *ibid*, p. 133.

107 Booth, *Life and Labour*, II. *Poverty*, pp. 46–48.

108 Quoted in Sir A. MacNalty, *The History of State Medicine* (1948), p. 21.

109 Reynolds, *A Poor Man's House*, p. 88.

110 Dowling, 'The Ladies' Sanitary Association', p. 171. For Kingsley, see especially, *Miscellanies*, II, p. 312.

111 Quoted in Dowling, 'The Ladies' Sanitary Association', p. 96.

112 Dr J. Challice, *How People Hasten Death. Plain Words for Plain Folk*; *The Power of Soap and Water*; *The 'Sick Child's Cry' and Other Household Verses*, Ladies' Sanitary Association Tracts (n.d.).

113 Quoted in Dowling, 'The Ladies' Sanitary Association', p. 103.

114 J. Haddon, 'Health and How to Preserve it', Manchester and Salford Sanitary Association, *Health Lectures for the People* (1875–76), pp. 34–5.

115 *Transactions of the Sanitary Institute of Great Britain*, IX (1887–8), p. 455.

116 Dowling, 'The Ladies' Sanitary Association', pp. 147, 202–3.

117 Quoted in *ibid.*, p. 123.

118 *Ibid.*, pp. 195, 216, 176, and *Transactions of the Sanitary Institute of Great Britain*, XXI (1900), p. 178.

119 *PP.* XXXII (1904), 'Inter-Departmental Committee on Physical Deterioration. II. Minutes of Evidence', p. 174.

120 A. Morrison, *A Child of the Jago* (1896), p. 45; *Public Health*, VIII, 92 (December 1895), p. 83. For Kerr see Hurt, *Elementary Schooling*, p. 103.

121 Another contributing factor might possibly have been the lessons in domestic science which were being taught in the board schools, although it was pointed out that since girls left school at 14 and did not marry until 18 or so, much of the learning may have been forgotten, Sir Alexander Patterson, *Across the Bridges, or Life by the South London Riverside* (1914), p. 21.

122 Dowling, 'The Ladies' Sanitary Association', p. 249; Mrs E. Eve, *Manual for Health Visitors and Infant Welfare Workers* (1921). See also Newman, *Infant Mortality*, p. 263, and Smith, *The People's Health*, p. 115.

123 C. Cameron, *A Manual of Hygiene* (Dublin, 1874), p. 174; see also *Public Health*, IV, 45 (January 1892), pp. 114–15.

124 Ipswich Council, *Third Annual Report of the Medical Officer of Health, for 1878*; Smith, *The People's Health*, p. 202.

125 Scannell, *Mother Knew Best*, pp. 38, 46.

126 Smith, *The People's Health*, pp. 202–3.

127 'However filthy a person may be', he wrote, 'there exists no power to compulsorily cleanse him', *Transactions of the Sanitary Institute of Great Britain*, XX (1889), pp. 32–3.

128 L. Wright, *Clean and Decent*, p. 242. In 1891 14 lbs of soap *per capita* were used annually. Smith, *The People's Health*, p. 218.

129 Quoted in L. Stevenson, ' "Science down the Drain", or the Hostility of Certain Sanitarians to Animal Experimentation, Bacteriology, and Immunology', *Bulletin of the History of Medicine*, XXIX, I (January–February 1955), p. 9; *Transactions of the Sanitary Institute of Great Britain*, II (1880), p. 196.

130 Kingsley, 'Great Cities and their Influence for Good and Evil', *Miscellanies*, II, p. 289.

131 *The Times*, 14 July 1848.

132 Gibson, *Journal of the History of Medicine and Allied Sciences*, IX, 4 (October 1954), p. 393.

133 *Ibid.*, p. 401.

134 *Lancet*, 27 June 1846, p. 712.

135 *PP*. LXIV (1875), 'A Digest of the Statutes relating to Urban Sanitary Authorities', p. 219.

136 B. Rathbone, ed., *Memoir of Kitty Wilkinson of Liverpool, 1786–1860* (Liverpool, 1927); White, *A History of the Corporation of Liverpool*, p. 46. She is commemorated by a stained glass window in the Liverpool Anglican Cathedral, T. McLaughlin, *Coprophilia, or a Peck of Dirt* (1971), p. 138.

137 *PP*. XLVII (1865), 'Return relating to Baths and Washhouses', pp. 1–5.

138 *Ibid.*, p. 9. Dublin did not build its one and only public bath in the nineteenth century until 1885, see J. V. O'Brien, *'Dear Dirty Dublin'. A City in Distress, 1899–1916* (Berkeley and Los Angeles, California, 1982), p. 29.

139 Ipswich Council, *Second Annual Report of the Medical Officer of Health, for 1875*, p. 26.

140 *PP*. XLVII (1865), 'Return relating to Baths and Washhouses', pp.1–5.

141 Gibson, *Journal of the History of Medicine and Allied Sciences*, IX, 4 (October 1954), p. 404. See also *Hansard*, Third Series, 88 (1846), 279.

142 *London*, 30 August 1893, p. 551 and *ibid.*, 4 June 1896, p. 530.

143 T. Wright, *Some Habits and Customs of the Working Classes* (1867), p. 188.

144 *London*, 9 July 1896, p. 655, and *Municipal Journal and London*, 17 March 1899, p. 327; N. Williams, *Powder and Paint* (1957), p. 95. This was true for swimming also, see *London*, 17 November 1898, p. 729.

145 *Ibid.*, 8 July 1897, p. 569.

146 *Municipal Journal and London* 6 October 1899, p. 1103.

147 *Ibid.*, 24 February 1899, p. 233.

148 London County Council, *Comparative Municipal Statistics*, I (1912–13), pp. 46–7. For maintenance costs see *ibid.*, pp. 134–5.

149 *Ibid.*, 6 October 1899, p. 1103. In Glasgow only 3,000 people used the

five municipal baths at the end of the century, *ibid.*, 10 November 1899, p. 1215. Liverpool at the end of the century was thinking of building 'people's baths', like Germany's, right in the heart of the slums, *ibid.*, 6 October 1899, p. 1103.

150 Scannell, *Mother Knew Best*, p. 44.

151 'At the bottom of our social ladder is a dirty shirt; at the top is fixed not laurels, but a tub', Reynolds, *A Poor Man's House*, p. 89.

152 *Ibid.*, p. 88.

153 T. Barclay, *Memoirs' Medley: the Autobiography of a Bottle Washer* (1939), quoted p. 137 of M. Elliott, 'The Leicester Board of Health, 1849–1872: A Study of Progress in the Development of Local Government', University of Nottingham M. Phil thesis (1971), p. 137.

154 P. Fitzgerald, *Memories of Charles Dickens* (1913) pp. 170–71, quoted in P. Collins, ed., G. A. Sala, *Twice Round the Clock* (Leicester, 1971), p. 19.

155 F. Tristan, *London Journal* (1840; trans. D. Palmer and G. Pincete, 1980), p.63 and Taine, quoted in Longmate, *Alive and Well* (1970), p. 12.

156 Of the contemporary artists the most dramatic and evocative was perhaps Frederick Barnard, who worked for the *Pictorial World*.

157 Both quoted in *PP.* XXI (1843), 'Fifth Annual Report of the Registrar-General, appendix, "Letter . . . by G. Farr" ', p. 214.

158 Quoted in M. Bruce, *The Coming of the Welfare State* (1966), p. 53.

159 Patterson, *Across the Bridges, or Life by the South London Riverside*, p. 39.

160 In Edinburgh, a cleaner city, the corresponding figure was only fourteen per cent. Edinburgh Charity Organisation, *Report on the Physical Condition*, p. 41.

161 Quoted in Bruce, *The Coming of the Welfare State*, p. 53.

162 Quoted in *London*, 17 August 1896, p. 810.

163 Rowntree *Poverty*, p. 214.

Chapter Four. 'The Valleys of the Shadow of Death'.

1 *Transactions of the Sanitary Institute of Great Britain*, V (1883–4), p. 247.

2 Bell, *Day and Night in the Wynds of Edinburgh*, p. 7. Lord Shaftesbury, after visiting the East End slums in 1841, wrote that the stench was indescribable – 'No pen nor paint brush could describe the thing as it is. One whiff of Cow-yard, Blue Anchor or Baker's Court outweighs ten pages of letter press,' quoted in A. Briggs, *Public Opinion and Public Health in the Age of Chadwick* (1946), p. 9.

3 *PP.* XXIX (1878–9), 'ARMOHLGB, for 1879', pp. xii; *ibid.*, pp. 42–43.

4 *PP.* XXXI (1874), 'ARMOHLGB, for 1873', p. 2.

5 Quoted in Robson, *The Government and Misgovernment of London*, p. 125, and *ibid*.

6 *Transactions of the Sanitary Institute of Great Britain*, XIX (1898), p. 53.

7 London also had to deal with the very ripe manure of the Atlantic cattle-ships and had depots for that purpose located in Feltham, Sunbury, Paddock Wood, Masden, Cookham, Egham, Welwyn, Maidstone, and Bexley, *PP*. XLII (1893–4), 'ARMOHLGB, for 1891', p. 88, and *ibid*., 'appendix IX, "Dr Parson's Report of an Inquiry concerning the Nuisances arising during the transport of manure from Towns to Agricultural Districts . . . ." ', pp. 105–6, 109–110.

8 *Transactions of the Sanitary Institute of Great Britain*, XXII (1901), p. 7.

9 Hill, *Victorian Lincoln*, p. 159.

10 Archer, 'A Study of Local Sanitary Administration', p. 67.

11 Engels, *The Condition of the Working Classes in England*, p. 106.

12 P. E. Malcolmson, 'Getting a Living in the Slums of Victorian Kensington', *The London Journal*, I, I (May 1975), pp. 53, 54.

13 *Ibid*., p. 36, n. 23. A local estimate claimed that at one time between 25 and 30 per cent of the heads of local families were professional pig-keepers, *ibid*., pp. 34, 54.

14 Ipswich Council, *Annual Report of the Medical Officer of Health, for 1874*, p. 19. Elliott, 'The Leicester Board of Health', pp. 26–27; R. Wood, *West Hartlepool, the Rise and Development of a Victorian New Town* (Hartlepool, 1969), p. 118; R. I. Penny, 'The Board of Health in Victorian Stratford-upon-Avon. Aspects of Environmental Control', *Warwickshire History*, I, 6 (Autumn, 1971), p. 7. Reading in 1847 had 378 pigsties, Smith, *The People's Health*, p. 198. For Southampton see D. Stanford and A. T. Patterson, *The Condition of the Children of the Poor in Mid-Victorian Portsmouth* (Portsmouth Papers, No. 21, Portsmouth, 1974).

15 McKichan, 'Stirling, 1780–1880', p. 229.

16 *PP*. XXXVII (1902), 'Supplement to the Twenty-ninth Annual Report of the Local Government Board for Ireland, for 1900–1901, "Supplement on the Sanitary Circumstances of Cities and Towns in Ireland . . . ." ', pp. 47, 60, 151.

17 H. P. Tait, *A Doctor and Two Policemen: the History of Edinburgh Health Department, 1862–1974* (Edinburgh, 1974), p. 205.

18 J. Toft, 'Public Health in Leeds', University of Manchester M. A. Thesis (1966), p. 99. Redford, *The History of Local Government in Manchester*, p. 289; London County Council, *Annual Report of the MOH, 1898*, appendix II, 'Slaughterhouses', pp. 6–7; *ibid*., 1892, p. 31.

19 *Tr nsactions of the Sanitary Institute of Great Britain*, XXI (1900), p. 302.

20 F. M. L. Thompson, *Victorian England: the Horse-drawn Society* (1970), p. 11.

21 *Transactions of the Sanitary Institute of Great Britain*, XXI (1900), p. 302.

22 *London*, 8 October 1896, p. 959.

23 *Ibid*, 3 May 1901, p. 326; *ibid.*, 14 January 1897, p. 19.

24 *Transactions of the Sanitary Institute of Great Britain*, IX (1887–8), p. 105.

25 *London* 1 July 1897, pp. 547, 550.

26 PP. XXX (1874), 'ARMOHLGB for 1873', p. 3; J. Fox, 'Defective Drainage as a Cause of Diseases', *Health Lectures for the People*, II (1878–9), p. 79.

27 *Public Health*, III, 27 (July 1890), p. 93.

28 L. Parkes, 'The Sanitary Condition of the Poor Districts in the Metropolis . . .', *Transactions of the Society of Medical Officers of Health* (1885–6), p. 97.

29 H. J. Smith, ed., *Public Health Act: Report to the General Board of Health on Darlington, 1850* (Durham, 1967), p. 35.

30 Quoted in M. Pelling, *Cholera, Fever, and English Medicine, 1825–1865* (1978), p. 25.

31 Smith, ed., *Public Health Act*, p. 35. One theory was that the 'noxious effluvia' was 'readily absorbed into the system by the skin' as well as through the lungs', *ibid.*, p. 69.

32 Flinn, ed., *Report on the Sanitary State*, p. 63. For a stimulating discussion of the differences of opinion between the supporters of the effluvia theory and the contagionists see Pelling, *Cholera, Fever, and English Medicine*, pp. 296ff.

33 PP. XXI (1843), 'Fifth Annual Report of the Registrar-General, Appendix', p. 207.

34 PP. XVII (1864), 'Twenty-fifth Annual Report of the Registrar-General, Appendix', p. 185.

35 A. Ransome, 'Long Life and the Causes that Prevent it', *Health Lectures for the People*, II (1878–9), p. 29.

36 For Simon's gradual acceptance of germ theory see Greenwood, *Epidemics and Crowd Diseases*, pp. 140ff.

37 E. Seaton, ed., *Public Health Reports by John Simon . . .* (1887) I, pp. 3–4, Simon's First Report, MOH, City of London, 1849.

38 *Ibid.*, p. 4. Quoted in Sheppard, *London, 1808–1870*, p. 255.

39 Toft, 'Public Health in Leeds', p. 13.

40 PP. XXXIII (1866), 'Eighth ARMOHPC, for 1865, Appendix V, "Report of Dr Edward Seaton on Circumstances endangering the Public Health of Chichester" ', p. 221.

41 *Sanitary Record*, 8 January 1876, p. 26.

42 Ipswich Council, *First Annual Report of the MOH* (1874), pp. 12, 18, 24; *Second Annual Report of the MOH* (1875), p. 33; *Third Annual Report of the MOH* (1876), p. 14; PP. XXXVII (1896), 'Twenty-fourth ARLGB, for 1894–5, Supplement, "Inland Sanitary Survey, 1893–5, by R. Thorne Thorne" ', p. 119.

43 *Transactions of the Sanitary Institute of Great Britain*, VI (1884–5), pp. 73–4.

44 *PP*. XXXIV (1890–1), 'ARMOHLGB, for 1890', p. 153. In Crewe the cesspools were cleaned out only twice a year, see Chaloner, *The Social and Economic Development of Crewe*, p. 125.

45 Archer, 'A Study of Local Sanitary Administration', p. 211.

46 Redford, *The History of Local Government in Manchester*, I p. 147; Toft, 'Public Health in Leeds', p. 125.

47 *PP*. XXVI (1865), 'Seventh ARMOHPC, for 1864, Appendix IX, "Sanitary State of Seacroft, by Dr Stevens" ', p. 509.

48 *Ibid*., 'Appendix IXg, "Sanitary State of Colliery Settlements at Gilesgate Moor" ', pp. 515, 516.

49 *PP*. XXXIII (1866), 'Eighth ARMOHPC, for 1865 Appendix IV, "Report by Dr George Buchanan on Epidemic Typhus at Greenock" ', pp. 214–15.

50 *Public Health*, VI, 66 (October 1893), p. 23; Redford, *The History of Local Government in Manchester*, I, p. 147.

51 *PP*. XXVI (1865), 'Seventh ARMOHPC, for 1864', p. 19.

52 *Ibid*., 'Appendix VI, "Inquiry into the State of Dwellings of Rural Labourers, by Dr H. J. Hunter" ', p. 159.

53 Brotherston, *Observations on the Early Public Health Movement*, p. 11. The value of the dung-heap features twice in Synge's *The Playboy of the Western World*.

54 *PP*. XXVI (1865), 'Seventh ARMOHPC, for 1864, Appendix VI, "Inquiry into the State of Dwellings of Rural Labourers, by Dr H. J. Hunter" ', p. 183.

55 C. Cameron, *A Brief History of the Municipal Public Health Administration in Dublin* (Dublin, 1914), p. 83.

56 R. C. W. Cox, 'The Old Centre of Croydon: Victorian Decay and Redevelopment', in A. Everitt, ed., *Perspectives in English Urban History* (1973), p. 192.

57 R. D. Till, 'Public Health and the Community in the Borough of Neath, 1835–60', *Welsh Historical Review*, 5 (1970–71), p. 379.

58 *PP*. XXVIII (1870), 'Twelfth ARMOHPC, for 1869', pp. 16, 17.

59 *PP*. XXI (1871), 'Thirteenth ARMOHPC, for 1870', p. 13.

60 *PP*. XXXI (1874), 'First ARMOHLGB, for 1873', pp. 17–18; *PP*. XXI (1874), 'Supplementary Report to the Local Government Board of some recent Inquiries under the Public Health Act, 1858', p. 7.

61 *Public Health*, VII, 85 (May 1895), p. 281.

62 Rowntree, *Poverty*, quoted p. 186.

63 *Public Health*, XIV, 5 (February, 1902), p. 282.

64 *PP*. XXXI (1874), 'ARMOHLGB, for 1873, Appendix VII, "Report by Mr J. Netten Radcliffe on certain means of preventing Excrement Nuisance in Towns and Villages" ', p. 178.

65 *Ibid*., pp. 143ff, and White, *A History of the Corporation of Liverpool*, p. 32. Liverpool did not systematically clean its pails until 1900.

Nottingham's pails were wooden until 1901 and leaked, see Smith, *The People's Health*, p. 222.

66 *PP*. XXXI (1874), 'ARMOHLGB, for 1873, Appendix VII, "Report by Mr J. Netten . . . ." ', pp. 156–158.

67 *Ibid*., p. 157.

68 Toft, 'Public Health in Leeds', p. 87; *PP*. XXV (1871), 'Third Report, RCRP', p. 7.

69 Toft, 'Public Health in Leeds', pp. 229, 232; *Transactions of the Sanitary Institute of Great Britain*, IX (1887–8), p. 105. Bolton spent £30,000 on its depot and another £30,000 on the processing plant, *ibid*.

70 Redford, *The History of Local Government in Manchester*, III, p. 156.

71 These cost between £3 and £10 to install, so it is not surprising that the landlord was reluctant to install them. F. Vigier, *Change and Apathy. Liverpool and Manchester during the Industrial Revolution* (Cambridge, Massachusetts, 1970) p. 196.

72 Redford, *The History of Local Government in Manchester*, II, p. 159.

73 *Ibid*., pp. 389, 398.

74 A. Sharratt and K. R. Farrar, 'Sanitation and Public Health in Nineteenth-Century Manchester', *Memoirs and Proceedings of the Manchester Literary and Philosophical Society*, 114 (1971–2), pp. 60–1, 64ff.

75 Redford, *The History of Local Government in Manchester*, II p. 426, and III, p. 128.

76 *PP*. XXXVIII (1870) 'Twelfth ARMOHPC, for 1869', pp. 125, 130.

77 A. Hill, 'Existing Methods of Refuse Disposal in Towns', *Transactions of the Society of Medical Officers of Health*, 1886–7, p. 3 and pp. 3–6; *PP*. XXXVIII (1876) 'Report of a Committee appointed by the President of the Local Government Board to Inquire into Several Modes of Treating Town Sewage', p. 33; and *PP*. XXXVIII (1870), 'Twelfth ARMOHPC, for 1869, Appendix IVb, "report by Dr Buchanan and Mr J. Netten Radcliffe on the System in use in various Northern Towns for dealing with Excrement" '. For a municipal tax on w.cs see E. P. Hennock, *Fit and Proper Persons. Ideal and Reality in Nineteenth-Century Urban Government* (1973), pp. 107–8.

78 *Transactions of the Sanitary Institute of Great Britain*, VI (1884–5), pp. 232–3. *Ibid*. IV (1882), p. 92. The amount, £102,839, was exceeded only by the cost of the main sewers (£172,370), and street cleaning (£104,460), *ibid*.

79 *Ibid*., pp. 248–9.

80 *Public Health*, VII, 85 (May 1895), p. 283. See *ibid*., p. 285 for Nottingham.

81 In Liverpool the 'nightmen' occasionally paid for the excrement they emptied from the middens, but with the introduction of guano from South America they began to charge for the cleaning operation, see J. H. Treble, 'Liverpool Working-Class Housing, 1801–1851', in S. D.

Chapman, ed., *The History of Working-Class Housing* (Newton Abbot, 1971), p. 185. For the attempt of the Native Guano Company to convert the excrement into a saleable commodity, and its failure in the late 1870s, see Smith, *The People's Health*, p. 220.

82 *PP*. XXXVIII (1870), 'Twelfth ARMOHPC, for 1869, Appendix IVa, "Dr Buchanan on the Dry Earth System of dealing with Excrement" ', p. 81; *PP*. XLII (1893–4), 'ARMOHLGB, for 1891', p. 79; for Tamworth see Archer, 'A Study of Local Administration', p. 244.
83 Sharrat and Farrar, *Memoirs and Proceedings*, 114 (1971–2), p. 54.
84 *London*, 12 November 1896, p. 1083. The cost of pail cleaning and removal had risen from 1¼d per pound on the rates to 7¹⁄₉d between 1850 and 1895. Carters' wages during the same period rose from 17s to 25s per week, *ibid*.
85 O'Brien, *'Dear Dirty Dublin'*, p. 32. In 1869 Glasgow grossed £18,000 from the sale of its excrement and this helped to defray the collection costs of £27,000, but generally it made less, *Transactions of the Sanitary Institute of Great Britain*, VI (1884–5), pp. 232–5; *London* 8 October 1896, p. 961; *PP*. XXXVIII (1870), 'Twelfth ARMOHPC, for 1869, Appendix IVb, "Report . . . dealing with Excrement" ', p. 133. For Nottingham see *Public Health*, VII, 85 (May 1895), p. 285.
86 'So far as our examinations extend, none of the manufactured manure made . . . with or without chemicals, pay the contingent costs of such treatment', *PP*. XXXVIII (1876), 'Report of a Committee . . . into the Several Modes of Treating Town Sewage', pp. xii, xiii.
87 *Ibid*., p. xii.
88 White, *A History of the Corporation on Liverpool*, p. 51; W. E. Townley, 'Urban Administration and Health: A Case Study of Hanley in the mid-Nineteenth Century', University of Keele, MA thesis (1969), pp. 112–13.
89 Ruskin, quoted in Stevenson, *Bulletin of the History of Medicine*, XXIX, I (January–February, 1955), p. 11.
90 Cameron, *A Brief History*, quoted p. 81.
91 The designer was N. Rigby, a bricklayer, see Smith, *The People's Health*, p. 221.
92 For a Freudian approach see R. L. Schoenwald, 'Training Urban Man: A Hypothesis about the Sanitary Movement', in Dyos and Wolff, eds., *The Victorian City*, II.
93 White, *A History of the Corporation of Liverpool*, p. 51; Sharrat and Farrar, *Memoirs and Proceedings*, 114 (1971–2), pp. 53, 60.
94 Smith, *The People's Health*, pp. 222–3.
95 White, *A History of the Corporation of Liverpool*, p. 50.
96 Sharrat and Farrar, *Memoirs and Proceedings*, 114 (1971–2), pp. 57, 58. *PP*. XXXVIII (1876), 'Report of a Committee . . . into the Several Modes of Treating Town Sewage', p. xxv and 'Appendix VI', pp. 105ff. For Birmingham see Hennock, *Fit and Proper Persons*, p. 110.

97   *Leeds Intelligencer*, 11 March 1848, quoted in Toft, 'Public Health in Leeds', p. 184. By 1855 the Leeds sewers had cost £137,000 and between 1850 and 1862 Leeds spent over £211,000 on its main sewerage, D. Fraser, *Power and Authority in the Victorian City* (Oxford, 1979), p. 65.

98   E. Smith, *Victorian Farnham. The Story of a Surrey Town, 1837–1901* (1971), pp. 64–222.

99   Sheppard *London, 1808–1870*, pp. 282–4. The London sewer scheme is discussed in great detail in D. Owen, *The Government of Victorian London, 1855–1889. The Metropolitan Board of Works, the Vestries, and the City Corporation*, edited by R. MacLeod (Cambridge, Massachusetts, 1982), Chapter 3.

100 *Punch*, 31 July 1858 and 14 August 1858, quoted in C. B. Chapman, 'The Year of the Great Stink', *The Pharos*, 35 (July 1972), p. 97.

101 *Ibid.*, p. 94.

102 *PP.* XXXVII (1867), 'Ninth ARMOHPC, for 1866, Appendix II, "Report by Dr Buchanan on the Results . . . of Regulation designed to promote the Public Health" ', p. 75.

103 E. Greenhow, *Papers Relating to the Sanitary State of the People of England . . .* (1858), p. 102.

104 *Transactions of the Sanitary Institute of Great Britain*, II (1880), p. 140. In 1871 the Royal Sanitary Commission concluded that 'most towns of any considerable size have already made or are making sewers and few (except in the north of England) retain the ashpits and scavenger system', *PP.* XXXV (1871), 'Second Report of the Royal Sanitary Commission', p. 42.

105 I base this generalization partly on the amount of loans requested from the central government, see *PP.* LXI (1880), 'Return showing . . . all the Local Visitations . . . with Regard to Prevalence of Disease . . . .', pp. 80–91.

106 *PP.* XXI (1886), 'ARMOHLGB, for 1885, Supplement, "On Cholera" ', *passim*, and especially p. 117. Barnsby, 'Social Conditions in the Black Country', p. 96.

107 For the comment of the Royal Sanitary Commission see note 104 above; for Leicester see *PP.* XXXVII (1867), 'Ninth ARMOHPC, for 1866, Appendix II, "Report by Dr Buchanan . . . Public Health" ', p. 75.

108 *PP.* XXXV (1871), 'Second Report of the Royal Sanitary Commission', p. 177, 48; *PP.* XXVI (1865), 'Seventh ARMOHPC, for 1864', p. 487.

109 Redford, *The History of Local Government in Manchester*, III, p. 128; and *PP.* XXXI (1874) 'ARMOHLGB, for 1873, Appendix VII, "Report by Mr J. Netten Radcliffe on . . . Excrement Nuisance in Towns and Villages" ', p. 178; Sharrat and Farrar, *Memoirs and Proceedings*, 114 (1971–2), p. 61.

110 Chaloner, *The Social and Economic Development of Crewe*, p. 183.

111 *PP*. XXXI (1874), 'ARMOHLGB, for 1873, Appendix VII, "Report by Mr J. Netten Radcliffe ... Excrement Nuisance in Towns and Villages" ', p. 156; and Macdonald, 'Public Health Legislation and Problems in Victorian Edinburgh', pp. 166, 182.

112 *PP*. XXXVIII (1870), 'Twelfth ARMOHPC, for 1869, Appendix B, "Report ... dealing with Excrement" ', pp. 112–133.

113 *PP*. XXXVIII (1876), 'Report of a Committee ... into the several Modes of Treating Town Sewage', pp. 33, 41. *Transactions of the Sanitary Institute of Great Britain*, XIX (1898), p. 407.

114 Quoted in Rowntree, *Poverty*, pp. 184–6. For similar conditions of the almost 10,000 'large, deep, and offensive' privy middens in Ipswich, see *PP*. XXXVI (1887), 'ARMOHLGB, for 1886, Appendix "Dr. Ballard and Dr. Blasall, On the Result of the Sanatory Survey made in anticipation of the Cholera, 1886" ', p. 118.

115 *PP*. XXXVII (1902), 'Supplement to the Twenty-ninth Annual Report of the Local Government Board for Ireland, 1900–1901: Reports on the Sanitary Circumstances and Administration of Cities and Towns in Ireland', p. 24.

116 *London*, 30 January 1896, p. 145.

117 *Municipal Journal and London*, 26 June 1899, p. 107; Hennock, *Fit and Proper Persons*, pp. 108–10. The situation in Birmingham caused the Corporation to press for the right to purchase land beyond its own boundaries. This was granted in the 1865 Sewage Utilization Act.

118 J. H. Stephen, *Water and Waste* (1967), pp. 55–61.

119 Redford, *The History of Local Government in Manchester*, II, p. 398; Sharrat and Farrar, *Memoirs and Proceedings*, p. 66; *London*, 12 November 1896, p. 1084.

120 Quoted in Toft, 'Public Health in Leeds', p. 163.

121 Robson, in Laski, Jennings, and Robson, eds., *A Century of Municipal Progress*, p. 313.

122 *Ibid.*, p. 302.

123 *Ibid.*, pp. 316, 317; Treble in Chapman, ed., *The History of Working-Class Housing*, p. 110. For Holme see Fraser, *Power and Authority in the Victorian City*, quoted p. 31.

124 Toft, 'Public Health in Leeds', p. 296; Robson, in Laski, Jennings, and Robson, eds., *A Century of Municipal Progress, p. 318*.

125 E. C. Midwinter, *Social Administration in Lancashire, 1830–1860, Poor Law, Public Health, and Police* (Manchester, 1969), p. 83.

126 *Ibid.*, p. 114.

127 H. Finer, *Municipal Trading. A Study of Public Administration* (1914), p. 20.

128 Redford, *The History of Local Government in Manchester*, II, p. 395. For problems of municipal ownership see Midwinter, *Social Administration in Lancashire*, pp. 107, 108.

129 W. E. Luckin, 'Typhus and Typhoid in London, 1851–1900', an unpublished paper given at the Urban History Group Annual Confer-

ence, at Cambridge University, 7–8 April 1976, p. 2. Luckin was referring to London but his observation applies equally to the large provincial cities.

130 *PP.* XL (1875), 'ARMOHLGB, for 1874', p. 11. These are exclusive of loans under private acts.

131 *PP.* XXVII (1872), 'ARMOHLGB, for 1871–72', p. xliv.

132 *PP.* XXXI (1875), 'ARLGB, for 1874–5', pp. xli, xlii. Sewerage accounted for £1,039,644; water supply for £1,399,606. Most of the remainder went on street improvements and markets.

133 *PP.* XXI (1876), 'ARLGB, for 1875', p. lvii.

134 See Chapter 6, below.

135 *PP.* XXXVIII (1892), 'ARLGB, for 1891–2', p. cv.

136 *Ibid.*, p. cx. Between 1873 and 1891 another £55,041,566 was raised for sanitary purposes under local acts, *ibid.*, p. cxi. See also *PP.* XXIX (1898), 'ARLGB, for 1897', pp. ciii, civ.

137 Cameron, *A Brief History*, p. 109, and Cameron, 'Results of Sanitary Work in Dublin', *Public Health*, IV, 45 (January 1892), p. 116. By 1892 Dublin had spent £607,000 in sanitary work, *ibid.* The 1878 Act enabled Dublin to borrow up to £620,000 for sanitary purposes. See O'Brien, *'Dear Dirty Dublin'*, p. 17.

138 *Transactions of the Sanitary Institute of Great Britain*, VI (1884–5), pp. 194, 214; *PP.* XXV (1900), 'Annual Report of the Local Government Board for Ireland for 1900', p. lxii; for Scotland, see *PP.* XXXVI (1900), 'Fifth Annual Report of the Local Government Board for Scotland', p. xli; most of Scotland's expenditure for sanitary improvements in the last quarter of the century was on waterworks. Between 1867 and 1880 Scotland received £782,509 from the Board of Supervision for sanitary purposes; *PP.* XXVIII (1880), 'Thirty-fifth Annual Report of the Board of Supervision . . . 1879–1880', pp. xx–xxi.

139 The urban administrations were forced, partly by the sheer scale of their public health work, to turn to the central government for low-cost loans.

140 *PP.* XXXI (1875), 'ARMOHLGB, for 1874–5', p. 462.

141 *Flying Post*, 27 October 1880, quoted in R. Newton, *Victorian Exeter, 1837–1914* (Leicester, 1968), p. 252; *ibid.*, p. 261. Expenses for a city of Liverpool's size could be formidable: between 1848 and 1858 Liverpool spent £63,000 on paving and flagging, £300,000 on sewerage, £210,000 on nuisances removal, and the cost of improving the water supply in the mid-1850s was around £1,500,000, A. T. McCabe, 'The Standard of Living on Merseyside, 1850–1875', in Bell, ed., *Victorian Lancashire*, p. 134.

142 Flinn, ed., *Report on the Sanitary Condition*, p. 423.

143 *PP.* XXXII (1904), 'Inter-Departmental Committee on Physical Deterioration. I. Report', p. 21.

144 Quoted in B. Barrows, *A County and its Health. A History of the*

Development of the West Riding Health Services, 1889–1974, (1974), p. 10; *PP*. XXX, Pt. 1 (1882), 'ARLGB, for 1881–2', p. cxix.

145 *PP*. XVIII (1902), 'Sixty-fourth Annual Report of the Registrar-General, for 1902', p. li. This was lower than deaths from pneumonia (37, 413) or consumption (58,930), *ibid.*, pp. liii, lv.

Chapter Five. 'Fever! 'Fever!'

1 See for example, Charlotte Yonge, *The Three Bridges* (1882), pp. 392, 397.

2 It is for this reason that public health has been handled by historians mainly in terms of political or administrative history.

3 Rosen, 'Disease, Debility, and Death', in Dyos and Wolff, eds., *The Victorian City*, II, pp. 635–6.

4 R. Morris, *Cholera, 1832. The Social Response to an Epidemic* (New York, 1976), p. 79. For different figures see Smith, *The People's Health*, p. 230 and W. M. Frazer, *A History of English Public Health, 1834–1939* (1950), p. 168, and Pelling, *Cholera, Fever, and English Medicine*, p. 2.

5 Morris, *Cholera, 1832*, p. 12. It may not be too fanciful to suggest that part of the fear of cholera lay in is foreign, Eastern origin – it had crossed God's "moat" which was supposed to protect England from invasion.

6 Sheppard, *London, 1808–1870*, pp. 247–8.

7 Quoted in Morris, *Cholera, 1832*, p. 16.

8 M. Durey, 'Popular Reactions to the 1832 Cholera Epidemic in Britain', unpublished paper given at the Annual Conference of the Urban History Group, at Cambridge University, 7–8 April 1976, pp. 1–3.

9 M. Barnet, 'The 1832 Cholera Epidemic in York', *Medical History*, XVI (January 1972), p. 27.

10 See both Durey, 'Popular Reactions' and Morris, *Cholera, 1832, passim*.

11 Durey, 'Popular Reactions', p. 5.

12 Morris, *Cholera, 1832*, pp. 106, 123; see also Durey, 'Popular Reactions', p. 5, and C. Yonge, *Three Brides*, p. 438.

13 Quoted in Morris, *Cholera, 1832*, p. 123.

14 Quoted in Longmate, *Alive and Well*, p. 30.

15 Morris, who used the cholera epidemic to test the 'symbiotic tension of class relationships', concluded, 'this lack of major panic and disorganisation in the face of cholera was another indication of the basic stability of British society', *Cholera, 1832*, pp. 17, 123–4.

16 *Ibid.*, p. 15, and Sir M. Burnet, *The Natural History of Infectious Diseases* (Cambridge, 1962), p. 332.

17 Pelling, *Cholera, Fever, and English Medicine*, p. 60.

18 Penny, *Warwickshire History*, I, 6 (Autumn, 1971), p. 2; Morris, *Cholera, 1832*, pp. 48–50.

19 Pelling, *Cholera, Fever, and English Medicine*, p. 60. Chadwick and Southwood Smith were determined to prevent the contagionists from gaining the day: 'That the correlation between smell and disease became an article of popular faith was a triumph of sanitary propaganda.' *ibid*. Pelling and Eyler both stress, however, that there was no really strict or clean division between contagionist and miasma theory.

20 *Lancet*, 12 November 1831.

21 Barnet, *Medical History*, XVI (January, 1972), p. 32. Other popular remedies ran the gamut from ice to hot compresses, opium, arsenic doses, tobacco, burnt cork, horse-radish, black pepper, and pounded ginger, see Longmate, *Alive and Well*, p. 35.

22 Morris, *Cholera, 1832*, pp. 133, 141, 149, 151.

23 Quoted in *ibid.*, pp. 142, 150–151.

24 Quoted in Simon, *English Sanitary Institutions* (1897), p. 218.

25 *Ibid.*

26 *Lancet*, 25 August 1832, pp. 652–657. Morris states that under the pressure of the cholera epidemic 'the Board was chosen for its bureaucratic skills and medical experience, not its social status or authority', *Cholera, 1832*, p. 32.

27 Macdonald, 'Public Health Legislation and Problems in Victorian Edinburgh', pp. 13, 14.

28 Quoted in Simon, *English Sanitary Institutions*, p. 176.

29 In Liverpool, for example, over 5000 people died in the 1848–9 cholera epidemic compared with 1,523 in the earlier visitation, see Midwinter, *Social Administration in Lancashire*, p. 71.

30 See for example, Townley, 'Urban Administration and Health', pp. 165ff.; Newton, *Victorian Exeter*, pp. 122ff., B. Jennings, ed., *A History of Harrogate and Knaresborough* (Huddersfield, 1970), p. 344.

31 *PP*. XXXI (1886), 'ARMOHLGB, for 1885, Appendix VII, "Dr Ballard, Supplement . . . on Cholera" ', pp. 110–111.

32 *PP*. XL (1894), 'ARMOHLGB, for 1893–4', p. xv.

33 *PP*. XXXVII (1896), 'Supplement to the Twenty-fourth Report of the Local Government Board, 1894–5: Supplement in Continuation of the Report by the MOH for 1894–5', p. v.

34 W. P. D. Logan, 'Mortality in England and Wales from 1848 to 1947', *Population Studies*, IV (1950–51), table 2a, p. 138.

35 Sheppard, *London, 1808–1870*, pp. 276–7. For Farr's slow conversion from the miasmic theory, see J. Eyler, 'William Farr on the Cholera: the Sanitarian's Disease Theory and the Statistician's Method', *Journal of the History of Medicine and Allied Sciences*, XXVIII, 2 (April 1973), and *Victorian Social Medicine*, pp. 97ff, 107, 119. For the remarkable contrast in cholera deaths between the customers of the Southwark and Vauxhall Company and those of the

Lambeth Company, which drew its water from the safe reaches above Teddington Lock, see *ibid*, pp. 117–18. Not until 1866 did the water-borne theory prove dominant, *ibid*, p. 119.

36   The specific reference is to Liverpool, but it is applicable to all large towns, *PP*. XXVI (1865), 'Seventh ARMOHPC, for 1864, Appendix VIII "Report by Dr Buchanan upon an Epidemic of Typhus in Liverpool" ', p. 69. M. Flinn writes, 'The history of British towns in the first half of the nineteenth century is, to a considerable extent, the history of typhus and consumption', *Report on the Sanitary Condition*, p. 8.

37   Rosen, in Dyos and Wolff, eds., *The Victorian City*, II, p. 633. MacNalty, *The History of State Medicine*, p. 50. The body louse was the vector for the micro-organism, Rickettsia.

38   Rosen, in Dyos and Wolff, eds., *The Victorian City*, II, p. 633; T. McKeown and R. G. Record, 'Reasons for the Decline of Mortality in England and Wales during the Nineteenth Century', *Population Studies*, XVI, Pt. 2 (November 1962), p. 119.

39   *Ibid*.

40   Frazer, *The History of English Public Health*, p. 184.

41   Luckin, 'Typhus and Typhoid in London', p. 1.

42   *Ibid*., pp. 4, 5. T. McKeown states, 'the epidemiology of the disease [typhus] is complex, and it is unlikely that any single influence accounted for its decline and eventual disappearance', *The Modern Rise of Population* (1976), p. 126.

43   Luckin, 'Typhus and Typhoid in London', p. 1.

44   *Ibid*., p. 8 n. 1.

45   Wright, *Clean and Decent*, p. 210; for Cambridge, see *PP*. XXXI (1874), 'ARMOHLGB, for 1873, Appendix III "Supplementary Report . . . on some Recent Inquiries under the Public Health Act, 1858" ', pp. 64ff.

46   *Public Health*, XI, 2 (November 1898), p. 139; see also Smith, *The People's Health*, p. 246.

47   *PP*. XXXI (1871), 'Thirteenth ARMOHPC, for 1870', p. 11.

48   Luckin speculates that 'mortality from typhus may only have been reduced at the social cost of a short-term increase in mortality from water-transmitted typhoid', 'Typhoid and Typhus in London', p. 3.

49   *Ibid*., p. 2.

50   *Ibid*., p. 6.

51   *PP*., XXXIX (1894), 'ARMOHLGB, for 1892, Appendix A, 6 "Introduction to Dr Barry's Report on Enteric Fever in the Tees Valley, 1890–91" ', pp. 40–44; Smith, *The People's Health*, p. 247.

52   *PP*. XXIV (1890–91), 'ARLGB, for 1890', p. 54; Greenwood, *Epidemics and Crowd Diseases*, pp. 146, 152.

53   Rosen, in Dyos and Wolff, eds., *The Victorian City*, II, p. 653.

54   MacNalty, *The History of State Medicine*, p. 59; Smith, *The People's Health*, p. 324.

55   Tait, *A Doctor and Two Policemen*, p. 43.

56 Smith, *The People's Health*, p. 137; London County Council, *Annual Report of the MOH*, 1892, p. 16.
57 *PP*. XXXVIII (1870), 'Twelfth ARMOHPC, for 1869', pp. 12–14.
58 Smith, *The People's Health*, p. 147.
59 *Ibid.*, p. 137.
60 *Public Health*, IV, 46 (February 1892), p. 446; Rosen in Dyos and Wolff, eds., *The Victorian City*, II, p. 652.
61 McKeown and Record, *Population Studies*, XVI, Pt. 2 (November 1962), pp. 97, 117.
62 Frazer, *The History of English Public Health*, p. 89.
63 Longmate, *Alive and Well*, p. 40; Smith, *The People's Health*, p. 151, says that there is no evidence of tracheotomies for diphtheria.
64 *Ibid.*, p. 114. Diphtheria actually increased in England and Wales between 1881 and 1890, see McKeown, *The Modern Rise of Population*, p. 98.
65 *Public Health*, VI, 75 (July 1894), p. 329. The issue was complicated by the fact that government grants to schools were tied to attendance figures. For a splendid discussion of school attendance and diseases see Rubinstein, *School Attendance in London*, pp. 76ff. In London, after 1883, children suffering from scarlet fever, diphtheria, smallpox, and typhus could not attend school until they produced a doctor's certificate of good health, *ibid*, p. 77.
66 Leff, *Social Medicine*, p. 154.
67 Rosen in Dyos and Wolff, eds., *The Victorian City*, II, pp. 641, 644.
68 Leff, *Social Medicine*, p. 154.
69 T. Ferguson, 'Public Health in Britain in the Climate of the Nineteenth Century', *Population Studies*, XVII (1963–4), Pt. 3 (March 1964), p. 214; *Transactions of the Sanitary Institute of Great Britain*, XV (1894), p. 432.
70 McKeown and Record, *Population Studies*, XVI, Pt. 2 (November 1962) p. 107.
71 Rosen in Dyos and Wolff, eds., *The Victorian City*, II, p. 648.
72 *Public Health*, IV, 50 (June 1892), p. 267; *ibid.*, XI, 5 (February 1899), pp. 317ff.
73 Sir Benjamin Richardson, quoted in Stevenson, *Bulletin of the History of Medicine*, XXIX, 1 (January-February 1955), p. 16.
74 Smith, *The People's Health*, p. 293.
75 T. McKeown, 'Medical Issues in Historical Demography', in E. Clarke, ed., *Modern Methods in the History of Medicine* (1971), p. 66.
76 MacNalty, *The History of State Medicine*, p. 56.
77 MacNalty, 'The Prevention of Smallpox ...', *Medical History*, 12 (January 1968), pp. 10, 11; Simon, *English Sanitary Institutions*, p. 167.
78 *The Graphic*, 8 April 1871, p. 323.
79 *Ibid*.
80 Rosen, in Dyos and Wolff, eds., *The Victorian City*, II, p. 654.

81 *Ibid.*, and Frazer, *The History of English Public Health*, pp. 16, 197. Guardians and single parents had up to four months to vaccinate the child.

82 Rosen, in Dyos and Wolff, eds., *The Victorian City*, II, pp. 654–655.

83 *Public Health*, 69, 8 (May 1896), p. 175.

84 The above section is based upon the excellent account in A. Beck, 'Issues in the Anti-Vaccination Movement in England', *Medical History*, 4 (October 1960), pp. 311–16. For opposition based upon fear or dislike of the Poor Law authorities, see Smith, *The People's Health*, pp. 161ff.

85 D. Ross, 'Leicester and the Anti-Vaccination Movement, 1853–1889', *The Leicester Archaeological and Historical Society Transactions*, XLIII (1967–8), pp. 36, 38. The only leading scientist among the anti-vaccination forces was Alfred Wallace, see Smith, *The People's Health*, p. 167.

86 *Public Health*, XI, 8 (May 1899), p. 601; *PP*. XXIX (1882), 'Report of the Commissioners . . . Smallpox and Fever Hospitals', pp. viii, x.

87 *PP*. XXXVIII (1899), 'ARMOHLGB, for 1898', p. ix. The Local Government Board stated that in 1898 some 61 per cent of all the infants in England and Wales were vaccinated within three months of birth, see Smith, *The People's Health*, p. 165.

88 Luckin, 'Typhus and Typhoid in London', p. 1.

89 Burnet, *Natural History of Infectious Diseases*, pp. 170, 171; see also *ibid.*, pp. 167, 169.

90 *PP*. XXXI (1874), 'ARMOHLGB, for 1873, "Supplementary Report to the Local Government Board on some recent Inquiries under the Public Health Act, 1858" ', p. 7.

91 *PP*. XXXII (1884–5), 'ARLGB, for 1884', p. cxviii.

92 *Public Health*, 69, 8 (May 1956), p. 179.

93 *Ibid.*, XI, 3 (December 1898), p. 314.

94 As late as 1882 a proposal to make notification of infectious diseases compulsory met with opposition from doctors who feared the extra work, *Transactions of the Sanitary Institute of Great Britain*, XVIII (1886–7), p. 128. In Edinburgh doctors, resenting the extra paper work, refused to rise to Dr Littlejohn's offer of 2s.6d for every report of infectious diseases they handed in, see Macdonald, 'Public Health Legislation and Problems in Victorian Edinburgh', p. 198.

95 *Transactions of the Sanitary Institute of Great Britain*, VIII (1886–7), p. 128.

96 *Public Health*, III, 34 (February 1891), p. 298, and *PP*. XXXIII (1890–91), 'ARLGB, for 1890–91', p. clxvii. Compulsory notification was not extended to Scotland until the Public Health (Scotland) Act of 1897.

97 *PP*. XXXVIII (1892), 'ARLGB, for 1891', p. clv; *PP*. XXXVIII (1894), 'ARLGB, for 1893', p. clix.

98 *Transactions of the Sanitary Institute of Great Britain*, XI (1890),

pp. 101, 106. For a conference between the Metropolitan MOH and the London School Board on this issue see, *Public Health*, III, 40 (August, 1891), p. 309.

99   Macdonald, 'Public Health Legislation and Problems in Victorian Edinburgh', p. 203. *PP*. XXIX (1882), 'Report of the Commissioners . . . Smallpox and Fever Hospitals', p. vi. For Windsor, see *Municipal Journal*, 12 October 1900, p. 798.

100 *Public Health*, VII (February 1895), p. 150.

101 *Ibid.*, p. 153.

102 *PP*. XXX (ii) (1882), 'ARLGB, for 1880–1881, "Supplement . . . on the Use and Influence of Hospitals for Infectious Diseases', p. 19. For Liverpool see *PP*. LXXXIV (1895), 'Return . . . Isolation Hospitals for Cases of Infectious Diseases.'

103 *PP*. XXXVII (1896), 'ARLGB, for 1894–5 "Supplement in Continuation of the Report of the MOH . . . Inland Sanitary Survey, 1893–4" ', pp. 28–132.

104 *Transactions of the Sanitary Institute of Great Britain*, IX (1887–8), p. 101. *PP*. LXXXIV (1895), 'Return . . . Isolation Hospitals for Cases of Infectious Diseases.'

105 White, *A History of the Corporation of Liverpool*, pp. 121, 122.

106 *PP*. LXXXIV (1895), 'Return . . . Isolation Hospitals for Cases of Infectious Diseases', *passim*. Among other towns and facilities were Newcastle (186,300 population), 105 beds; Cardiff (129,000), twenty-four beds; Swansea (90,000), twenty-six beds; Sunderland (131,000), fifty beds; Wolverhampton (83,000), thirty-six beds. Not all these were free. Liverpool, for example, charged 42s per week for beds in first-class wards, 21s per week in second-class wards, and 10s a week in third-class wards.

107 Sheppard, *London, 1808–1870*, pp. 293ff.

108 London County Council, *Annual Report of the MOH, 1893*, p. 60, and London County Council, *Annual Report of the MOH, 1895*, pp. 24, 33. It was not until 1899 that, at the request of the Local Government Board, the restrictions on Poor Law Board hospitals in London were removed and non-paupers were accepted, *Transactions of the Sanitary Institute of Great Britain*, XVII (1896), pp. 44–5.

109 Barrows, *A County and its Health*, p. 10. Partly as a result (anti-toxins also played a role), the death rate from zymotic diseases in the West Riding of Yorkshire fell from 2.03 deaths per thousand in 1889–1893 to 1.93 (1894–8) and 1.85 (1899–1903), *ibid*. The County MOH was assisted by the Isolation Hospitals Acts of 1893 and 1901, which enabled county councils to provide isolation hospitals. For the provision of fever hospitals in Ireland see *PP*. XXXVII (1902), 'Supplement to the Twenty-ninth Annual Report of the Local Government Board for Ireland, for 1900–1901'.

Chapter Six: 'State Medicine'

1 Still most comprehensively by Frazer, *A History of English Public Health*, and most recently by Smith, *The People's Health*. The main legislative developments in public health are splendidly analyzed in S. E. Finer, *The Life and Times of Sir Edwin Chadwick* (1952), R. A. Lewis, *Edwin Chadwick and the Public Health Movement, 1832–1854* (1952), and R. Lambert, *Sir John Simon, 1816–1904, and English Social Administration* (1963).

2 Despite Disraeli's electioneering emphasis on good sanitation, this is equally true of his ministry of 1874–80.

3 There has been a disappointing use of central archives and local MOH and other reports by Ph.D candidates.

4 S. E. Finer, 'The Transmission of Benthamite Ideas, 1820–50', in G. Sutherland, ed., *Studies in the Growth of Nineteenth Century Government* (1972), pp. 13ff. See also J. J. Clarke, *The History of Local Government in the United Kingdom* (1953), p. 63. Chadwick was not a member of the Health of Towns Commission but he wrote most of the report.

5 Quoted in Cullen, *The Statistical Movement*, pp. 34ff. Farr has been superbly analyzed by John Eyler, who states that among Farr's several remedies were careful comparative statistical tastes of mortality and morbidity, the teaching of the principles of personal hygiene, changes in the education of doctors, exercise, vaccination and the provision of pure water, see *Victorian Social Medicine*, chapter six and *ibid.*, p. 142 for the statistics for 1851–60.

6 G. Newman, *The Building of a Nation's Health* (1939), p. 18. Simon, *English Sanitary Institutions*, pp. 211–12. It was Duncan's use of the Registrar-General's statistics which brought him into prominence in Liverpool as a possible future MOH, see W. M. Frazer *Duncan of Liverpool* (1947), p. 28.

7 *PP*. XXXI (1843), 'Fifth Annual Report of the Registrar-General', p. 215. In its obituary of Farr the *British Medical Journal* wrote that he 'had done more to forward the progress of sanitation' than 'any other man who could be named', although it also singled out Simon for praise, Eyler, *Victorian Social Medicine*, p. 193.

8 Frazer, *A History of English Public Health*, pp. 33–4.

9 Cullen, *The Statistical Movement*, p. 146.

10 *Ibid.*, p. 178.

11 See especially Charles Dickens's *Bleak House*, Chapter 8, for an attack on the do-gooder, Mrs Pardiggle. For a superb analysis of Dickens's attitude towards and co-operation with the evangelicals and his participation in social reform, see Pope, *Dickens and Charity*.

12 Quoted in A. Briggs, 'Public Health: the "Sanitary Idea" ', *New Society*, 15 February 1968, p. 229.

13 Hodgkinson, *The Origins of the National Health Services*, p. 630.

Southwood Smith maintained that one-third of the paupers in Bethnal Green and one-half in Whitechapel were fever cases, *ibid*.

14 By 'fever' was meant primarily typhus and typhoid fevers. Quoted in Sheppard, *London, 1808–1870*, p. 252; Hodgkinson, *The Origins of the National Health Service*, p. 630.

15 *Ibid*., p. 628.

16 *Public Health*, VII, 87 (July 1895), p. 350.

17 Flinn, ed., *Report on the Sanitary Condition*, pp. 192, 193, 194. Flinn provides an excellent introduction to the *Report*.

18 For a summary of the *Report* see *PP*. XXXV (1871), 'Second Report of the Royal Sanitary Commission. I. Report', p. 6.

19 See the Nuisances Removal and Diseases Prevention Act, 1846 (9 and 10 Vict.C.96).

20 The Act was supplemented by a stronger Nuisances Removal Act, 1848 (11 and 12 Vict.C.123).

21 Simon, *English Sanitary Institutions*, p. 223.

22 *Ibid*., p. 208.

23 *Ibid*., p. 215.

24 *Ibid*.

25 Midwinter, *Social Administration in Lancashire, 1830–1860*, pp. 83–4.

26 In short, the indictment of the London vestries, 'jostling, jarring, unscientific, cumbrous, and costly', might be applied with equal force to many local authorities throughout Britain, see H. Jephson, *The Sanitary Evolution of London* (1907), p. 2. J. L. Hammond, 'The Social Background, 1835–1935', in Laski, Jennings, and Robson, eds. *A Century of Municipal Progress*, p. 45.

27 Under the Act it became unlawful to erect houses without drains and adequate w.cs, ashpits, or privies; and cellars for human habitation had to be at least 7′ high.

28 Smith, ed., *Public Health Act*, pp. 30, 31, 35.

29 Archer, 'A Study of Local Sanitary Administration', pp. 51ff, 70.

30 Penny, *Warwickshire History*, I, 6 (Autumn, 1971), pp. 4ff, 9.

31 Townley, 'Urban Administration and Health', pp. 119ff.

32 R. MacLeod, 'The Anatomy of State Medicine: Concept and Application', in F. N. L. Poynter, ed., *Medicine and Science in the 1860s* (1968). See also Simon, *English Sanitary Institutions*, pp. 215, 216, 224.

33 *Ibid*., p. 233.

34 Flinn, ed., A. P. Stewart and E. Jenkins, *The Medical and Legal Aspects of Sanitary Reform* (Leicester, 1969), p. 9.

35 Quoted in *ibid*., p. 14.

36 *PP*. XXXV (1871), 'Second Report of the Royal Sanitary Commission. II. Minutes of Evidence', p. 233.

37 Morris, *Cholera, 1832, passim*.

38 Briggs, *New Society*, 15 February 1968, p. 229.

39 R. MacLeod gives this title to the period 1860–75, see MacLeod in Poynter, ed., *Medicine and Science in the 1860s*, p. 225. See Archer, 'A Study of Local Sanitary Administration', p. 221 for the way towns like Burton and Derby would turn to the central government for advice on the smallest details.

40 Newton, *Victorian Exeter, 1837–1914*, pp. 123ff.

41 Simon, *English Sanitary Institutions*, pp. 299–300.

42 *PP.* XXXVII (1867), 'Ninth ARMOHPC, for 1866', p. 28.

43 Simon, *English Sanitary Institutions*, pp. 277–80, 380.

44 See for example, *PP.* XXIX (1860), 'Second ARMOHPC for 1859', p. 36.

45 *PP.* XXXVIII (1870), 'Twelfth ARMOHPC, for 1869', p. 15. Hennock, *Fit and Proper Persons*, pp. 207, 208. Hunter's report is in *PP.* XXXIII (1866), 'Eighth ARMOHPC, for 1865, Appendix VI, "Report by Dr Henry Julian Hunter on Circumstances endangering the Public Health of Leeds"'.

46 Simon, *English Sanitary Institutions*, p. 317.

47 Frazer, *A History of English Public Health*, p. 43.

48 *PP.* XXXII (1868–9), 'Eleventh ARMOHPC, for 1868', p. 21 (my italics).

49 The first two have been reprinted, with a splendid introduction in Flinn, ed., *The Medical and Legal Aspects of Sanitary Reform*.

50 Simon, *English Sanitary Institutions*, quoted pp. 328–9. *PP.* XXXV (1871), 'Second Report of the Royal Sanitary Commission. I. Report', p. 36.

51 Frazer, *A History of English Public Health*, pp. 117, 120. The 1875 Act remained in force until 1936.

52 J. Brand, 'John Simon and the Local Government Board Bureaucrats, 1871–1876', *Bulletin of the History of Medicine*, XXXVII 2 (March–April 1963), quoted p. 191; MacLeod, 'The Frustration of State Medicine . . .', *Medical History*, XI (January 1967), pp. 19, 21, 22.

53 The request for £100 would have brought the total for 'auxiliary Scientific Investigation' back up to the original £2,000 pa Simon had enjoyed, but the estimates were in fact cut by £800, *ibid.*, p. 24.

54 *Ibid.*, p. 25.

55 *Ibid.*, p. 29.

56 Simon, *English Sanitary Institutions*, p. 40. For Simon's criticism of Stansfeld see *ibid.*, pp. 389ff. By 1880 the Board had visited only 375 separate districts, but many of them several times, *PP.* LXI (1880), 'Return showing all the local visitations which have been made by Medical Inspectors under the Direction of the Local Government Board . . .', pp. 118–19. In addition, between October 1878 and February 1881 the Medical Department drafted, discussed, and issued 119 circulars and memoranda to local sanitary authorities, MacLeod, *Medical History*, XI (January 1967), p. 19, and *PP.* XXXVIII (1899), 'ARLGB, for 1898', pp. 548–61.

57 MacLeod, *Medical History*, XI (January 1967), p. 31.

58 *Ibid.*, pp. 31, 37. In view of all the difficulties in its way, the efforts of the Local Government Board hardly deserves the censure (however mild) of the Inter-Departmental Committee on Physical Deterioration, see G. Slater, *Poverty and the State* (1930), pp. 170ff.

59 *PP.* XXXI (1875), 'ARLGB, for 1874–5', pp. xli, xlii. The work amounted, *in toto*, to £3,728, 182, of which over £1,000,000 was spent in sewerage systems and £1,399,000 on water supply, *ibid.*, p. xliii.

60 *PP.* XXI (1876), 'ARLGB, for 1875–6', p. lvii.

61 *PP.* XXIX (1873), 'ARLGB, for 1872–3', p. lxix; *PP.* LXI (1880), 'Return . . . showing all the Local Visitations . . . Local Government Board', pp. 118–19. See also *PP.* XL (1875), 'ARLGB, for 1874', p. 11. *PP.* XXVII (1872), 'ARLGB, for 1871–2', p. xliv.

62 *PP.* XXXVIII (1899), 'ARLGB, for 1898', pp. 548–61; also *PP.* XXIX (1898), 'ARLGB, for 1897', p. ciii.

63 *Ibid.*, p. civ.

64 Quoted in MacLeod, in Poynter, *Medicine and Science*, p. 20, Large loans frequently followed hard on the heels of an inspection; thus Sunderland received £64,000 and Bradford £50,000 shortly after a Board inspection, *PP.* LXI (1880), 'Return . . . showing all the Local Visitations . . . Local Government Board', p. 6; *PP.* XXXI (1876), 'ARLGB, for 1875–6', p. lvii.

65 R. Hodgkinson, 'The Social Environment of British Medical Science and Practice in the Nineteenth Century', in W. C. Gibson, ed., *British Contributions to Medical Science* (1971), p. 51.

66 *PP.* XXXIII (1890), 'ARMOHLGB, for 1889–90', p. cxxxvi. For model by-laws, see *PP.* XXXVII (1878), 'ARLGB, for 1877–8', pp. 171–4.

67 Quoted in MacNalty, *The History of State Medicine*, p. 32.

68 See Lambert, *Sir John Simon*, *passim*, MacLeod in Poynter, ed., *Medicine and Science*, MacNalty, *The History of State Medicine*, *passim*, and R. Thorne Thorne, *The Progress of Preventive Medicine during the Victorian Period* (1888), pp. 30ff.

Chapter Seven. 'Local Affairs'

1 Hennock, *Fit and Proper Persons*, p. 10. My debt to this outstanding work will be apparent throughout the first part of this chapter.

2 *Ibid.*, p. 11.

3 In no town in the nineteenth century did the figure go above 20 per cent, *ibid.*, p. 12.

4 For the franchise see *ibid.*, pp. 11, 12, and *PP.* LXIV (1875), 'A Digest of the Statutes Relating to Urban Sanitary Authorities', p. 13. See also

Hennock, 'Finance and Politics in Urban Local Government in England, 1835–1900', *Historical Journal*, VI, 2 (1967), p. 216, and Midwinter, *Social Administration in Lancashire*, pp. 89, 91.

5 *Transactions of the Sanitary Institute of Great Britain*, VIII (1886–7), quoted, p. 210. The investigation was by T. H. Harrison and was entitled, 'On an Account of an Investigation into the Classes who Administer the Public Health Act.' For above see pp. 210–11. See also Hennock, *Fit and Proper Persons*, p. 33.

6 *Ibid.*, pp. 314, 315, 316. For Chamberlain's appeal to the shopkeepers, see *ibid.*, pp. 127–8. For the *Salford Weekly News*, see Fraser, *Power and Authority in the Victorian City*, quoted p. 151.

7 Hennock, *Fit and Proper Persons, passim.*

8 *Transactions of the Sanitary Institute of Great Britain*, VIII (1886–7), p. 210.

9 *Ibid.* In Birmingham doctors composed 6.3, 9.7, and 6.9 per cent of the town council in the years 1882, 1892, and 1896 respectively. Hennock, *Fit and Proper Persons*, p. 34, see also *ibid.*, pp. 37, 207.

10 *Transactions of the Sanitary Institute of Great Britain*, VIII (1886–7), pp. 210, 212. Builders comprised some nine per cent of the Exeter City Council between 1868 and 1877, see Hennock, *Fit and Proper Persons*, p. 49.

11 *PP.* XXXI (1886), 'ARMOHLGB, for 1885, Appendix VII, "Supplement . . . on Cholera" ', pp. 123–4.

12 *Ibid.*, p. 124.

13 Hennock, *Fit and Proper Persons*, p. 112.

14 Hole, quoted in Toft, 'Public Health in Leeds', p. 207. Fraser characterizes the 'economists' as 'the petty bourgeoisie, inured by occupation to meagreness', *Power and Authority in the Victorian City*, p. 96. By contrast, he argues, big businessmen often 'brought business accumen, and enlarged municipal vision and organizational talent' to urban government, *ibid.*, p. 159. See also *ibid.*, p. 128 for an impassioned attack on the 'economists' by Robert Rawlinson, the government inspector.

15 Hennock, *Fit and Proper Persons*, pp. 190–2. The Corporation was now the authority for paving, drainage, streets, housing standards, nuisances, etc.

16 *Ibid.*, pp. 197–9, and Townley, 'Urban Administration and Health', pp. 226, 237.

17 Hennock, *Fit and Proper Persons*, p. 197; Fraser, *Power and Authority in the Victorian City*, p. 128 and Fraser, *Urban Politics in Victorian England* (Leicester, 1979), p. 175.

18 Hennock *Fit and Proper Persons*, pp. 96, 316, 319.

19 Hennock, *Historical Journal*, VI, 2 (1967), p. 216.

20 Hill, *Victorian Lincoln*, p. 167.

21 In Hanley, where the 'mass of ratepayers, obsessed with questions of expense, usually acted as a retarding influence on the expansion and

improvement of local government services in the town', the inspector of nuisances and the surveyor did not become full-time employees until 1886, Townley, 'Urban Administration and Health', pp. 79, 112–13, 327. For Oldbury see *Transactions of the National Association for the Promotion of Social Science*, 1868, p. 474.

22 Hennock, *Fit and Proper Persons*, p. 31. See *ibid.*, pp. 31–3 for the composition of the 'Economy party' and the freezing of the rates at 2s.6d in the £.

23 *Ibid.*, pp. 210, 211; and for Liverpool see Fraser *Power and Authority in the Victorian City*, p. 45 and *ibid.*, quoted p. 70 for the *Leeds Mercury*.

24 Redford, *The History of Local Government in Manchester*, II, pp. 145ff.

25 *PP.* XXIX (1860), 'Second ARMOHPC, for 1859', p. 46.

26 Hennock, *Fit and Proper Persons*, pp. 105–6. For an interesting analysis of Avery's concept of 'efficiency' in municipal affairs, see Fraser, *Power and Authority in the Victorian City*, p. 99.

27 This argument was applied most vigorously to the question of air and water pollution. See below, Chapters 8 and 9.

28 For Leicester (led by Joseph Whetstone, the Mayor and Chairman of the Highways and Sewage Committee), see Elliott, 'The Leicester Board of Health', p. 25. The Leicester by-laws were models for other towns to copy.

29 Hennock, *Fit and Proper Persons*, pp. 231, 232.

30 See Chapter 6, above.

31 See for example, Hennock, *Fit and Proper Persons*, p. 115; for London and the Royal Commission on housing see Wohl, *The Eternal Slum*, especially Chapter 8.

32 See for example, Hennock *Fit and Proper Persons*, pp. 107, 213, and also below Chapter 9.

33 Townley, 'Urban Administration and Health', p. 327.

34 Redford, *The History of Local Government in Manchester*, II, p. 267.

35 *Ibid.*, III, p. 391.

36 Hennock, *Fit and Proper Persons*, pp. 119ff.

37 *Ibid.*, pp. 72ff. See especially pp. 61–79.

38 Dawson in a speech in 1869, quoted in *ibid.*, p. 75.

39 *Ibid.*, p. 77. For the efforts of this group see pp. 77ff.

40 *Ibid.*, pp. 70ff., 139ff., 154ff.

41 *Ibid.*, pp. 125ff.

42 Wohl, *The Eternal Slum*, Chapter 8.

43 Quoted in K. Inglis, *The Churches and the Working Classes in Victorian England* (1963), p. 68.

44 Wohl, *The Eternal Slum*, pp. 215ff. See also M. Richter, *The Politics of Conscience. T.H.Green and his Age* (1964).

45 B. Webb, *My Apprenticeship* (1926), pp. 179–180.

46 R. W. Dale, 'Political and Municipal Duty', in *The Laws of Christ for*

Common Life (1884), pp. 198–200, quoted in Hennock, *Fit and Proper Persons*, pp. 161–2. The phrase, 'the sacredness of what is called secular business' is from Dale's *The Evangelical Revival, and other Sermons* (1880), quoted in *ibid*., p. 161.

47   See for example, the 'civic gospel' in Bristol, Fraser, *Power and Authority in the Victorian City*, pp. 117ff. Smith, ed., *Public Health Act*, pp. 3, 8; Elliott, 'The Leicester Board of Health', *passim*; Hennock, *Fit and Proper Persons*, *passim*.

48   See for example, *ibid*., pp. 249–50.

49   For the *Leicester Chronicle* see D. Ross, *The Leicester Archaeological and Historical Society, Transactions*, XLIII (1967–8), pp. 35ff; for the *Flying Post*, Newton, *Victorian Exeter*, p. 255; for the *Warwick Advertiser*, Penny, *Warwickshire History*, I, 6 (Autumn, 1971), pp. 4–5, for the *Darlington and Stockton Times*, see Smith, ed., *Public Health Act* pp. 2–5; for the *Leeds Mercury*, Toft, 'Public Health in Leeds', p. 214; for the *City Press* and local London papers, Wohl, *The Eternal Slum*, *passim*. and for the *Porcupine* and *Town Crier*, see Fraser, *Power and Authority in the Victorian City*, pp. 40, 43. See also Hennock, *Fit and Proper Persons*, *passim*.

50   Midwinter, *Social Administration in Lancashire*, pp. 71–2.

51   One could argue that a table of death rates at various dates would give a graphic indication of the rates of progress in sanitary reform but, as we have mentioned, many other factors besides public health reforms and sanitary administration influence death rates.

52   Once again it is pertinent to point out what disappointing use local historians and Ph.D candidates have made of the MOH records.

53   *Public Health*, VI, 73 (May 1894), p. 25.

54   *Lancet*, 23 September 1843, p. 1902.

55   For Leicester's appointment of Drs Buck and Barclay see Elliott, 'The Leicester Board of Health', pp. 25, 186.

56   Frazer, *Duncan of Liverpool* is the standard biography, see also his *A History of English Public Health*, p. 37.

57   See section 122 of the Liverpool Sanitary Act.

58   *PP*. XXXVII (1867), 'Ninth ARMOHPC, for 1866', p. 14. In 1865 Bath, Berwick, Hull, Derby, Dudley, Grimsby, Hull, Greenock, Portsmouth, Preston, and Swansea were among the important towns without MOH, *PP*. XXXIII (1866), 'Eighth ARMOHPC, for 1865, Appendix II, "Report by Dr Henry Julien Hunter on the Housing of the Poorer Parts of the Population of Towns . . ." ', pp. 97, 121, and *ibid*., 'Appendix IV, "Report by Dr George Buchanan on Epidemic Typhus at Greenock" ', p. 209.

59   For Manchester, Sharrat and Farrar, *Memoirs and Proceedings*, 114 (1971–2), p. 60, for Wolverhampton, West Bromwich and Smethwick, Barnsby, 'Social Conditions in the Black Country', pp. 96–7; for Leeds and Birmingham, Hennock, *Fit and Proper Persons*, pp. 111, 114.

60 The staff consisted of a sanitary inspector, a bacteriologist, and three clerks, Barrows, *A County and its Health*, p. 7. By 1917 the staff had grown to 172!, *ibid.*, p. 18.

61 For an example of this see the Norfolk County MOH, J. M. Mackintosh, *Trends of Opinion about the Public Health, 1901–1951* (1953), p. 34.

62 *Public Health*, III, 25 (May 1890), p. 10.

63 Barrows, *A County and its Health*, p. 9. As a result of his constant pressure, the number of local authorities in the West Riding adopting the Notification of Diseases Act rose from sixteen (end of 1889) to ninety-six (1891), *ibid*. For an interesting brief discussion of the role of a County MOH, see J. D. Marshall, *The History of Lancashire County Council, 1889 to 1974* (1977).

64 *PP.* XXXI (1875), 'ARLGB, for 1874–5', p. xxxix. The total was 727 MOH.

65 *PP.* XXXVII (1877), 'ARLGB, 1876–7', p. liii; *PP.* XXVIII (1878–9), 'ARLGB, for 1878–9', p. xci.

66 J. L. Brand, *Doctors and the State* (Baltimore, Maryland, 1965), p. 109.

67 *Public Health*, VI, 73 (May 1894), pp. 244ff.

68 *Lancet*, 3 February 1872, p. 166, quoted in Brand, *Doctors and the State*, p. 109.

69 *PP.* XXIX (1878–9), 'ARLGB, for 1878', p. ix; 1880 Report quoted in Brand, *Doctors and the State*, p. 113.

70 See for example, *Public Health*, VI, 73 (May 1894), p. 243. In 1876 the Local Government Board issued a memorandum on the subject, calling for statistical comparisons between districts rather than mere descriptive material, *PP.* VII (1876–7), 'Sixth ARLGB, for 1876, Appendices XXI–XXIII, pp. 27–31. For model annual reports, see *PP.* XLVI (1881), 'Tenth ARLGB, for 1880–81, Appendix B" '.

71 Simon played an important role in the creation of the post, see C. F. Brockington, *Public Health in the Nineteenth Century* (Edinburgh, 1965), pp. 197, 199. See also H. C. Thomson, *The Story of the Middlesex Hospital Medical School* (1935).

72 *Transactions of the Sanitary Institute of Great Britain*, XV (1894), p. 390.

73 *Public Health*, VI, 73 (May 1894), p. 244.

74 *Ibid.*, pp. 242–3. See *ibid.*, pp. 242–7 for the debate on the appropriate qualities of the MOH and his qualifications.

75 Quoted in Brand, *Doctors and the State*, p. 110.

76 Blyth was MOH for St Marylebone and one of the most articulate and industrious MOH.

77 *Public Health*, VI, 73 (May 1894), pp. 242–3. The MOH for combined rural districts were exempt from the requirements of the General Medical Council. During the six months' apprenticeship the candidate was to concentrate on outdoor sanitary work.

78 Frazer, *Duncan of Liverpool*, pp. 45, 47.

79 Hennock, *Fit and Proper Persons*, p. 214.

80 *Transactions of the National Association for the Promotion of Social Science*, 1868, p. 474. Even at the low salary the Oldbury MOH was ousted by the Local Ratepayers' Protection Society.

81 J. F. B. Firth, *Municipal London* (1876), pp. 307, 408. *PP*. XLIII (1875), 'Copy of Reports of Local Government Inspectors on the Workings of the Public Health Act, 1872, Appendix I', pp. 98–9. For Southampton see H. C. M. Williams, *Public Health in a Seaport Town by the Medical Officer of Health* (Southampton 1962), p. 1. *Lancet*, 22 March 1856, p. 322.

82 Chaloner, *The Social and Economic Development of Crewe*, pp. 122, 124. See also U. R. Q. Henriques, *Before the Welfare State. Social administration in early industrial Britain* (1979), p. 143.

83 Frazer, *Duncan of Liverpool*, p. 122, and Hennock, *Fit and Proper Persons*, p. 235.

84 For a complete list of the salaries of London MOH at the end of the century, see London County Council, *Annual Report of the MOH*, 1898, p. 10.

85 Hennock, *Fit and Proper Persons*, p. 235.

86 *Public Health*, XII, 2 (November 1899), p. 66. For salaries which could be earned in private practice, see M. J. Peterson, *The Medical Profession in Mid-Victorian London* (Berkeley and Los Angeles, California, 1978), p. 214. At mid-century a successful young doctor, after eight years or so in practice, could hope to earn between £500 and £1,000. In 1871 Poor Law MOH earned an average of only £180 pa. Hodgkinson, *The Origins of the National Health Service*, p. 399.

87 *Public Health*, II (January 1869); Simon, *English Sanitary Institutions*, p. 366.

88 The complaints were usually voiced in the MOH's own journals and meetings, rarely in their reports of course.

89 *Public Health*, II (January 1869), pp. 1–2.

90 E. Hart, *Local Government as it is and as it ought to be* (1885), p. 45; *Lancet*, 22 February 1868, p. 265.

91 Farr, quoted in Jephson, *The Sanitary Evolution of London*, p. 189. *Public Health*, XII, I (October 1899).

92 Quoted in V. Zoond, 'Housing Legislation in England, 1851–1867, with special reference to London', London University, MA thesis (1932), p. 57.

93 *Pall Mall Gazette*, 11 February 1884.

94 Zoond, 'Housing Legislation in England', p. 133.

95 *PP*. XXVI (1865), 'Seventh ARMOHPC, for 1864', p. 20. In Sheerness, which was very insanitary, the Privy Council inspector, Henry Austin, could not even locate the local inspector of nuisances, *PP*. XXIX (1860), 'Second ARMOHPC, for 1859', p. 46.

96 *PP*. XXX (1884–5), 'Royal Commission on the Housing of the Working Classes. II. Minutes of Evidence', p. 12.

97 Quoted in Rev Mearns, *Contemporary Review*, XLIX (October 1883), p. 928.

98 G. Sims, *How the Poor Live and Horrible London* (1898), pp. 43, 129.

99 G. Haw, *No Room to Live: the Plaint of Overcrowded London* (1900), pp. 134–5.

100 *Transactions of the National Association for the Promotion of Social Science* (1865), p. 74. The condemnation of 'inquisitorial legislation' was by Roger Paget, vestry clerk of Clerkenwell, a vestry composed of small property owners, *PP*. XXX (1884–5), 'Royal Commission on the Housing of the Working Classes. II. Minutes of Evidence', pp. 656, 662.

101 Metropolitan Association of MOH, *Papers*, 1878–9, p. 16. In the view of the MOH for St Giles, 'the duty of making these sanitary improvements should be imperative instead of permissive' quoted in Jephson, *The Sanitary Evolution of London*, p. 218.

102 On the other hand some MOH were denied permission to appear before their boards. One MOH was told that his reports were 'too elaborate' and his request for money to print and circulate them was met with an inadequate grant of £5, see *Public Health*, IX, 63 (June 1950), p. 176. Particularly vulnerable were the MOH of combined rural sanitary districts, *Lancet*, 12 July 1879, p. 55.

103 Two hundred and thirty MOH were appointed from two to five years, and 112 held their appointments at the pleasure of the local authority, *Public Health*, VI, 73 (May 1894), p. 247.

104 *Lancet*, 23 December 1899, p. 1760.

105 *Public Health*, XI, I (October 1898), pp. 15–16. Metropolitan MOH were given tenure under the Public Health (London) Act of 1891.

106 Mackintosh, *Trends of Opinion about the Public Health*, pp. 25–6.

107 Jephson, *The Sanitary Evolution of London*, p. 189. Rendle attacked the vestries in his *London Vestries and their Sanitary Work* (1865); for Godrich see P. E. Malcolmson, 'The Potteries of Kensington: a Study of Slum Development in Victorian London', University of Leicester, M. Phil thesis (1970), p. 129.

108 *Public Health*, XII, 2 (November 1899), pp. 66–76. For a summary of these dismissals see *Lancet*, 23 December 1899, p. 1760.

109 The phrase is John Sykes's (MOH, St Pancras), see *Public Health*, VI, 73 (May 1894), p. 245.

110 See for example the position of the MOH for Crewe, in Chaloner, *The Social and Economic Development of Crewe*, p. 122.

111 For Thorne Thorne's concern, at the Local Government Board, for the status of the MOH, see *Lancet*, 23 December 1899, pp. 1748, 1762.

112 *Public Health*, LXI, 11 (August 1948), p. 210.

113 For the most part the relationship, from the local MOH's point of view, consisted of submitting reports and getting guide lines.

114 It is for this reason that some of the early Metropolitan MOH were reluctant to meet in Simon's office at the General Board of Health, see *ibid.*, LXIII, 9 (June 1950), p. 178.

115 Hennock, *Fit and Proper Persons*, p. 114. In 1875, when it adopted a much more progressive policy, Birmingham did accept the offer. For Leeds, see *ibid.*, p. 214.

116 *Public Health*, LXI, 11 (August 1848), p. 210. Eventually over half the local authorities accepted the subsidy from the Local Government Board, see Simon, *English Sanitary Institutions*, p. 371.

117 When it first advertised for a MOH Leeds received 67 applicants; Salford received 42, Manchester, Nottingham, Sunderland, and South Shields between twenty and thirty applicants, *Public Health*, LXI, 11 (August 1948), p. 211.

118 *The Times*, 7 December 1855. See *Lancet* 29 December 1855, pp. 632–3, and 12 January 1856, p. 37 for advice to vestries on certain kinds of candidate to avoid.

119 Quoted in *Public Health*, LXIII, 9 (June 1950), p. 176.

120 *The Times*, 7 December 1855.

121 *Public Health*, XVIII (1906: Jubilee number), p. 237 and LXIII, 9 (June 1950), pp. 176–7.

122 Macdonald, 'Public Health Legislation', p. 69. For Wandsworth see J. Roebuck, 'London Government and some aspects of Social Change in the Parishes of Lambeth, Battersea, and Wandsworth, 1838–1888', London University, Ph.D thesis (1968), p. 144; for Manchester, Redford, *The History of Local Government in Manchester*, II, pp. 266–7.

123 Quoted in Mackintosh, *Trends of Opinion*, p. 38.

124 For doctors on local boards and their committees see Hennock, *Fit and Proper Persons*, pp. 34, 44, 49, 50.

125 Hill, *Victorian London*, p. 167; Penny, *Warwickshire History*, I, 5 (Autumn 1971), p. 13.

126 For the founding and original purpose of the Institute see *Transactions of the Sanitary Institute of Great Britain,* 1880, p. xvii.

127 *Public Health*, III, 25 (May 1890), p. 30; see also *London*, 15 June 1893, p. 307.

128 Mansion House Council on the Dwellings of the Poor, *Report for the Year ending 1889* (1890), p. 11; see also Gibbon and Bell, *History of the London County Council*, p. 59 and *PP*. XXXI (1886); 'ARLGB for 1885, Appendix VII, "Supplement . . . on Cholera" ', p.126.

129 *PP*. XXX (1884–5), 'Royal Commission on the Housing of the Working Classes. II. Minutes of Evidence', p. 63.

130 W. Blyth, *A Manual of Public Health* (1890), p. 602.

131 Zoond, 'Housing Legislation in England', pp. 129–30, *PP*. XXX (1884–5), 'Royal Commission on the Housing of the Working Classes. II. Minutes of Evidence', p. 16.

132 The fifty-one MOH in London had between them 256 inspectors; Gibbon and Bell, *History of the London County Council*, p. 59;

Mansion House Council on the Dwellings of the Poor, *Report for the Year ending 1889* (1890), p. 5. The two exceptions were St Olave's and St Martin-in-the-Fields.

133 The nature of these house inspections can be gathered from the annual reports of the London MOH.

134 *Transactions of the Sanitary Institute of Great Britain*, 1882–3, pp. 90, 122; *ibid.*, 1892, p. 60; *ibid.*, 1895, p. 266; *ibid.*, 1897, p. 16, and *ibid.*, 1898, p.53. For an important analysis of the attempt of doctors to gain control of the public health movement see S. J. Novak, 'Professionalism and Bureaucracy: English Doctors and the Victorian Public Health Administration', *Social History*, VI, 4 (Summer, 1976).

135 The Poor Law MOH formed their Association in 1868.

136 *Public Health*, LXIX, 8 (May 1956), pp. 177ff.

137 In 1884 it still had only 123 full members, forty associate, and twenty-three honorary members; by 1900 it had attracted roughly one-half of all the MOH in the country. Brand, *Medicine and the State*, p. 114. Their pamphlets generally sold for 2s for a hundred copies, *Public Health*, LXIX, 8 (May 1956), p. 71.

138 Macdonald, 'Public Health Legislation', pp. 169, 187–8.

139 Redford, *The History of Local Government in Manchester*, II, p. 279.

140 *Ibid.*, pp. 280, 283.

141 *Ibid.*, pp. 436–7. Unfortunately no attempt was made to train the committee members or the subordinate officials, *ibid.*, p. 440.

142 See for example, Hennock, *Fit and Proper Persons*, pp. 208, 235. In Manchester, within a few years of his appointment, Dr Leigh had filled in 4,000 cesspools, introduced a system of cleaning ash-closets twice a week, and had reconstructed 40,000 privy closets and pail closets, see Sharrat and Farrar, *Memoirs and Proceedings*, 114 (1971–72), pp. 60–1.

143 Quoted in Lambert, *Sir John Simon*, p. 152.

144 *PP*. XXXVII (1867), 'Ninth ARMOHPC, for 1866', p. 28. By 1899 the seven MOH and fourteen sanitary inspectors of Cork, to take one example, had conducted 61,000 inspections, *PP*. XXXVII (1902), 'Twenty-ninth Annual Report of the Local Government Board for Ireland, 1900–1901, Supplement, "Report on the Sanitary Circumstances and Administration of Cities and Towns in Ireland"', p. 30.

145 The Nuisances Removal Act of 1855 permitted MOH to enter homes on the order of a JP, and Torrens's Housing Act of 1868 first enabled them to enter on their own initiative. After that, they no longer had to wait until a house was unfit for human habitation, but could enter on mere suspicion of a nuisance or sanitary defect.

146 Quoted in Toft, 'Public Health in Leeds', p. 23, and in Fraser, *Power and Authority in the Victorian City*, p. 105.

147 See Wohl, *The Eternal Slum*, p. 119. Until biographical studies of the MOH are undertaken we can only guess at the inspiration and motives

which lay behind their work. For the MOH and poverty see Chapters 11 and 12.

148 Blyth, *A Manual of Public Health*, p. 593.
149 Frazer, *A History of English Public Health*, p. 125 writes, 'when the long account of the benefits conferred by the medical profession on the modern community has been finally computed, it will assuredly be acknowledged that the debt owing to the Medical Officers of Health of the past is a great one', yet he devotes only five pages to an analysis of their accomplishments.
150 Quoted in Mackintosh, *Trends of Opinion*, p. 37.
151 See for example Macdonald 'Public Health Legislation', *passim*, and Brotherston, *Observations on the Early Public Health Movement*, *passim*.
152 The Board of Supervision became the Local Government Board for Scotland under the Local Government Act of 1889.
153 *Public Health*, XI, 1 (October 1898), pp. 14ff.
154 *PP.* XXIV (1871), 'Second Report of the Royal Sanitary Commission. II. Minutes of Evidence', p. 189.
155 It could (and did) require local authorities to appoint MOH, and it could approve or disapprove of their selections.
156 F. McKichan, 'Stirling, 1780–1880: the Response of Burgh Government to the Problems of Urban Growth', University of Glasgow, M. Litt thesis (1972), p. 228.
157 Quoted in *ibid.*, p. 230.
158 Quoted in *ibid.*, p. 182. It was only after three years of debate that the rate was passed.
159 *Ibid.*, pp. 222ff.
160 Under the General Police and Improvement Act, see Tait, *A Doctor and Two Policemen*, p. 19.
161 Of the total amount of £2,070,949, £1,353,632 was for waterworks, £414,171.11.3, for drainage, £52,712, for water and drainage, £241,809 for hospitals, £3,500 for public baths, and £5,125 for public slaughter houses, *PP.* XXXVI (1899) 'Fifth Annual Report of the Local Government Board for Scotland, 1900', p. lxi.
162 *PP.* XXXV (1900), 'Annual Report of the Local Government Board for Ireland, 1900', p. lxii.
163 *Transactions of the Sanitary Institute of Great Britain*, VI (1884–5), pp. 109, 115.
164 Some of the relevant Acts were the Public Health Act, 1848; Diseases Prevention Act, 1858; Nuisances Removal and Diseases Prevention Act, 1860; Local Government Act, 1858, Amendment Act, 1861, Sewage Utilization Act, 1865, Nuisances Removal Act, 1863, Sanitary Act, 1866, Sanitary Act, 1868 and Sanitary Act, 1870.
165 Cameron, *A Brief History*, pp. 19, 32.
166 *Ibid.*, p. 68. *PP.* XXXVII (1902), 'Twenty-ninth Annual Report of the Local Government Board for Ireland, 1900–1901, Supplement,

"Report on the Sanitary Circumstances and Administration of Cities and Towns in Ireland" ', p. 3.

167 Cameron, *A Brief History*, pp. 42, 50.
168 *Ibid.*, p. 108.
169 Wohl, *The Eternal Slum*, pp. 320, 323, 324.
170 Hennock, *Fit and Proper Persons*, pp. 250–1.
171 *Ibid.*, p. 254. Among the other nine points were the extension of cheap tramways, more labour representation on local committees, and 'economy in the administration of all departments of City affairs by the Council, with due regard to efficiency'.
172 *Public Health*, VI, 73 (May 1894), pp. 245–6.

Chapter Eight. ' "The Black Canopy of Smoke": Atmospheric Pollution'.

1 T. C. Barker and J. R. Harris, *A Merseyside Town in the Industrial Revolution: St Helens, 1750–1900* (1959), p. 318.
2 *PP.* XXXVII (1902), 'Twenty-ninth Annual Report of the Local Government Board for Ireland, 1900–1901. Supplement, "Report on the Sanitary Circumstances and Administration of Cities and Towns in Ireland" ', p. 33.
3 K. Woodward, *Jipping Street* (1929), pp. 24–5.
4 *PP.* XLIV (1878), 'RCNV. II. Minutes of Evidence', pp. 524–5.
5 *PP.* VII (1843), 'SCSP. II. Minutes of Evidence', pp. 64, 79.
6 *PP.* XXV (1920), 'Interim Report of the Committee on Smoke and Noxious Vapours Abatement', p. 3.
7 L. Faucher, *Manchester in 1844; it's Present Condition and Future Prospects* (1844), p. 16.
8 *PP.* VII (1843), 'SCSP. II. Minutes of Evidence', p. 62.
9 *PP.* XLIV (1878), 'RCNV. II. Minutes of Evidence', p. 29.
10 *PP.* XIII (1845), 'SCSP. II. Minutes of Evidence', p. 32.
11 Flinn, ed., *Report on the Sanitary Condition*, p. 356.
12 *PP.* VII (1843), 'SCSP. I. Report', pp. 28, 33. *Punch*, XX (January–June 1851), p. 83.
13 *Blackwood's Magazine*, March 1842, pp. 380–1.
14 *PP.* VII (1843), 'SCSP. II. Minutes of Evidence', p. 80.
15 *Ibid.*, p. 187.
16 C. Dickens, *Bleak House* (Signet Classics ed., 1964), p. 141.
17 *PP.* XLIV (1878), 'RCNV. I. Report', pp. 20, 24. Residents of Plymouth complained of nausea, depression, and loss of appetite resulting from the smoke and smells of the local soap, manure, vitriol, sugar, and tar distilling works, *ibid.*, pp. 25, 26.
18 *Ibid.*, p. 23. *PP.* XIII (1845), 'SCSP. II. Minutes of Evidence', pp. 38ff.
19 Dickens, *Bleak House*, p. 1.

20   *Ibid.*, p. 44.

21   Ministry of Health, *Miscellaneous Papers*, 1921, 'Committee on Smoke and Noxious Vapours: Final Report', p. 5.

22   Flinn, ed., *Report on the Sanitary Condition*, p. 350.

23   G. Wyld, *Notes on My Life* (1903), p. 100.

24   *PP*. XLIV (1878), 'RCNV. II. Minutes of Evidence', p. 233.

25   *Transactions of the Sanitary Institute of Great Britain*, XIII (1892), pp. 61, 62. Parkes called for the use of only anthracite as a domestic fuel, *ibid.*, p. 63.

26   *Ibid.*, p. 61.

27   Wyld, *Notes on My Life*, p. 101, and *PP*. XII (1887), 'Select Committee of the House of Lords on the Smoke Nuisances (Abatement Metropolis) Bill', p. 48.

28   *PP*. XXV (1920), 'Interim Report of the Committee on Smoke and Noxious Vapours Abatement', p. 2.

29   *PP*. XXIII (1887), 'Forty-ninth Annual Report of the Registrar-General, for 1886', pp. 118–19: for a normal year see *PP*. XXX (1888), 'Fiftieth Annual Report of the Registrar-General, for 1887', pp. 118–19 and *PP*. XVII (1886) 'Forty-eighth Annual Report of the Registrar-General, for 1885', pp. 118–19. For the London fog see Stedman Jones, *Outcast London*, pp. 291ff.

30   *PP*. XII (1887), 'Select Committee of the House of Lords on the Smoke Nuisance Abatement (Metropolis) Bill', p. 10.

31   *Ibid.*, p. 12.

32   *PP*. XLIV (1878), 'RCNV. II. Minutes of Evidence', p. 21.

33   *Ibid.*, p. 20.

34   *Ibid.*, p. 22.

35   *Ibid*, p. 326.

36   *PP*. XIII (1845), 'SCSP. II. Minutes of Evidence', pp. 38ff.

37   J. L. and B. Hammond, *The Rise of Modern Industry* (1925, eighth edition, 1951), p. 232.

38   W. Cooke Taylor, *Notes on a Tour in the Manufacturing Districts of Lancashire* (1842), quoted in J. T. Ward, *The Factory System*, II, *The Factory System and Society* (New York, 1970), p. 62.

39   Smith, ed., *Public Health Act*, p. 11.

40   Quoted in Barker and Harris, *A Merseyside Town*, p. 404. The authors conclude that 'noxious vapours and offending smells' were 'an integral part of the prosperity of the town', *ibid*. See also Toft, 'Public Health in Leeds', p. 103. For an interesting contemporary choice between stagnation and pollution see the Mobil advertisement in the *New York Times* for 20 March 1980: 'Stagnation is still the worst form of pollution', and 'Pollution takes many forms. In the American experience by far the most damaging form has been economic stagnation.'

41   *PP*. XLIV (1878), 'RCNV. II. Minutes of Evidence', p. 452.

42   *Ibid.*, 'I. Report', p. 29.

43   *PP*. XIV (1862), 'Report from the Select Committee of the House of Lords on Injury from Noxious Vapours:, pp. 45, 55.

44   38 and 39 Vict.C.55, clause 91.

45   *PP*.X (1873), 'Select Committee on Noxious Businesses. II. Minutes of Evidence'. p. 169. This was the evidence of E. Knight, the owner of a small tallow melting and soap concern. There were some thirty soap manufacturers in London, turning out between them 47,000 tons of soap a year, *ibid*., p. 128.

46   *PP*. VII (1843), 'SCSP. II. Minutes of Evidence', pp. 82, 187.

47   *PP*. XIII (1845) 'SCSP. II. Minutes of Evidence', p. 31.

48   *PP*. XLIV (1878), 'RCNV. II. Minutes of Evidence', pp. 450, 452.

49   A. Beck, 'Some Aspects of the History of Anti-Pollution Legislation in England, 1819–1954', *Journal of the History of Medicine and Allied Sciences*, XIV (October 1959), p. 477.

50   *PP*. VII (1843), 'SCSP. I. Report'', pp. iii, iv.

51   *PP*. XII (1887), 'Select Committee of the House of Lords on the Smoke Nuisance Abatement (Metropolis) Bill, pp. 3ff. For the use of the police see *ibid*., p. 27.

52   *PP*. LX (1866), 'Summaries of Replies of Letters sent by the Secretary of State . . .', pp. 2ff.

53   *Ibid*., pp. 1–2. See also Ministry of Health, *Miscellaneous Papers*, 1921, 'Committee on Smoke and Noxious Vapours. First Report', pp. 11ff.

54   Redford, *The History of Local Government in Manchester*, I, p. 84.

55   By 1880 about half the furnaces inspected in Leeds had some form of smoke-consuming device, see Toft, 'Public Health in Leeds', p. 136.

56   *PP*. LXI (1854), 'Copy of a Letter . . . with a Digest of . . . inventions for the Consumption of Smoke', pp. 4, 7.

57   *PP*. L (1861), 'Returns . . . Smoke Consuming Furnaces', p. 1. Of these the largest number were in Lambeth (1,238), Southwark (1,672), Stepney (933), and Wandsworth (796), *ibid*.

58   Clause 91. My italics.

59   *PP*. XLIV (1878), 'RCNV. I. Report', pp. 3, 4.

60   Thus up to 1855 the local authorities in London, operating under the various smoke and nuisances acts, had imposed fines totalling some £614, but court costs were almost £900, excluding lawyers' fees, *PP*. LIII (1854–5), 'Return of the number of prosecutions . . . under the Smoke Nuisance (Abatement) Act', p. 1. For the National Smoke Abatement Society see *PP*. LXIII (1884), 'Copy of Correspondence . . . on the Defective Administration of the Smoke Nuisance Act in the Metropolis', p. 6. The Society was headed by the Duke of Westminster and Ernest Hart, editor of the *British Medical Journal* from 1866 to 1898.

61   *PP*. LXI (1854), 'Copy of a Letter . . . with a Digest of . . . Inventions for the Consumption of Smoke', p. 5. *PP*. XLIV (1878), 'RCNV. II. Minutes of Evidence', pp. 31, 37.

62   *Ibid*., p. 528.

63   *Ibid*., p. 506.

64   *PP.* XXXII (1904), 'Inter-Departmental Committee on Physical Deterioration. I. Report', p. 20, 'II. Minutes of Evidence', p. 176.

65   Definition in *American Heritage Dictionary*. For much of the following I am indebted to R. MacLeod, 'The Alkali Acts Administration, 1863–84: the Emergence of the Civil Scientist', *Victorian Studies*, IX, 2 (December 1965).

66   *Ibid.*, p. 87.

67   *PP.* XLIV (1878), 'RCNV. II. Minutes of Evidence', pp. 12–13.

68   *Ibid.*

69   MacLeod, *Victorian Studies*, IX, 2 (December, 1965), p. 87.

70   *PP.* XLIV (1878), 'RCNV. II. Minutes of Evidence', pp. 6–7.

71   MacLeod, *Victorian Studies*, IX, 2 (December 1965), p. 88.

72   *PP.* XLIV (1878), 'RCNV. II, Minutes of Evidence', pp. 4–6.

73   *Ibid.*, p. 13.

74   MacLeod, *Victorian Studies*, IX, 2 (December 1965), p. 99.

75   *PP.* XLIV (1878), 'RCNV. II. Minutes of Evidence', p. 14.

76   *Transactions of the Sanitary Institute of Great Britain*, XVI (April 1895), p. 78.

77   *PP.* XLIV (1878), 'RCNV. II. Minutes of Evidence', p. 7.

78   D. Hunter, *The Diseases of Occupations* (1978), p. 660.

79   *PP.* XLIV (1878), 'RCNV. II. Minutes of Evidence', p. 10.

80   Quoted in Beck, *Journal of the History of Medicine and Allied Sciences*, XIV (October 1959), p. 484.

81   *PP.* XLIV (1878), 'RCNV. II. Minutes of Evidence', pp. 7–8.

82   *PP.* XIV (1862), 'Select Committee of the House of Lords on Injury from Noxious Vapours. I. Report', pp. 16ff.

83   MacLeod, *Victorian Studies*, IX, 2 (December 1965), p. 89.

84   *Ibid.*, pp. 92, 93. For an interesting analysis of Smith and his theories of disease, see J. M. Eyler, 'The Conversion of Angus Smith: the Changing Role of Chemistry and Biology in Sanitary Science, 1850–1880', *Bulletin of the History of Medicine*, 54, 2 (Summer, 1980).

85   MacLeod, *Victorian Studies*, IX, 2 (December 1965), pp. 94, 97.

86   *Ibid.*, quoted, p. 97.

87   *Ibid.*, p. 100.

88   *Ibid.*, p. 107.

89   *Ibid.*, pp. 107, 108.

90   Barker and Harris, *A Merseyside Town*, p. 404.

91   MacLeod, *Victorian Studies*, IX, 2 (December 1965), p. 108, n. 65.

92   *Ibid.*, pp. 111ff.

93   *Ibid.*, p. 95 and pp. 103ff for Smith's relations with 'the severely bureaucratic' Lambert.

94   *PP.* XLIV (1878) 'RCNV. I. Report', p. 27.

95   MacLeod writes that Simon 'appears not to have demonstrably encouraged this important branch of public health', *Victorian Studies*, IX, 2 (December 1965), p. 95. See also p. 99.

96   W. Morris, *A Factory as it might be* (1907), p. 7.

Chapter Nine: ' "Reservoirs of Poison": River Pollution'.

1 *PP*. XXXIII (1867), 'RCRP. Third Report (Aire and Calder). I Report', p. xli. In the statement which heads this chapter the Commission was referring to the West Riding of Yorkshire, but the statement is applicable to much of Britain.

2 *PP*. XXXIII (1866), 'RCRP. First Report (Thames). I. Report', pp. 11–12.

3 *Ibid*., p. 16.

4 *Ibid*., p. 19.

5 Smith, *The People's Health*, p. 219, and Parkes, *Hygiene and Public Health*, p. 162.

6 *PP*. LXII (1884), 'Return showing the number of Human Corpses found in the River Lea . . . 1882 and 1883', pp. 2–3; *PP*. LIV (1882), 'Return showing the number of Human Corpses found in the Regent's Canal and River Lea, 1877–1881', pp. 1ff.

7 *PP*. XXXIII (1867), 'RCRP. Second Report (Lee). 1. Report', p. xi.

8 Redford, *The History of Local Government in Manchester*, II, p. 380.

9 Barker and Harris, *A Merseyside Town*, p. 416; *PP*. XXXIX (1894) 'ARMOHLGB, for 1892, Appendix A, No. 6, ". . . Report on Enteric Fever in the Tees Valley . . ." ', pp. 41, 42, 44.

10 *PP*. XL (1894), 'ARMOHLGB, for 1893–4, Appendix A, No. 9, "Report on the Circumstances of the River Trent and . . . the Occurrence of Enteric Fever" ', p. 106.

11 Quoted in Toft, 'Public Health in Leeds', p. 31.

12 *PP*. XXV (1871), 'RCRP. Third Report (Woollen Towns). I. Report', p. 7; *PP*. XXXIII (1867), 'RCRP. Third Report (Aire and Calder). I. Report', p. xi; 'II. Minutes of Evidence', p. 46; and 'I. Report', p. x.

13 *Hansard*, Third Series, 223 (1875), 1886.

14 *PP*. XXV (1871), 'RCRP. Third Report (Woollen Towns), I. Report', p. 5; *PP*. XXXIII (1867), 'RCRP. Third Report (Aire and Calder), I. Report, p. xxxviii.

15 *Ibid*., p. xxi.

16 *Ibid*., pp. xxix, xxv.

17 *PP*. XXV (1871), 'RCRP. Third Report (Woollen Towns), I. Report', p. 35; for the Irk see Faucher, *Manchester in 1844*, p. 17; for the Don, *PP*. XXXIV, Pt. I (1901), 'Interim Report of the Commission appointed in 1898 to Inquire into . . . Treating and Disposing of Sewage' II. Minutes of Evidence', p. 62.

18 *PP*. XXXIII (1867), 'RCRP. Third Report (Aire and Calder). I. Report', p. xxxix.

19 *PP*. XLVII (1865), 'Copy of all Memorials . . . Pollution of Rivers . . .', p. 2; Hennock, *Fit and Proper Persons*, pp. 107–10.

20 *PP*. XXXIII (1867), 'RCRP. Third Report (Aire and Calder). I. Report', pp. xlvi ff.

21 *PP*. XXXIV (1872), 'RCRP. Fourth Report (Scotland), II. Minutes of Evidence', pp. 99, 102.

22 *PP*. XXXVII (1896), 'ARLGB, for 1895, Appendix XII "Report... of certain Valleys ... with Special Reference to ... the Pollution of Streams" ', pp. 11, 115; *PP*. XXXIII (1874), 'RCRP. Fifth Report (Pollution arising from Mining Operations and Metal Manufactures), I. Report', pp. vii–viii. In Dublin, the Liffey, a notoriously filthy river, continued to receive the city's sewerage down to the end of the century. See O'Brien, *'Dear Dirty Dublin'*, p. 20.

23 *Hansard*, Third Series, 223, (1875), 1884–1885.

24 *PP*. XXXIV, Pt. I (1901), 'Interim Report of the Commission appointed in 1898 to Inquire into ... Treating and Disposing of Sewage II. Minutes of Evidence', p. 62. If the idea was that the tidal flow would take care of the sewage it was often a mistaken one. A marked object was once observed for three weeks floating back and forth between Vauxhall and London Bridge before it disappeared, see *The Times*, 4 August 1862, quoted in Chapman, *The Pharos*, 35 (July 1972), p. 92.

25 *Quoted* in *ibid*., p. 92.

26 *PP*. XXXIII (1874), 'RCRP. Fifth Report (Pollution arising from Mining Operations and Metal Manufacturers), I. Report', p. xi.

27 *PP*. XXXVIII (1876), 'Report ... purification of the Clyde', p. 50.

28 *Hansard*, Third Series, 223 (1875), 1886.

29 For the Princess Alice incident see Owen, *The Government of Victorian London*, pp. 69–70, and *The Times*, 19 September 1878, and *Saturday Review*, 20 October 1878, p. 428. There was a similar scandal in Manchester, when a woman who had tried to drown herself was fished out of the Irwell and some five days later died, it was said of poisoning from the river water, see Smith, *The People's Health*, p. 219.

30 *Hansard*, Third Series, 224 (1875), 1886. Salisbury was here quoting a letter from R. Duncombe Shaft to the Royal Commission on the Prevention of River Pollution.

31 *PP*. XXXIII (1867), 'RCRP. Third Report (Aire and Calder), I. Report', p. xxvi.

32 *PP*. XXXIII (1866), 'RCRP. First Report (Thames), II. Minutes of Evidence', p. 82.

33 *PP*. XXVIII (1876), 'Report ... the Clyde', p. 50.

34 *PP*. XXXIV, Pt. 1 (1901), 'Interim Report of the Commission appointed in 1898 to Inquire into... Treating and Disposing of Sewage', II. Minutes of Evidence, p. 22.

35 Quoted in *ibid*., p. 6.

36 *Hansard*, Third Series, 224 (1875), 550.

37 *PP*. LIX (1888), 'Report ... for Scotland ... Rivers Pollution Prevention Act, 1874', p. 4. 'Cases often occur where the local authority and

those who have influence with it are themselves the offender. It is evident that in such cases the [1876 River Pollution Prevention] Act is inoperative', *ibid*.

38   *PP*. XXXV (1871), 'Second Report of the Royal Sanitary Commission', p. 4.

39   Flinn, ed., *Report on the Sanitary Condition*, p. 68.

40   *PP*. XXXIV, Pt. 1 (1901), 'Interim Report of the Commission appointed in 1898 to Inquire into . . . Treating and Disposing of Sewage, II. Minutes of Evidence', pp. 1–2.

41   *Ibid*., p. 2; *Hansard*, Third Series, 223 (1875), 1884.

42   *PP*. XXXIX, Pt. 1 (1860), 'ARMOHPC, for 1859', pp. 60, 160.

43   For a complete summary see *PP*. XXXIV, Pt. 1 (1901), 'Interim Report of the Commission appointed in 1898 to Inquire into . . . Treating and Disposing of Sewage', pp. 2, 6.

44   *PP*. XXXIII (1867), 'RCRP. Third Report (Aire and Calder), I. Report', p. li.

45   *Ibid*., pp. lii, liii.

46   *Ibid*., p. liii.

47   *PP*. XXXIII (1866), 'RCRP. First Report (Thames). II. Minutes of Evidence', pp. 182, 213, 214, 246. *Sanitary Record*, 12 July 1878, p. 17. See also *PP*. XXVII (1904), 'Fourth Report of the Commission . . . Trade Effluents', p. x.

48   *PP*. XXXIV, Pt. 1 (1901), 'Interim Report of the Commission appointed in 1898 to inquire into . . . Treating and Disposing of Sewage', II Minutes of Evidence pp. 9, 10, 12. See also Redford, *The History of Local Government in Manchester*, II, p. 382.

49   *Hansard*, Third Series, 224 (1875), 554.

50   *Ibid*., 556.

51   *Ibid*., 552, 553.

52   *Ibid*., 225 (1875), 773–4.

53   P. Smith, *Disraelian Conservatism and Social Reform* (1967), p. 226. Smith plays down the element of Tory Democracy in the bill, *ibid*., pp. 258–60.

54   *Hansard*, Third Series, 231 (1876), 283.

55   *Ibid*., 557, 558.

56   Ministry of Health, *Second Report of the Joint Advisory Committee on River Pollution*, pp. 4–5.

57   *Transactions of the Society of MOH* (1886), p. 81; *PP*. XXXIV, Pt. 1 (1901), 'Interim Report of the Committee appointed in 1898 to Inquire into . . . Treating and Disposing of Sewage', p. 19. Ten years after its passage only two corporations in England had adopted the Act, Smith, *The People's Health*, pp. 219–20.

58   *PP*. LXXII (1898), 'Report to H.M. Secretary for Scotland . . . Rivers Pollution Act of 1876', pp. iv, 20. See also *PP*. XXXIV, Pt. 1 (1901), 'Interim Report of the Committee appointed in 1898 to Inquire into . . . Treating and Disposing of Sewage', p. 100. For the Tay see *Public*

Health IV 51 (July 1892), p. 303; *PP.* LIX (1888), 'Report . . . Rivers Pollution Act of 1876', p. 6.

59 *PP.* LIX (1888), 'Report to H.M. Secretary for Scotland on the Alleged Pollution of the Water of Loch Long and Loch Gail . . .', p. 3. It was generally held that over the past fifteen years or so fishing had become less productive, *ibid*. In Scotland the Act was supplemented by the Public Health (Scotland) Act of 1897 and the Burgh Police (Scotland) Act of 1892.

60 *PP.* XXXIV, Pt. 1 (1901), 'Interim Report of the Committee appointed in 1898 to Inquire into . . . Treating and Disposing of Sewage. I. Report', p. xi.

61 *Ibid*. To William Morris, factories in general were 'hot houses of rheumatism', *Factory Work as it is and might be* (New York, 1922), p. 12.

62 Redford, *The History of Local Government in Manchester*, II, p. 389.

63 These issues and the Thames Conservators are discussed in Owen, *The Government of Victorian London*, p. 66 and pp. 70ff.

64 *PP.* XXXIV, Pt. 1 (1901), 'Interim Report of the Committee appointed in 1898 to Inquire into . . . Treating and Disposing of Sewage. II. Minutes of Evidence', p. 19.

65 *Ibid*., p. 20.

66 *Ibid*. The inspector was R. A. Tatton.

67 *Ibid*., p. 22. Nevertheless the Huddersfield Millowners' Association was founded to fight the Board, *PP.* XXXI (1903), 'Third Report of the Commission . . . Trade Effluents, II. Minutes of Evidence', p. 18.

68 *PP.* XXXIV, Pt. 1 (1901), 'Interim Report of the Committee appointed in 1898 to Inquire into . . . Treating and Disposing of Sewage. II. Minutes of Evidence', p. 22.

69 *Ibid*., pp. 61, 66.

70 *Ibid*., p. 66.

71 *Ibid*., p. 58.

72 *Ibid*., p. 1. Evidence of Alfred Austin.

73 *PP.* XXX (1903), 'Third Report of the Trade Commission . . . Trade Effluents, I. Report', p. xiii. Sixteen authorities accepted trade effluents into their sewers unconditionally, and another four did so but without conditions imposed on the manufacturers, *ibid*., p. 26.

74 *Ibid*., p. 13.

75 *PP.* XXXVII (1904), 'Fourth Report . . . Trade Effluents, I. Report', p. xi.

76 *Ibid*.

77 *Ibid*., pp. xvii, xv.

78 *PP.* XLVII (1865), 'Copy of all Memorials . . . Pollution of Rivers or the Utilization of Sewage', p. 2.

79 *PP.* XXXV (1914–16), 'Tenth and Final Report of the Royal Commission on the Treating and Disposing of Sewage', *passim*. It was tentatively suggested that different standards should be applied to different

industries – four parts of suspended solids per 10,000 for quarries, tin, lead, and zinc mines; six parts of suspended solids per 10,000 for the paper industry and so forth. The leading chemist in these investigations was Frankland.

Chapter Ten: 'The Canker of Industrial Diseases'.

1   Woodward, *Jipping Street*, p. 71
2   *PP.* LXII (1884), 'Report on the Effects of Heavy Sizing in Cotton Weaving upon the Health of the Operatives Employed', p. 9.
3   *PP.* XXVII (1862), 'Fourth ARMOHPC, for 1861', pp. 13–14.
4   *Ibid.*, p. 28.
5   As early as 1795 Dr Thomas Percival had argued that:

> the large factories are generally injurious to the constitution of those employed in them, even when no particular diseases prevail, from the close confinement which is enjoined, from the debilitating effects of hot and impure air, and from the want of the active exercises which nature points out as essential in childhood and youth to invigorate the system, and to fit our species for the employments and for the duties of manhood.

quoted in B. L. Hutchins and A. Harrison, *A History of Factory Legislation* (New York, 1903), p. 10.
6   It is perhaps understandable that dramatic industrial disasters attracted far more attention than the insidious effects of industrial diseases. Between 1851 and 1881 there were 34,000 known deaths from mining accidents, and these were more widely publicized than the many deaths of miners from silicosis and other pulmonary diseases, see *PP.* XVIII (1882), 'Report of the Chief Inspector of Factory Workshops, for 1881', p. xxi.
7   See especially F. Hayek, *Capitalism and the Historians* (Chicago, 1954). The origins of occupational medicine in the modern era are to be found in the work of the Italian Ramazzini, who published a treatise on the connection between work and illness in 1700.
8   Faucher, *Manchester in 1844*, pp. 72, 119.
9   *Lancet*, 27 April 1833, p. 149, and 11 May 1833, p. 220.
10   T. Holman, 'Historical Relationship of Mining, Silicosis, and Rock Removal', *British Journal of Industrial Medicine*, 4 (January 1974), p. 4.
11   Dr Holland, *Diseases of the Lungs from Mechanical Causes and Inquiries into the Condition of the Artizans exposed to the Inhalation of Dust* (1843), *passim* For an interesting review of this work see the *Lancet*, 10 February 1844, p. 657.
12   Flinn, ed., *Report on the Sanitary Condition*, p. 252.
13   Quoted in W. R. Lee, 'Occupational Medicine', in Poynter, *Medicine and Science in the 1860s*, p. 153. Farr's work was not published until 1864, *ibid.*

14 Quoted in Lambert, *Sir John Simon*, p. 235.

15 *Ibid.*, p. 263. The Statistical Society of London also had many articles on the subject.

16 For a complete list of the towns see *ibid.*, p. 331 and Rosen in Dyos and Wolff, eds., *The Victorian City*, II, p. 644.

17 Lambert, *Sir John Simon*, p. 334.

18 *PP*. XVI (1861), 'Third ARMOHPC for 1860, p. 30 and Appendix VI, "Dr Greenhow's Report on Districts with Excessive Mortality from Lung Diseases" ', pp. 105ff.

19 Quoted in Rosen, in Dyos and Wolff, eds., *The Victorian City*, II, p. 644.

20 Quoted in Lambert, *Sir John Simon*, pp. 331–2. It is in this report that Simon wrote that 'the canker of industrial diseases gnaws at the very root of our national strength', *PP*. XXVII (1862), 'Fourth ARMOHPC, for 1861', pp. 31–2.

21 *Transactions of the National Association for the Promotion of Social Science* (1862), pp. 670ff. A motion to call for a royal commission on industrial diseases failed, *ibid.*, p. 675. See also Lambert, *Sir John Simon*, p. 373.

22 *Ibid.*, p. 374 for Simon's role in the passage of the 1864 Factory Act.

23 Simon, *English Sanitary Institutions*, p. 301.

24 W. R. Lee, 'Emergence of Occupational Medicine in Victorian Times', *British Journal of Industrial Medicine*, 30 (April 1973), pp. 120ff. Hutchins and Harrison, *A History of Factory Legislation*, p. 230.

25 *Transactions of the Sanitary Institute of Great Britain*, XIV (1893), p. 133.

26 W. R. Lee, 'The History of Statutory Control of Mercury Poisoning in Great Britain', *British Journal of Industrial Medicine*, 25, 1 (January 1968), pp. 52ff; Lee, *ibid.*, 30 (April 1973), pp. 120ff.

27 Hunter, *The Diseases of Occupations*, p. 702. *PP*. XVII (1897), 'Report of the Departmental Committee . . . Wool Sorting and other Kindred Trades'; *PP*. XII (1899), 'Annual Report of the Chief Inspector of Factories and Workshops, for the Year 1898', p. 332.

28 J. T. Arlidge, *The Hygiene Diseases and Mortality of Occupations* (1892), pp. 411–18.

29 Quoted in Hunter, *The Diseases of Occupations*, pp. 348–9. Arsenic was also bought across the counter at pharmacists and used as a skin beautifier by woman – a use which provided dramatic material for murder melodramas.

30 Arlidge, *The Hygiene Diseases* p. 435.

31 *Ibid.*, pp. 437–8.

32 *Ibid.*, p. 434. Although in 1899 only one case of death due to arsenical poisoning was reported, the side effects of its use in industry continued to disfigure, *PP*. XII (1899), 'Annual Report of the Chief Inspector of Factories and Workshops, for the year 1898', p. 332.

33 *PP*. XII (1899), 'Reports to the Secretary of State . . . on the Use of

Phosphorus . . . Lucifer Matches. . . .', p. 123. For the practice of using matches to cure toothache see *PP*. XVIII (1863), 'First Report of the Royal Commission on Children's Employment. I. Report. Appendix, "Evidence Collected by Mr J. E. White upon the Lucifer Match Manufacture" ', p. 84.

34 *Ibid.*, p. 48. My attention was drawn to this statement by an anonymous unpublished article on match-making.

35 *PP*. XII (1899), 'Reports . . . Matches', p. 150. Cunningham is quoting Dr John Bristowe.

36 Quoted in *ibid.*, p. 152; see Arlidge, *The Hygiene Diseases*, p. 458.

37 *Ibid.*, p. 459.

38 *Ibid.*, pp. 459–60.

39 In 1862 there were fifty-seven factories employing 2,500 people in Great Britain; in 1897 the figures were twenty-five and 4,152 respectively, *PP*. XII (1899), 'Reports . . . Matches', pp. vi, 130.

40 Of the thirty-eight cases only three were fatal, and these were men engaged in the dipping process, *ibid*. pp. vi, vii. For an interesting description of conditions in the domestic manufacture of matches and also in the Bryant and May factory in the 1890s see M. Williams, *Round London. Down East and Up West* (1892), Chapter 2.

41 The Salvation Army venture was directed towards publicity and not profit: their matches sold for 4d. a gross, compared to 2¼d a gross of other brands, see Hunter, *The Diseases of Occupations*, p. 376.

42 *PP*. XII (1899), 'Reports . . . Matches', p. v.

43 Arlidge, *The Hygiene Diseases* pp. 423, 431; *PP*. XXXIII (1896), 'Interim Report of the Departmental Committee appointed to Inquire into and Report upon certain Miscellaneous Dangerous Trades', pp. 10–12; *PP*. XVII (1897), 'Annual Report of the Chief Inspector of Factories and Workshops, for the year 1896', p. 23.

44 *Transactions of the Sanitary Institute of Great Britain*, XIV (1893), pp. 157–8, 161.

45 *PP*. XVIII (1882), 'Report of Alexander Redgrave . . . Inspector of Factories . . . Whitelead Works', pp. 2, 4.

46 Arlidge, *The Hygiene Diseases*, p. 430.

47 *Ibid.* Workmen were also criticized for not washing or changing out of their work-clothes after work, *ibid.*, p. 425.

48 Hunter, *The Diseases of Occupations*, p. 252.

49 *Transactions of the Sanitary Institute of Great Britain*, XIV (1893), p. 122.

50 Arlidge, *The Hygiene Diseases*, p. 337.

51 *PP*. XII (1899), 'Third Interim Report of the Department Committee to Inquire into and Report upon Certain Miscellaneous Dangerous Trades', p. 7. It is interesting to note that the London and Newcastle authorities were worried that plumbism, by throwing people out of work, was causing a strain on the poor rates, see *PP*. XVIII (1883), 'Copy of Communications . . . Whitelead Poisoning', pp. 2–4.

52 Almost one-half died in the age group 20–30; the death rate for

fork-grinders was three times higher than the national average, see Arlidge, *The Hygiene Diseases*, p. 343.

53 *PP*. XII (1899), 'Third Interim Report ... Dangerous Trades', pp. 7–8. At the end of the century many of the shops were well under the 250 cubic feet in size required by the law. See also, Hutchins and Harrison, *A History of Factory Legislation*, pp. 206–7.

54 *PP*. XII (1899), 'Third Interim Report ... Dangerous Trades, Appendix II', p. 35; see also Arlidge, *The Hygiene Diseases*, p. 335; *PP*. XXI (1897), 'Supplement to the Fifty-fifth Annual Report of the Registrar-General, Pt. II (1897), "Letter to the Registrar-General on the Mortality of Males engaged in Certain Occupations, 1890–1892" ', p. xxi.

55 *PP*. XXVII (1862), 'Fourth ARMOHPC, for 1861', p. 14.

56 *Ibid*. p. 18.

57 E. Gaskell, *North and South* (Penguin edition, 1979), p. 146.

58 Arlidge, *The Hygiene Diseases*, p. 306. Arlidge was the first President (1868) of the Association of Certifying MOH of Great Britain and Ireland and later became mayor of Newcastle-under-Lyne, see E. Posner, 'John Thomas Arlidge, (1822–1899) and the Potteries', *British Journal of Industrial Medicine*, 30 (July 1973), p. 267.

59 *Ibid*., p. 308.

60 *Ibid*., pp. 310, 311.

61 *PP*. XVI (1861), 'Third ARMOHPC, for 1860', pp. 112ff.

62 Arlidge, *The Hygiene Diseases*, p. 312. Apparently the use of respirators provoked the scorn of fellow workers and in any case the respirators quickly became clogged and so made breathing difficult, *ibid*.

63 *Ibid*., p. 318.

64 *Transactions of the Sanitary Institute of Great Britain*, XVI (1895), pp. 72–95

65 Hunter, *The Diseases of Occupations*, p. 407.

66 Arlidge, *The Hygiene Diseases*, p. 449.

67 Lee, *British Journal of Industrial Medicine*, 25, 1 (January 1968), pp. 52, 54. Arsenic was also involved in the making of hats.

68 Arlidge, *The Hygiene Diseases*, p. 439, and *Transactions of the Sanitary Institute of Great Britain*, XVI (1895), pp. 65–66.

69 *Ibid*., pp. 84, 87. Hunter, *The Diseases of Occupations*, p. 66. For high temperatures see Hutchins and Harrison, *A History of Factory Legislation*, p. 137.

70 *PP*. XXXIII (1896), 'Interim Report of the Departmental Committee ... Miscellaneous Dangerous Trades', p. 17.

71 *Ibid*., p. 79.

72 R. Tressell, *The Ragged Trousered Philanthropists* (Panther Books edition, 1973), p. 392.

73 *Transactions of the Sanitary Institute of Great Britain*, XIV (1893), p. 153.

74 Arlidge, *The Hygiene Diseases*, p. 359.
75 *PP*. XXI (1897), 'Supplement to the Fifty-fifth Annual Report of the Registrar-General, pt. 11, "Letter to the Registrar-General on the Mortality of Males engaged in Certain Occupations, 1890–1892" ', pp. xix, lxxviii, lxxx.
76 Arlidge, *The Hygiene Diseases*, p. 272.
77 *Transactions of the Sanitary Institute of Great Britain*, XVI (1895), p. 107; but see *ibid.*, p. 110.
78 Arlidge, *The Hygiene Diseases*, p. 274.
79 J. Bullock, *Bower's Row; Recollections of a Mining Village* (Wakefield, 1976), quoted p. 461 of J. Benson, 'British Coalminers in the Nineteenth Century. A Social History', unpublished ms.
80 'Forty-fifth Annual Report of the Registrar-General, for 1897', p. 23, quoted in Arlidge, *The Hygiene Diseases*, p. 15.
81 Adapted from *PP*. XXI (1897), 'Supplement to the Fifty-fifth Annual Report of the Registrar-General, Pt. 11 (1897), "Letter to the Registrar-General . . ." ', pp. cxix ff.
82 For an indictment of the lives and habits of the publicans see Arlidge, *The Hygiene of Diseases*, pp. 152–5.
83 *PP*. XXI (1897), 'Supplement to the Fifty-fifth Annual Report of the Registrar-General, Pt. 11 (1897), "Letter to the Registrar-General . . ." ', pp. lv, lvii, lxxv.
84 *Ibid.*, p. xxi. These figures should be compared with those in *PP*. XXVIII (1864), 'Sixth ARMOHPC, for 1863', p. 24, in which Simon showed that the female death rate from phthisis and other lung diseases at ages 15–25 was two-and-a-half times higher in Macclesfield and Leek (where many women worked in the silk factories) than among female workers as a whole. See also Parkes, *Hygiene and Public Health* p. 207.
85 *PP*. XII (1899), 'Third Interim Report of the Departmental Committee appointed to Inquire and Report upon Certain Dangerous Trades', p. 7. See also n. 51 above.
86 *PP*. XXXII (1904), 'Report of the Inter Departmental Committee on Physical Deterioration, I. Report', p. 30.
87 J. Simmons, *Life in Victorian Leicester* (Leicester, 1971), p. 77.
88 Even the 1901 Factory Act made domestic industry comply with the various factory and workshop acts only if the activities carried on there were certified as dangerous, see Hutchins and Harrison, *A History of Factory Legislation*, pp. 208, 238–9.
89 *PP*. XXXII (1904), 'Inter-Departmental Committee on Physical Deterioration, I. Report', p. 29.
90 *Ibid.*, see especially the evidence of Miss Adelaide Mary Andersen, the Principal Lady Inspector of Factories, pp. 63ff.
91 Hutchins and Harrison, *A History of Factory Legislation*, p. 253.

Chapter Eleven: 'Home Sweet Home'

1   See Wohl, *The Eternal Slum*, J. Burnett, *A Social History of Housing, 1815–1970* (Newton Abbot, 1978), E. Gauldie, *Cruel Habitations: a History of Working-Class Housing, 1780–1918* (1974), and Chapman ed., *The History of Working-Class Housing*.

2   *Transactions of the National Association for the Promotion of Social Science*, 1862, p. 681. The speaker, a Mr Prideaux, was attacking the atmospheric pollution of towns which led to closed windows and hence the lack of ventilation he deplored.

3   C. Dickens, *Hard Times*, quoted in F. Schwarzbach, *Dickens and the City* (1979), p. 145. Southwood Smith, *A Treatise on Fever* (1830), quoted in C. Lewes, *Dr Southwood Smith, A Retrospect* (1898), pp. 25–6. By definition a slum was a closed-in, hidden, low place, see Wohl, *The Eternal Slum*, p. 5.

4   E. Seaton, ed., *Public Health Reports* (1887); this was in Simon's Eighth Annual Report as MOH to the Privy Council (1865).

5   *PP*. VII (1881), 'Select Committee on Artizans' and Labourers' Dwellings Improvement, II. Minutes of Evidence', p. 25, and *PP*. XXIV (1871), 'Second Report of the Royal Sanitary Commission, II. Minutes of Evidence', p. 40. The witness was Dr Robert Druitt.

6   *Transactions of the National Association for the Promotion of Social Science*, 1860, p. 788.

7   C. Dickens, *Bleak House*, quoted in Schwarzbach, *Dickens and the City*, p. 130; *Nottingham Review*, 17 April 1829, quoted in Chapman, 'Working-Class Housing in Nottingham during the Industrial Revolution', in Chapman, ed., *The History of Working-Class Housing*, p. 151.

8   Duncan, quoted in Treble, *ibid.*, p. 108; Shaftesbury, quoted in J. Bready, *Lord Shaftesbury and Socio-Industrial Progress* (1926), p. 118. For Farr's views on population density and mortality, see Eyler, *Victorian Social Medicine*, pp. 131ff. To Farr, the significant factor was the density of air-borne organic material.

9   F. J. Ball, 'Housing in an Industrial Colony in Ebbw Vale, 1778–1914', in Chapman, ed., *The History of Working-Class Housing*, p. 293; E. Smith, *The Peasant's House, 1760–1865* (1876), quoted in Burnett, *A Social History of Housing*, p. 44.

10 Leff, *Social Medicine*, p. 103.

11 Thus Edward Smith wrote that 'it is his sleeping accommodation which produces the most insidious (and often fatal) results upon his health', *The Peasant's Home*, quoted in Burnett, *A Social History of Housing*, p. 44.

12 For these see the bibliography in my *The Eternal Slum*, pp. 350–2.

13 Sunderland, *A History of Darlington*, p. 89.

14 London County Council, *Annual Report of the MOH*, 1892, p. 10. Figures are for people living more than two to a room in tenements of

less than five rooms, for the years 1885–92, for London only. The MOH, Shirley Murphy, held that there was a direct correlation between overcrowding and infant mortality, *Public Health* (Jubilee No. 1906), p. 244.

15 Dr T. J. MacNamara, 'The Physical Condition of the People', in W. T. Stead, ed., *Coming Men on Coming Questions* (1905), p. 6.

16 *PP.* XVIII (1905), 'Supplement to the Sixty-fifth Annual Report of the Registrar-General, Pt. 1 (1905)', taken from Table 5, p. lxix.

17 *Public Health*, III, 28 (August 1890), p. 103.

18 *Transactions of the Sanitary Institute of Great Britain*, VI (1884–5), p. 91, from table iv.

19 *PP.* XC (1901), '1901 Census', table 10, pp. 202ff.

20 Gauldie, *Cruel Habitations*, p. 145.

21 I. C. Taylor, 'The Insanitary Housing Question and Tenement Dwellings in Nineteenth-Century Liverpool', in A. Sutcliffe, ed., *Mutli-Storey Living: the British Working-Class Experience* (1974), p. 45. A square mile is 640 acres, an acre is 4,840 sq. yards.

22 J. Russell, *Life in One Room, or Some Serious Considerations for the Citizens of Glasgow* (Glasgow, 1888), p. 10. All these densities were higher than in the 1860s, see *Public Health*, I (January, 1868), p. 26.

23 *PP.* XXXIII (1866), 'Eighth ARMOHPC, for 1865, Appendix IV, "Report by Dr George Buchanan on Epidemic Typhus in Greenock" ', p. 23; Taylor in Sutcliffe, ed., *Mutli-Storey Living*, p. 45; J. Butt, 'Working-Class Housing in Glasgow, 1851–1914', in Chapman, ed., *The History of Working-Class Housing*, p. 58. The City of London as a whole had a density of 180 people to the acre, see Lambert, *Sir John Simon*, p. 81.

24 Godwin, quoted in Burnett, *A Social History of Housing*, p. 86. For the phrase, 'embryo slums', see Rev A. Mearns, 'The Outcast Poor. II. Outcast London', *Contemporary Review*, XLVI (December, 1883), p. 924.

25 T. H. Lloyd, 'The Cholera Epidemic in 1849 in Leamington Spa and Warwick', *Warwickshire History*, II, 4 (Winter, 1973–4), p. 20.

26 Chapman, in Chapman, ed., *The History of Working-Class Housing*, p. 52.

27 Treble, in *ibid.*, p. 176; Midwinter, *Social Administration in Lancashire*, p. 15.

28 *PP.* XXXIII (1866), 'Eighth ARMOHPC, for 1865, Appendix II, "Report by Dr Henry Julian Hunter . . ." ', p. 77; *ibid.*, 'Appendix IV, "Report by Dr George Buchanan on Epidemic Typhus in Greenock" ', p. 211.

29 *PP.* XXVI (1865), 'Seventh ARMOHPC, Appendix VIII "Report by Dr George Buchanan on an Epidemic of Typhus in Liverpool" ', p. 476.

30 Quoted in Lambert, *Sir John Simon*, p. 149. This was Simon's first report as MOH to the City of London.

31 Sutcliffe, 'Introduction', in Sutcliffe, ed., *Multi-Storey Living*, p. 13. For the term, 'honeycomb', see T. S. Ashton, *Economic and Social Investigations in Manchester, 1833–1933* (Hassocks, Sussex, 1977), p. 46.

32 Burnett, *A Social History of Housing*, pp. 74, 163; see *ibid.*, pp. 70ff. for an excellent discussion of the architecture of back-to-backs.

33 M. W. Beresford, 'The Back-to-Back in Leeds, 1787–1937', in Chapman, ed., *The History of Working-Class Housing*, p. 121.

34 *Ibid.*, p. 96.

35 *Ibid.*, pp. 112, 119.

36 *Public Health*, IV, 46 (February 1892), pp. 145, 148. The MOH for Bradford, however, thought that they were not 'radically insanitary', *ibid.*, p. 145.

37 *Ibid.*, VII, 8 (July, 1895), p. 426.

38 *Transactions of the Sanitary Institute of Great Britain*, XV (1894), p. 449, and Beresford, in Chapman, ed., *The History of Working-Class Housing*, p. 116.

39 Burnett, *A Social History of Housing*, pp. 155, 168, and Sutcliffe, 'A Century of Flats in Birmingham, 1875–1973', in Sutcliffe, ed., *Multi-Storey Living*, p. 181.

40 Beresford, in Chapman, ed., *A History of Working-Class Housing*, p. 119.

41 *Ibid.*, p. 112, and Chapman in *ibid.*, pp. 156–7; Treble in *ibid.*, pp. 193–4. White, *The History of the Corporation of Liverpool*, p. 62; Redford, *The History of Local Government in Manchester*, I, p. 363.

42 *PP.* XXI. 3 (1850), 'Report of the General Board of Health . . .', p. 424, and Weir, 'St Giles', Past and Present', in C. Knight, ed., *London*, III (1842), p. 266.

43 Engels had argued that 'the majority of cellar-dwellers are nearly always Irish in origin', *The Condition of the Working-Classes in England*, p. 105.

44 P. Gaskell, *The Manufacturing Population of England* (1833), quoted in Burnett, *A Social History of Housing*, p. 58.

45 Anon, *A General and Descriptive History of the Antient and Present State of the Town of Liverpool* (1797), quoted in Treble, in Chapman, ed., *The History of Working-Class Housing*, pp. 168, 178, 179.

46 Flinn, ed., *Report on the Sanitary Condition*, pp. 6, 105.

47 Treble, in Chapman, ed., *The History of Working-Class Housing*, p. 179.

48 Duncan, quoted in Flinn, ed., *Report on the Sanitary Condition*, pp. 104–5. A similar description appears in Elizabeth Gaskell's *Mary Barton* (Penguin edition, 1979), p. 98.

49 *PP.* XVIII (1845), 'Royal Commission on the State of Large Towns and Populous Districts', p. 22, quoted in Treble, in Chapman, ed., *The History of Working-Class Housing*, pp. 179–80.

50 Midwinter, *Social Administration in Lancashire*, p. 72. In 1831 Not-

tingham had under two hundred cellars, Birmingham had none, and Leeds had 'only' 555 cellar dwellings out of a total of almost 18,000 dwellings, Burnett, *A Social History of Housing*, p. 61.

51 Taylor in Sutcliffe, ed., *Multi-Storey Living*, p. 48; see also *PP*. XXVI (1865), 'Seventh ARMOHPC, for 1864, Appendix VIII, "Report by Dr Buchanan on an Epidemic of Typhus in Liverpool" ', p. 479.

52 Redford, *A History of Local Government in Manchester*, I, pp. 140, 362, and *ibid*., II, p. 145.

53 *Ibid*., p. 403. R. Thorne Thorne, *The Progress of Preventive Medicine During the Victorian Era* (1888), p. 18.

54 *PP*. XXVI (1865), 'Seventh ARMOHPC, for 1864, Appendix VIII, "Report by Dr George Buchanan on an Epidemic of Typhus in Liverpool" ', p. 479. See p. 89.

55 For rent riots and the Workmen's National Housing Council see Wohl, *The Eternal Slum*, pp. 306, 317, and 320ff.

56 *PP*. XXI (1843), 'Fifth Annual Report of the Registrar-General', p. 214. *Justice*, 5 August 1889 and 2 December 1889; *Housing Journal*, 7 (February 1901) and 70 (June 1907).

57 Quoted in Burnett, *A Social History of Housing*, pp. 31, 32.

58 *PP*. XXVI (1865), 'Seventh ARMOHPC, for 1864, Appendix IX, "Dr Hunter on the Death Rate of the Population of South Wales" ' p. 499; Gauldie, *Cruel Habitations*, p. 23.

59 Quoted in *ibid*.

60 Quoted in *ibid*., p. 54.

61 Flinn ed., *Report on the Sanitary Condition*, p. 83; *ibid*., p. 54.

62 *PP*. XXVI (1865), 'Seventh ARMOHPC, for 1864, Appendix VI, "Inquiry on the State of Dwellings of Rural Labourers, by Dr H. J. Hunter" ', p. 161.

63 *Ibid*., p. 148.

64 *Public Health*, IV, 52 (August 1892), pp. 341–2. The Royal Commission on the Housing of the Working Classes was told that the condition of houses in some parts of Scotland varied with the seasons:

> If your visit is in July, you make an unexpected descent of a foot down to the earthen floor. If your visit is in March, the inside level is higher than the surface of the ground, for you step upon a thick mass of cattle-bedding and dung, which has accumulated since the last summer.

quoted in Gauldie, *Cruel Habitations*, p. 32.

65 Burnett, *A Social History of Housing*, pp. 34, 35.

66 *PP*. XXVI (1865), 'Seventh ARMOHPC, for 1864, Appendix VI, "Inquiry into the State of Dwellings of Rural Labourers, by Dr H. J. Hunter" ', table B, p. 192. Hunter called for the construction of cottages to rent at 1s a week. He maintained that these could be built for £50, *ibid*., p. 139.

67 *Ibid*., pp. 146, 147.

68 *PP*. XXVI (1865), 'Seventh ARMOHPC, for 1864', pp. 9, 13.

69 Burnett, *A Social History of Housing*, pp. 123ff. See also Lambert, *Sir John Simon*, pp. 346ff.
70 Burnett, *A Social History of Housing*, p. 124.
71 Quoted in *ibid.*, p. 132.
72 *Ibid.*, p. 52.
73 *Ibid.*, p. 119. Burnett's is far and away the best account of rural housing and my debt to him is obvious.
74 For the connection housing reformers made between drink and slums, see Wohl, *The Eternal Slum*, pp. 15, 61–3, 106–7.
75 White, *A History of the Corporation of Liverpool*, p. 5.
76 *PP.* XXXIII (1866), 'Eighth ARMOHPC, for 1865, Appendix II, "Report on the Housing of the Poorer Parts . . . of Towns" ', pp. 50, 13.
77 Burnett, *A Social History of Housing*, p. 143. Overcrowding was defined as occupation of a single room by two adults (with children under ten years of age counting as half an adult), with children under one year old not included.
78 *PP.* XVIII (1905), Supplement to the Sixty-fifth Annual Report of the Registrar-General, Pt. I (1905), taken from Table 1, pp. cxxxvi. ff. With the exception of the figure for England and Wales the figures refer to the percentage of one-to-four roomed tenements with more than two people to a room.
79 London County Council, *Comparative Municipal Statistics*, I *1912–13* (1915), table 5, pp. 6–7. The figures are for tenements of one to five rooms.
80 *Supplement to the Sixty-fifth Annual Report of the Registrar-General*, table I, pp. cxxx ff.
81 *The Working Man: A Weekly Record of Social and Industrial Progress*, 3 March 1866, p. 136.
82 This forms one of the themes of my *The Eternal Slum, passim*. For a strong statement see Dr J. Russell, *Life in One Room, or Some Serious Considerations for the Citizens of Glasgow* (Glasgow, 1888), p. 30.
83 Quoted in Jephson, *The Sanitary Evolution of London*, pp. 5–6.
84 See Flinn's splendid introduction to Flinn, ed., *Report on the Sanitary Condition*; for the biases, see Cullen, *The Statistical Movement, passim*.
85 M. Gore, *On the Dwellings of the Poor and the Means of Improving Them* (1851), pp. iv–v.
86 For details of these various acts see Gauldie, *Cruel Habitations, passim*, and Burnett, *A Social History of Housing, passim*.
87 *The Times*, 10 July 1851. For the Shaftesbury Act see Wohl, *The Eternal Slum*, pp. 75–8.
88 Kingsley, *Miscellanies*, II, p. 312.
89 *PP.* XXXIII (1866), 'Eighth ARMOHPC, for 1865, Appendix II, "Report on the Housing of the Poorer Parts . . . of Towns . . ." ', p. 60.

90 *Ibid.*, p. 421; Lambert, *Sir John Simon*, quoted pp. 348–9.

91 Quoted in *ibid.*, p. 349; E. Smith, *Manual for Medical Officers of Health* (1873), p. 210.

92 The two Acts and their amendments are dealt with extensively in my *The Eternal Slum*, Chapter 4.

93 *Hansard*, Third Series, 189 (1867), 754. S. Gaselee.

94 Royal College of Physicians, *A Memorial on the Condition of the Poor in London* (1874).

95 *Hansard*, Third Series, 222 (1875), 95ff.

96 *Ibid.*, 743; see also *ibid.*, 754–5.

97 *Law Times*, quoted in the *Building News*, 17 September 1875.

98 The new housing was to 'be situate within the limits of the same area or in the vicinity thereof'.

99 White, *A History of the Corporation of Liverpool*, pp. 82ff, 131–2; Taylor in Sutcliffe, ed., *Multi-Storey Living*, p. 51.

100 Gauldie, *Cruel Habitations*, p. 86; Butt, in Chapman, ed., *The History of Working-Class Housing*, p. 59.

101 *Ibid.*, p. 68. For the registration of houses in London see Wohl, *The Eternal Slum*, pp. 122, 274.

102 Gauldie, *Cruel Habitations*, pp. 279–80.

103 Sutcliffe, 'A Century of Flats . . .', in Sutcliffe, ed., *Multi-Storey Living*, pp. 186, 190.

104 Quoted in Redford, *The History of Local Government in Manchester*, II, p. 413. The Manchester MOH said in 1876 that 'the exigencies of commerce' had done far more than anything else to 'sweep away the old fever dens', *ibid.* See also *ibid.*, p. 150.

105 *Ibid.*, pp. 414ff.

106 Macdonald, 'Public Health Legislation and Problems', pp. 139, 161, and appendix, p. 304.

107 Gauldie, *Cruel Habitations*, p. 279.

108 Taylor in Sutcliffe, ed., *Multi-Storey Living*, p. 80.

109 *The Eternal Slum, passim.*

110 G. Gibbon and R. Bell, *History of the London County Council, 1889–1939* (1939), p. 38. London County Council, *The Housing Question in London between the Years 1855 and 1900*, (1900), pp. 113, 133, 152.

111 The subsidy is discussed in Wohl, *The Eternal Slum*, Chapter 6.

112 *Ibid.*, p. 260

113 Treble in Chapman, ed. *The History of Working-Class Housing*, p. 199.

114 *PP.* XVIII, Pt. II (1845), 'Second Report of the Commissioners for Inquiring into the State of Large Towns and Populous Districts', p. 45, quoted in *ibid.*, p. 196.

115 P. Edwards, *London Street Improvements*, pp. 136–7; G. Godwin, *Town Swamps and Social Bridges* (1859), p. 3.

116 London County Council, *Housing* 2/2 item 69.

117 *PP*. VII (1882), 'Select Committee on Artizans' and Labourers' Dwellings, II. Minutes of Evidence', p. 128.

118 Rev A. O. Jay, *A Story of Shoreditch: Being the Sequel to 'Life in Darkest London'* (1896), p. 11.

119 London County Council, *London Statistics*, XXV (1914–15), pp. 164, 165.

120 *Transactions of the Society of MOH* (1883–4), pp. 33–7.

121 *Public Health*, XII, 8 (May 1900), p. 577. The MOH was Dr J. Priestley.

122 Charity Organisation Society, *Dwellings of the Poor. Report of the Dwellings' Committee of the Charity Organisation Society* (1881), p. 141. *Transactions of the Society of MOH* (1883–4), pp. 36–7

123 *Hansard*, Third Series, 245 (1879), 1937, 1939.

124 *Transactions of the Society of MOH*, (1883–4), pp. 36–7.

125 For the model dwelling movement see J. Tarn, *Five Per Cent Philanthropy* (1973) and Wohl, *The Eternal Slum*. Chapter 6.

126 *Ibid*., Appendix III, tables (a) and (b). The figure is for both housing and re-housing.

127 See Gauldie, *Cruel Habitations*, *passim*, and Sutcliffe, ed., *Multi-Storey Living*, *passim*.

128 *PP*. VII (1881), 'Select Committee on Artizans' and Labourers' Dwellings Improvement. II. Minutes of Evidence', p. 20. William Morris called them 'Bastilles', see *Justice*, 10 September 1887 and *ibid*., 14 July 1884 and 21 July 1884.

129 Quoted in D. J. Olsen,. *Town Planning in the Eighteenth and Nineteenth Century* (New Haven, Connecticut, 1964), pp. 142, 192. St Saviour's Board of Works, *Annual Report of the MOH* (1858), p. 9.

130 Whitechapel Borough Council, *Annual Report on the Sanitary Condition of the Whitechapel District* (1891), p. 16; Shoreditch Borough Council, *Annual Report of the MOH* (1914), p. 88.

131 *PP*. VII (1881), 'Select Committee on Artizans' and Labourers' Dwellings Improvement. II. Minutes of Evidence', pp. 103–4.

132 *Pall Mall Gazette*, 27 April 1882.

133 *The Times*, 11 January 1866, quoted in Tarn, *Five Per Cent Philanthropy*, p. 47.

134 *Journal of the Statistical Society of London*, XXXVIII (March 1875), pp. 36–7, 41. This is perhaps less impressive when it is placed within the context of the careful screening of tenants, the job security and relatively high and stable wages of the tenants of the model blocks.

135 Sutcliffe, 'Introduction', in Sutcliffe, ed., *Multi-Storey Living*, pp. 14–15.

136 Butt, in Chapman, ed., *The History of Working-Class Housing*, p. 59; Cameron, *A Brief History*, p. 62; O'Brien, '*Dear Dirty Dublin*', pp. 129–30; Macdonald 'Public Health Legislation', p. 266; Gauldie, *Cruel Habitations*, pp. 298–9. For the totals of Liverpool, Manchester, and Glasgow see London County Council, *Comparative Municipal*

Statistics, 1912–13 (1915), p. 38. For London see London County
Council, *London Statistics*, XXV (1914–15), pp. 155–61.

137 London County Council, *Comparative Municipal Statistics, 1912–13*
(1915), p. 38.

138 Quoted in Gauldie, *Cruel Habitations*, p. 303.

139 For loans for housing purposes see *PP*. XXXVIII (1892), 'ARLGB for
1891–2', p. cvii. Perhaps the local authorities feared that subsidized
housing would attract an influx of immigrants to their towns, see Butt,
in Chapman, ed., *The History of Working-Class Housing*, p. 86. See
also Burnett, *A Social History of Housing*, p. 181.

140 Wohl, *The Eternal Slum*, pp. 336ff.

141 *Hansard*, Fifth Series, Commons, 35 (1912), 1449.

142 J. P. Dickson-Poynder, *The Housing Question* (1908), p. 2.

143 *Municipal Journal*, 9 August 1907, p. 683.

144 *The Times*, 26 November 1883.

145 H. Gavin, *The Habitations of the Industrial Classes* (1851), p. 49.

146 Butt in Chapman, ed., *The History of Working-Class Housing*, p. 82.

147 Simon, *English Sanitary Institutions*, pp. 433, 444. *Public Health*,
XXI (January 1890), p. 277, *ibid*., XVII (February 1905), p. 28.

148 Bethnal Green, *Tenth Annual Report of the Chief Inspector* (1905), p. 7;
Eleventh Annual Report . . . (1906), p. 20; *Twelfth Annual Report . . .*
(1907), pp. 3–4; *Sixteenth Annual Report . . .* (1911), pp. 2–3.

149 *Medical Times and Gazette*, 9 (February 1884), p. 196. *Public Health*,
II, 21 (January 1890), p. 277.

150 G. Sims, *In London's Heart* (1900), pp. 49–50.

151 Macnamara, in Stead, ed., *Coming Men on Coming Questions* (1905),
p. 5.

152 Gauldie, *Cruel Habitations*, p. 168.

153 Barnsby, 'Social Conditions in the Black Country', p. 133. See also H.
J. Dyos, 'The Slum Attacked', *New Society*, 8 February 1968, p. 195.

154 Bell, *Blackfriars Wynd Analyzed*, p. 22, in *Day and Night in the
Wynds of Edinburgh and Blackfriars Wynd Analyzed*.

Chapter Twelve: 'A Nation of Good Animals'?

1 *PP*. XVIII (1902), 'Sixty-fourth Annual Report of the Reigstrar-
General (1901)', table 12, p. xci; between 1856–60 and 1896–1900
the corrected death rate declined from 20.7 to 17.6, *ibid*.

2 O. N. Anderson, 'Age Specific Mortality in Selected Western European
Countries with Particular Emphasis on the Nineteenth Century', *Bulletin of the History of Medicine*, XXIX, 3 (May–June 1955), table 5,
p. 252. In the age group 45–54 there was only a 1.2% improvement,
ibid. As we saw in Chapter 5 the improvement was partly the consequence of a spontaneous decline in the virulence of certain diseases.

3 The life expectancy rates are for males only; there were similar improvements for women, see *PP*. XVIII (1902), 'Sixty-fourth Annual Report of the Registrar-General (1901)', table 31, p. cxliv. See also D. V. Glass, 'Some Indications of Differences between Urban and Rural Mortality in England and Wales and Scotland', *Population Studies*, XVII (1963–4), Pt. 3 (March 1964), table 1, p. 264. The decline in the ratio of urban to rural deaths is remarkable in view of increasing urban densities but less so when we take into account the fact that the young and hearty left the countryside for the towns, leaving behind an older population.

4 See above, Chapter 1, p. 9.

5 C. F. G. Masterman, 'Realities at Home', in *The Heart of Empire. Discussion of Problems of Modern City Life in England*, edited by B. G. Gilbert (Brighton, 1973), pp. 6–7.

6 Chapter 8, p. 207.

7 Masterman, *The Heart of Empire*, p. 7.

8 H. G. Wells, *The New Machiavelli* (1911), p. 46.

9 Masterman, *The Heart of Empire*, p. 7.

10 Gavin quoted a Dr Jackson, whom he described as 'the most eminent . . . medico-military philosopher that the world has ever seen' to the effect that whereas 'manufacturers and artisans' were 'ill-calculated for the business of war', peasants and 'particularly the shepherds and the hunters' were 'familiar with the situations and hardships which fall to the lot of soldiers in war.' Gavin, *The Habitations of the Industrial Classes*, pp. 63–4.

11 Kingsley, quoted in Simon, *English Sanitary Institutions*, p. 242, and Farr, *Journal of the Statistical Society of London*, XV (April 1852), p. 178. See Chapter 10, page 260 for similar views of Chadwick.

12 *City Press*, 5 September 1857; W. Cooper, quoted in *The Times*, 15 October 1859.

13 In his *The Englishman's Castle* (n.d.), p. 20, the popular journalist, George Haw, argued that England had been saved from disgrace in the Boer War by the fit soldiers from the Empire.

14 The entire discussion was conducted in an unscientific fashion. There were few reliable anthropometric studies (but see Chapter 2, n. 14), and the class of volunteer varied enormously from good to bad times. The British Association had established an Anthropometric Committee, chaired by William Farr, see Eyler, *Victorian Social Medicine*, p. 155.

15 'National Health and Military Service', *British Medical Journal*, 25 July 1903, p. 202.

16 B. Gilbert, 'Health and Politics: the British Physical Deterioration Report of 1904', *Bulletin of the History of Medicine*, XXXIX, 2 (March–April, 1965), p. 145, and p. 143, n.l.

17 G. F. Shee, 'The Deterioration in the National Physique', *Nineteenth Century*, 53 (May 1903), p. 799.

18 Gilbert, *Bulletin of the History of Medicine*, XXXIX, 2 (March–April, 1965), p. 113. n.l.
19 Quoted in Shee, *Nineteenth Century*, 53 (Mary 1903), p. 805.
20 'Where to Get Men' (under the pseudonym, 'Miles'), *Contemporary Review*, LXXXI (Jan 1902); 'National Health: a Soldier's Study', *ibid.*, LXXXIII (January 1903).
21 W. Wilkins, *The Alien Invasion* (1892), p. 95. For the Jews and the alleged physical threat to England see B. Gainer, *The Alien Invasion* (1972), L. Gartner, *The Jewish Immigrant in England, 1870–1914*, (Detroit, 1960), and J. Garrard, *The English and Immigration, 1880–1910* (1971).
22 One of the few MOH who did think that physical determination had occurred was H. Beale Collins, MOH for Kingston-on-Thames. He argued that over the past five years some 113,884 recruits had been rejected as unfit and 'the sources of recruiting were nearly exhausted. Where could we find men to fight a nation of soldiers with a bigger population than our own?'; in a paper entitled, 'Health and Empire', *Public Health*, XVI, 7 (April 1904), p. 390. For the debate, see especially, *Public Health*, XVII, 5 (February 1905), *Lancet*, 6 August, 1904, pp. 390ff, and the series of articles in the *British Medical Journal*, 25 July 1903, 28 November 1903, 5 December 1903, 12 December 1903, 19 December 1903, and 26 December 1903. For the Royal College of Surgeons and the Royal College of Physicians, see *ibid.*, 21 November 1903, p. 1338.
23 *Public Health*, XVII, 5 (February 1905), pp. 293ff.; 301.
24 Shee, *Nineteenth Century*, 53 (May 1903), p. 797. Hobhouse ridiculed this type of argument; a declining death rate was obviously a clear indication, he argued, of an 'improvement of general health', L. T. Hobhouse, *Social Evolution and Political Theory* (New York, 1922), p. 50.
25 *Public Health*, I, 72 (April 1894), p. 232.
26 'The whole purpose of nature', wrote Herbert Spencer, was to 'clear the world' of the unfit and to 'make room for better. . . . If they are not sufficiently complete to live, they die, and it is best that they should die', quoted in P. Abrams, *The Origins of British Sociology, 1834–1914* (Chicago, 1968), p. 74.
27 Quoted in *ibid.*, p. 91. For the Eugenics Laboratory lecture and for *The Times* (26 May 1909) see Hobhouse, *Social Evolution and Political Theory*, pp. 55, 72. The correspondent to *The Times*, a Martin Conway, wrote that 'we calmly sit by and watch the . . . degeneration of our race', and, he asked rhetorically, 'Which is wrong – the breeder or racehorses, or Mr Lloyd-George? . . . If English racing men adopted our Governmental system, is it not certain that English racehorses would be beaten everywhere by horses bred by selection?' For an interesting analysis of the eugenicists see P. M. H. Mazumdar, 'The Eugenicists and the Residuum: the Problem of the Urban Poor',

Bulletin of the History of Medicine, 54, 2 (Summer, 1980). For the views of Newman and Farr on Eugenics, see Chapter 2, note 33, above.

28   For the Liberty and Property Defence League see Wohl, *The Eternal Slum*, pp. 231–3. The phrase 'maudlin sentiment' is Hobhouse's, in criticism, of course, of the school of social Darwinians, *Social Evolution and Political Theory*, p. 21.

29   *Ibid.*, pp. 21, 22. See also Abrams, *The Origins of British Sociology*, p. 91.

30   Sykes, *Public Health Problems*, p. 28. For a splendid discussion of Social Darwinism and its failure to capture 'the central bastions of English social thought,' see M. Freeden, *The New Liberalism. An Ideology of Social Reform* (Oxford, 1978), p. 11 and *passim*.

31   Masterman, *The Heart of Empire*, p. 7.

32   *Ibid.*, p. 8. Shee wrote that:

> While their forefathers lived, for the most part, in the country, where light, air, exercise, and contact with the woods and fields of English pastoral life had a healthy and invigorating effect on body and mind alike, the vast majority of the people now lived in large towns, where light, air, space, and all that goes to make a 'healthy and happy human being' are greatly lacking.

Nineteenth Century, 53 (May 1903), p. 798. See also the *British Medical Journal*, 28 November 1903, p. 1431 for the connection between urban densities and general 'physical weakness and debility'.

33   See for example the proposal of the Earl of Meath in his article on 'The Deterioration of British Health and Physique', *Public Health*, XVI, 7 (April 1904), p. 390.

34   *Public Health*, XVII, 5 (February 1905), p. 316, J. S. Nettlefold, Chairman of the Birmingham Town Planning Committee, argued that it was 'necessary to empty the slums into the country', *Practical Town Planning* (1914), quoted in G. F. Cherry, *Urban Change and Planning. A History of Urban Development in Britain since 1750* (Henley-on-Thames, 1972), p. 125.

35   The streets were to be washed daily and all houses would have back gardens to assist cross ventilation; there were to be 20 model hospitals, no alcohol, no industrial grime or smoke, and the factories were to be located on the outskirts. See Cherry, *ibid.*, q. p. 103. *Hygeia, a City of Health* was published in 1876.

36   For a brief discussion of these see *ibid.*, pp. 103ff. Cherry, *Urban Change and Planning*, pp. 103ff. and J. N. Tarn, 'Housing Reform and the Emergence of Town Planning . . .', in A. Sutcliffe, ed., *The Rise of Modern Urban Planning 1880–1914* (1980).

37   Howard was the author of *To-morrow: a Peaceful Path to Real Reform* (1898), revised and published in 1903 as *Garden Cities of To-morrow*; Howard, quoted in Cherry, *Urban Change and Planning*, p. 121.

38   *British Medical Journal*, 28 November 1903, p. 1431; it also recom-

mended that town children should attend day schools in the country, *ibid*.

39   *The Times*, 25 September 1909. By the end of 1913 50 urban authorities were preparing schemes, but only 2 town planning schemes had actually been accepted by the Local Government Board, A. Sutcliffe, *Towards the Planned City*, (Oxford 1981), pp. 64ff.

40   A. Barrington and K. Pearson, quoted in Hobhouse, *Social Evolution and Political Theory*, p. 61.

41   The Committee was originally appointed as a far more acceptable committee of inquiry than a select committee or a royal commission. It was primarily composed of civil servants, and not a single MOH sat on it, which is strange in view of the fact that it was called supposedly to determine how the medical profession could help in the formation of social policy. It did have on it J. M. Legge, Chief Inspector of Reformatories and Schools and Dr John Tatham, of the Registrar-General's Office. See *Lancet*, 6 August 1904, p. 392.

42   *PP.* XXXII (1904), 'Inter-Departmental Committee on Physical Deterioration. I. Report', *passim*. These suggestions were remarkably close to those of the Earl of Meath, see *Public Health*, XVI, 7 (April 1904), pp. 389–90. The Inter-Departmental Committee, it is true, also advocated a policy of labour colonies for the children of the degenerate and casual poor, but this was not its main emphasis or recommendation. See Stedman Jones, *Outcast London*, pp. 281, 314; see also Gilbert, *Bulletin of the History of Medicine*, XXXIX, 2 (March–April, 1965), p. 148, and Slater, *Poverty and the State*, pp. 173ff.

43   Dr J. C. McVail in *Public Health*, XVII, 5 (February 1905), p. 286. In Brighton the local authorities gave away 600 free breakfasts a day, *ibid.*, p. 287. For an excellent discussion of the feeding of schoolchildren and the legal responsibilities of parents, see Hurt, *Elementary Schooling*, pp. 128ff, see also Freeden, *The New Liberalism*, pp. 224ff., and Rubinstein, *School Attendance in London*, pp. 80ff.

44   The London School Board had a MOH from 1891; by 1905 there were 85 school MOH, but only London, Bradford, and Manchester appear to have had full-time MOH before 1908, see *ibid.*, p. 128. It was not until 1919, as part of the post-war reconstruction, that a Ministry of Health was established. It took over the functions for health of the Local Government Board, the Office of the Registrar-General, the Privy Council (for the Midwives Act) and the Home Office (Infant life protection). Its first MOH was George Newman, and Sir Robert Morant became the Permanent Secretary of the Ministry.

45   Smith, *Manual for MOH*, p. 71; Simon in *PP.* XXVII (1864), 'Sixth ARMOHPC, for 1863', p. 15; *PP.* XXXI (1871), 'Thirteenth ARMOHPC, for 1870', p. 9. See also his *English Sanitary Institutions*, pp. 434, 444.

46   Rev S. A. Barnett, 'The Duties of the Rich to the Poor', in H. Jones, ed., *Some Urgent Questions in Christian Lights, Being a Selection from*

some Sunday Afternoon Lectures . . . (1889), p. 68. In her *Family Life on a Pound a Week*, p.17 Mrs Pember Reeves evoked the reality of life at the poverty level and concluded that it was particularly hard on the children:

> The children of the poor suffer from want of light, want of air, want of warmth, want of sufficient and proper food, and want of clothes, because the wage of their fathers is not enough to pay for these necessaries. They also suffer from want of cleanliness, want of attention to health, want of peace and quiet, because the strength of their mothers is not enough to provide these necessary conditions.

47   For York and these statistics see Chapter 3, notes 8 and 9.

Bibliography

The wide variety of original and secondary sources available for a study of Victorian public health can be gauged by the footnotes. The following is not a comprehensive bibliography; it includes only those sources which I have found most useful and which will enable the reader to study in greater depth topics handled in this book. It does not include Hansard's Parliamentary Debates, articles in *The Times* and in the Victorian periodicals, or a list of the many Parliamentary Papers ('Blue Books') which I have consulted. I have not included Victorian and Edwardian sources on working-class housing and slum conditions, and for these the reader should consult my bibliography in *The Eternal Slum, Housing and Social Policy in Victorian London* (1977). The following bibliography can be most usefully supplemented by the excellent bibliographies in R. Lambert, *Sir John Simon, 1816–1904, and English Social Administration* (1963), F. B. Smith, *The People's Health, 1830–1910* (1979), and J. M. Eyler *Victorian Social Medicine. The Ideas and Methods of William Farr* (Baltimore, 1979). Except where otherwise indicated place of publication is London.

Original Sources

1 Parliamentary Papers

In addition to the minutes of evidence and reports of the many select committees and royal commissions (see footnotes), the most important body of information is that contained in the annual reports of the Privy Council and Local Government Board and the separate annual reports of the MOH to the Privy Council and the MOH to the Local Government Board. Also of great value are the annual reports of the Registrar-General of Births, Deaths and Marriages (1838–1907).

2 Papers of Specialized bodies and specialized journals

British Medical Journal (1857–1914).
The Health of Towns Association. See especially: *The Unhealthiness of Towns, its Causes and Remedies* (1845), *On the Moral and Physical Evils resulting from the Neglect of Sanitary Measures* (1847), and *The Sanitary Condition of the City of London* (1848).

Ladies' National Association for the Diffusion of Sanitary Knowledge, *Tracts*.

Lancet (1823–1914)

London. A Journal of Civic and Social Progress [later the Municipal Journal] (1893–1914)

London County Council, *Comparative Municipal Statistics*, I. 1912–1913 (1915)

Manchester and Salford Sanitary Association, *Health Lectures for the People* (1875–1887).

Medical Times [later *Medical Times and Gazette*] (1839–1885)

Public Health. A Record and Review of Sanitary, Social, and Municipal Affairs (1868–69)

Public Health. The Journal of the Society of Medical Officers of Health (1888–1914).

The Sanitary Record. A Journal of Public Health (1874–1880).

Transactions of the National Association for the Promotion of Social Science (1857–86).

Transactions of the Sanitary Institute of Great Britain [later *Journal . . .*] (1874–1914).

Transactions of the Society of Medical Officers of Health (1874–1886).

3 Autobiographies

B. C. Bloomfield, ed., *The Autobiography of Sir James Kay Shuttleworth* (1964)

M. L. Davies, ed., *Life as We have Known it, by Co-operative Working Women* (1931, reprinted, New York, 1975)

E. Flint, *Hot Bread and Chips* (1963).

E. Hall, ed., *Canary Girls and Stockpots* (Luton, 1977).

A. S. Jasper, *A Hoxton Childhood* (1969).

M. Loane, *The Next Street but One* (1907).

F. Petty, *The Pudding Lady. A New Departure in Social Work* (1910).

H. R. Rathbone, ed., *Memoir of Kitty Wilkinson of Liverpool, 1786–1860* (Liverpool, 1927).

S. Reynolds, *A Poor Man's House* (1908, reprinted, 1980).

R. Roberts, *The Classic Slum. Salford Life in the First Quarter of the Century* (1971).

D. Scannell, *Mother Knew Best* (1974).

E. Wallace, *People. A Short Autobiography* (1927).

T. Willis, *Whatever Happened to Tom Mix?* (1970).

K. Woodward, *Jipping Street* (1928).

G. Wyld, *Notes on My Life* (1903).

4 Books and Tracts

J. T. Arlidge, *The Hygiene Diseases and Mortality of Occupations* (1892)

G. Bell, *Day and Night in the Wynds of Edinburgh and Blackfriars Wynd Analyzed* (1849–50, reprinted, Wakefield, 1973).

W. Blyth, *A Dictionary of Hygiene and Public Health* (1876).

W. Blyth. *A Manual of Public Health* (1890).

W. Booth, *Life and Labour of the People of London* (1902–3).

S. Brown, *Notes on Sanitary Reform: the Health of Towns* (1870).

H. Burdett, *Help to Health: the Habitations, the Nursery, the School-Room and the Person, with a Chapter on Pleasure and Health Resorts* (1885).

C. A. Cameron, *A Brief History of the Municipal Public Health Administration in Dublin* (Dublin, 1914)

C. A. Cameron, *A Manual of Hygiene. Public and Private Compendium of Sanitary Laws* (Dublin, 1874).

C. A. Cameron, *The Prevention of Contagious Diseases. A Practical Treatise on Disinfectants, Antiseptics, and other Sanitary Agents* (1871).

E. Chadwick, *Report on the Sanitary Condition of the Labouring Population of Great Britain* (1842, reprinted, M. W. Flinn, ed., Edinburgh, 1965).

City of Edinburgh Charity Organisation Society, *Report on the Physical Condition of Fourteen Hundred School Children in the City, together with some Account of their Homes and Surroundings* (1906).

C. Creighton, *A History of Epidemics in Britain*, 2 vols. (Cambridge, 1891, 1894).

F. Engels, *The Condition of the Working Classes in England* (1842, trans. W. O. Henderson and W. H. Chaloner, Oxford, 1958).

E. Eve, ed., *Manual for Health Visitors and Infant Welfare Workers* (1921).

L. Faucher, *Manchester in 1844; its Present Condition and Future Prospects* (1844).

H. Gavin, *The Unhealthiness of London and the Necessity of Remedial Measures* (1847).

Rev C. Girdlestone, *Letters on the Unhealthy Condition of the Lower Classes of Dwellings, especially in Large Towns* (1845).

E. Greenhow, *Papers relating to the Sanitary State of the People of England* (1858).

W. Guy, *On the Health of Towns, as influenced by Defective Cleansing and Drainage, and on the Application of the Refuse of Towns to Agricultural Purposes* (1846).

E. Hart, *Local Government as it is and as it ought to be* (1885).

E. Hart, *London, Old and New. A Sanitary Contrast* (1885).

J. Hollingshead, *Ragged London in 1861* (1861).

International Health Exhibition (1884).

H. Jephson, *The Sanitary Evolution of London* (1907).

C. Kingsley, *Miscellanies*, 2 vols. (1859).

C. F. G. Masterman, ed., *The Heart of Empire. Discussion of Problems of Modern City Life in England* (1901, reprinted, B. G. Gilbert, ed., Brighton, 1973).

R. Metcalfe, *Sanitas Sanitatum et Omnia Sanitas* (1877).

G. Newman, *Infant Mortality. A Social Problem* (1906).

L. C. Parkes, *Hygiene and Public Health* (1889).

L. C. Parkes, *Jubilee Retrospect on the Royal Sanitary Institute, 1876–1926* (1926).

A. Patterson, *Across the Bridges, or Life by the South London River-side* (1914).

M. Pember Reeves, *Family Life on a Pound a Week* (1912).

B. Richardson, *Hygeia, A City of Health* (1876).

B. Seebohm, Rowntree, *Poverty. A Study of Town Life* (1902).

J. B. Russell, *Life in One Room or Some Serious Considerations for the Citizens of Glasgow* (Glasgow, 1888).

J. Simon, *English Sanitary Institutions* (1890).

J. Simon, *Public Health Reports*, 2 vols (E. Seaton, ed., 1887).

E. Smith, *Handbook for Inspectors of Nuisances* (1873).

E. Smith, *Manual for Medical Officers of Health* (1873).

St. John Smith, ed., *Public Health Act, Report to the General Board of Health on Darlington, 1850* (Durham, 1969).

W. T. Stead, ed., *Coming Men on Coming Questions* (1905).

A. P. Stewart and E. Jenkins, *The Medical and Legal Aspects of Sanitary Reform* (1866, M. Flinn, ed., Leicester, 1969).

J. F. J. Sykes, *Public Health and Housing* (1901).

J. F. J. Sykes, *Public Health Problems* (1892).

R. Thorne Thorne, *The Progress of Preventive Medicine during the Victorian Era* (1888).

F. Tristan, *London Journal* (1840, trans. D. Palmer and G. Pincete, 1980).

M. Williams, *Round London. Down East and Up West* (1892).

[T. Wright], *The Great Unwashed* (1868, reprinted, 1970).

T. Wright, *Some Habits and Customs of the Working Classes* (1867).

T. Wright 'The Riverside Visitor', *The Pinch of Poverty, Sufferings and Heroism of the London Poor* (1892).

Secondary Sources

1 Specialized Journals

British Journal of Industrial Medicine

Bulletin of the History of Medicine (organ of the American Association for the History of Medicine and the Johns Hopkins Institute of the History of Medicine).

Journal of the History of Medicine and Allied Sciences.

Journal of the Royal Institute of Public Health and Hygiene.

Medical History (organ of the British Society for the History of Medicine).

Population Studies.

World Health Organization (especially *Technical Report Series*).

2 Books

T. S. Ashton, *Economic and Social Investigations in Manchester, 1833–1933* (1934, reprinted 1977).

T. C. Barker and J. R. Harris, *A Merseyside Town in the Industrial Revolution. St. Helens, 1750–1900* (1959).

T. C. Barker, J. C. McKenzie, and J. Yudkin, *Our Changing Fare. Two Hundred Years of British Food Habits* (1966).

B. Barrows, *A County and its Health. A History of the Development of the West Riding Health Services, 1889–1979* (West Riding of Yorks, 1974).

S. P. Bell, ed., *Victorian Lancashire* (Newton Abbot, 1974).

H. G. Birch and J. D. Gussow, *Disadvantaged Children. Health, Nutrition and School Failure* (New York, 1970).

J. Boget, G. M. Briggs and D. H. Calloway, *Nutrition and Physical Fitness* (Philadelphia, 1973).

J. Brand, *Doctors and the State. The British Medical Profession and Government Action in Public Health, 1870–1912* (Baltimore, 1965).

A. Briggs, *Public Opinion and Public Health in the Age of Chadwick* (1946).

C. F. Brockington, *A Short History of Public Health* (1956).

C. F. Brockington, *Public Health in the Nineteenth Century* (Edinburgh, 1965).

C. Brook, *Battling Surgeon* (Glasgow, 1945).

J. H. F. Brotherston, *Observations on the Early Public Health Movement in Scotland* (1952).

M. Bruce, *The Coming of the Welfare State* (1966).

A. Burgess and R. F. Dean, eds., *Malnutrition and Food Habits* (1962).

M. Burnet, *The Natural History of Infectious Diseases* (Cambridge, 1962).

J. Burnett, *A History of the Cost of Living* (1969).

J. Burnett, *A Social History of Housing, 1815–1970* (Newton Abbot, 1978).

J. Burnett, *Plenty and Want. A Social History of Diet in England from 1815 to the Present Day* (1966).

W. H. Chaloner, *The Social and Economic Development of Crewe* (Manchester, 1950).

S. D. Chapman, ed., *The History of Working-Class Housing* (Newton Abbot, 1971).

J. Charles, *Research and Public Health* (1961).

E. Clarke, ed., *Modern Methods in the History of Medicine* (1971).

J. J. Clarke, *The History of Local Government in the United Kingdom* (1955).

D. M. Connan, *A History of the Public Health Department in Bermondsey* (1935).

M. J. Cullen, *The Statistical Movement in Early Victorian Britain* (Brighton, 1975).

J. S. Curl, *The Victorian Celebration of Death* (Newton Abbot, 1972).

J. Donnison, *Midwives and Medical Men. A History of Interprofessional Rivalries and Women's Rights*, (1977).

Bibliography

J. C. Drummond and A. Wilbraham, *The Englishman's Food* (1950).

H. J. Dyos and M. Wolff, eds., *The Victorian City. Images and Realities.* 2 vols. (1973).

G. E. Evans, *Where Beards Wag All. The Relevance of the Oral Tradition* (1970).

J. Eyler, *Victorian Social Medicine. The Ideas and Methods of William Farr* (Baltimore, 1979).

T. Ferguson, *Scottish Social Welfare, 1864–1914* (Edinburgh, 1958).

H. E. Finer, *Municipal Trading. A Study of Public Administration* (1914).

S. E. Finer, *The Life and Times of Sir Edwin Chadwick* (1952).

M. Flinn, *Public Health Reform in Britain* (New York, 1968).

D. Fraser, *Power and Authority in the Victorian City* (Oxford, 1979).

D. Fraser, *The Evolution of the British Welfare State. A History of Social Policy since the Industrial Revolution* (1973).

D. Fraser, *Urban Politics in Victorian England. The Structure of Politics in Victorian Cities* (Leicester, 1976).

W. M. Frazer, *Duncan of Liverpool* (1947).

W. M. Frazer, *A History of English Public Health, 1834–1939* (1950).

M. Freeden, *The New Liberalism. An Ideology of Social Reform* (Oxford, 1978).

E. Gauldie, *Cruel Habitations. A History of Working-Class Housing, 1780–1918* (1974).

W. C. Gibson, ed., *British Contributions to Medical Science* (1971).

M. Greenwood, *Epidemics and Crowd Diseases. An Introduction to the Study of Epidemiology* (1935).

B. Haley, *The Healthy Body and Victorian Culture* (Cambridge, Mass., 1978).

B. Harrison, *Drink and the Victorians. The Temperance Question in England, 1815–1872* (1971).

J. F. C. Harrison, *Social Reform in Victorian Leeds. The Work of James Hole 1820–1895* (Leeds, 1954).

D. Hartley, *Water in England* (1964).

J. D. J. Havard, *The Detection of Secret Homicide* (1960).

E. P. Hennock, *Fit and Proper Persons. Ideal and Reality in Nineteenth-Century Urban Government* (1973).

U. R. Q. Henriques, *Before the Welfare State. Social Administration in early industrial Britain* (1979).

M. Hewitt, *Wives and Mothers in Victorian Industry* (1958).

F. Hill, *Victorian Lincoln* (Cambridge, 1974).

R. Hodgkinson, *The Origins of the National Health Service* (1967).

P. Horn, *Labouring Life in the Victorian Countryside* (Dublin, 1976).

P. Horn, *The Victorian Country Child* (1974).

D. Hunter, *The Diseases of Occupations* (1978).

J. S. Hurt, *Elementary Schooling and the Working Classes, 1860–1918.* (1979).

B. Jennings, ed., *A History of Harrogate* (Huddersfield, 1970).

L. G. Jones, *Health, Wealth and Politics in Victorian Wales* (Swansea, 1979).

J. M. M. Kerr, R. W. Johnstone, and M. H. Phillips, *Historical Review of British Obstetrics and Gynaecology* (Edinburgh, 1954).

C. C. Knowles, *A History of the Regulation of Buildings in London and of the District Surveyors, 1189–1914* (1955).

R. Lambert, *Sir John Simon, 1816–1904, and English Social Administration* (1963).

H. J. Laski, W. Ivor Jennings and W. A. Robson, eds., *A Century of Municipal Progress, 1835–1935* (1935).

S. Leff, *Social Medicine* (1953).

C. Lewes, *Dr. Southwood Smith. A Retrospect* (1898).

R. A. Lewis, *Edwin Chadwick and the Public Health Movement 1832–1854* (1952).

N. Longmate, *Alive and Well. Medicine and Public Health, 1830 to the Present Day* (1970).

N. Longmate, *The Waterdrinkers. A History of Temperance* (1968).

G. F. McCleary, *The Early History of the Infant Welfare Movement* (1933).

T. McKeown and C. R. Lowe, *An Introduction to Social Medicine* (1966).

T. McKeown, *The Modern Rise of Population* (1976).

J. M. Mackintosh, *Trends of Opinion about the Public Health, 1901–1951* (1953).

G. Maclachlan and T. McKeown, eds., *Medical History and Medical Care* (1971).

T. McLaughlin, *Coprophilia, or a Peck of Dirt* (1971).

A. S. MacNalty, *The History of State Medicine in England* (1948).

J. D. Marshall, ed., *The History of Lancashire County Council, 1889 to 1974* (1977).

S. Meacham, *A Life Apart. The English Working Class, 1890–1914* (1977).

E. C. Midwinter, *Social Administration in Lancashire, 1830–1860. Poor Law, Public Health, Police* (Manchester, 1969).

C. E. Mingay, ed., *The Victorian Countryside*, 2 vols (1981).

R. Morris, *Cholera 1832. The Social Response to an Epidemic* (New York, 1976).

G. Newman, *The Building of a Nation's Health* (1939).

G. Newman, *The Rise of Preventive Medicine* (1932).

A. Newsholme, *Evolution of Preventive Medicine* (1927).

A. Newsholme, *The Last Thirty Years in Public Health* (1936).

R..Newton, *Victorian Exeter, 1837–1914* (Leicester, 1968).

J. V. O'Brien, *'Dear Dirty Dublin'. A City in Distress, 1899–1916* (Berkeley and Los Angeles, California, 1982).

D. Oddy and D. Miller, eds., *The Making of the Modern British Diet* (1976).

T. Ogawa, ed., *Public Health, Proceedings of the Fifth International Symposium on the History of Medicine – East and West* (Tokyo, 1981).

D. Owen, *The Government of Victorian London, 1855–1889. The Metropolitan Board of Works, the Vestries, and the City Corporation* (R. MacLeod, ed., Cambridge, Massachusetts, 1982).

R. Palmer, *The Water Closet. A New History* (Newton Abbot, 1973).

A. T. Patterson, *Radical Leicester. A History of Leicester, 1780–1850* (Leicester, 1954).

M. Pelling, *Cholera, Fever, and English Medicine, 1825–1865* (1978).

M. J. Peterson, *The Medical Profession in Mid-Victorian London* (Berkeley and Los Angeles, California, 1978).

F. N. L. Poynter, ed., *Medicine and Science in the 1860s* (1968).

W. Radcliffe, *Milestones in Midwifery* (Bristol, 1967).

A. Redford, *The History of Local Government in Manchester*, 3 vols. (1939).

R. Reynolds, *Cleanliness and Godliness* (1943).

M. Riley, *Brought to Bed* (1968).

W. A. Robson, *The Government and Misgovernment of London* (1939).

L. Rose, *Health and Hygiene* (1975).

G. Rosen, *A History of Public Health* (New York, 1958).

D. Rubinstein, *School Attendance in London, 1870–1904: A social History* (University of Hull, Occasional Papers in Economic and Social History, No. I, Hull, 1969).

R. Salaman, *The History and Social Influence of the Potato* (Cambridge, 1949).

F. Schwarzbach, *Dickens and the City* (1979).

F. Sheppard, *London, 1808–1870: the Infernal Wen* (1971).

T. S. Simey, *Principles of Social Administration* (1937).

J. Simmons, *Life in Victorian Leicester* (Leicester, 1971).

G. Slater, *Poverty and the State* (1930).

E. Smith, *Victorian Farnham. The Story of a Surrey Town, 1837–1901* (1971).

F. B. Smith, *The People's Health, 1830–1910* (1979).

W. D. Smith, *Stretching their Bodies. The History of Physical Education* (Newton Abbot, 1974).

D. Stanford and A. T. Patterson, *The Conditions of the Children of the Poor in Mid-Victorian Portsmouth* (Portsmouth Papers, No. 21, Portsmouth, 1974).

J. H. Stephens, *Water and Waste* (1967).

N. Sunderland, *A History of Darlington* (Manchester, 1972).

A. Sutcliffe, ed., *Multi-Storey Living. The British Working-Class Experience* (1974).

A. Sutcliffe, ed., *The Rise of Modern Urban Planning, 1800–1914* (1980).

A. Sutcliffe, *Towards the Planned City. Germany, Britain, the United States and France, 1780–1914* (Oxford, 1981).

G. Sutherland, ed., *Studies in the Growth of Nineteenth-Century Government* (1972).

H. P. Tait, *A Doctor and Two Policemen: the History of the Edinburgh Health Department, 1862–1974* (Edinburgh, 1974).

J. M. Tanner, *Growth at Adolescence* (Oxford, 1955).

P. Thane, *The Foundations of the Welfare State* (1982).

F. Vigier, *Change and Apathy, Liverpool and Manchester during the Industrial Revolution* (Cambridge, Mass., 1970).

M. E. M. Walker, *Pioneers of Public Health. The Story of some Benefactors of the Human Race* (1930).

B. D. White, *A History of the Corporation of Liverpool, 1835–1914* (Liverpool, 1951).

H. C. Maurice Williams, *Public Health in a Seaport Town by the Medical Officer of Health* (Southampton, 1962).

J. H. Williams, *A Century of Public Health in Britain, 1832–1929* (1932).

N. Williams, *Powder and Paint* (1957).

A. S. Wohl, *The Eternal Slum. Housing and Social Policy in Victorian London* (1977).

R. Wood, *West Hartlepool. The Rise and Development of a Victorian New Town* (West Hartlepool, 1967).

J. H. Woodward and D. Richards, eds. *Health, Care and Popular Medicine in Nineteenth-Century England: Essays in the Social History of Medicine* (1977).

L. Wright, *Clean and Decent. The Fascinating History of the Bathroom and Water Closet* (1926).

J. C. Wylie, *The Wastes of Civilization* (1959).

A. J. Youngson, *The Scientific Revolution in Victorian Medicine* (1979).

3 Articles

British Journal of Industrial Medicine.

W. R. Lee, 'The History of Statutory Control of Mercury Poisoning in Great Britain', 25 (January 1968).

W. R. Lee, 'Emergence of Occupational Medicine in Victorian Times', 30 (April 1973).

E. Posner, 'John Thomas Arlidge, (1822–1899) and the Potteries', 30 (July 1973).

Bulletin of the History of Medicine

O. N. Anderson, 'Age-Specific Mortality in Selected Western European Countries, with Particular Emphasis on the Nineteenth Century', 29, 3 (May–June 1955).

J. Brand, 'John Simon and the Local Government Board Bureaucrats, 1871–1876', 37, 2 (March–April 1963).

J. M. Eyler, 'Mortality Statistics and Victorian Health Policy: Program and Criticism', 50, 3 (Fall 1976).

J. M. Eyler, 'The Conversion of Angus Smith: the Changing Role of Chemistry and Biology in Sanitary Science, 1850–1880', 54, 2 (Summer, 1980).

B. B. Gilbert, 'Health and Politics: the British Physical Deterioration Report of 1904', 39, 2 (March–April 1965).

E. Lomax, 'The Uses and Abuses of Opiates in Nineteenth Century England', 47, 1 (January–February 1973).

G. Rosen, 'What is Social Medicine? A Genetic Analysis of the Concept', 21, 5 (September–October 1947).

T. L. Savitt, 'Smothering and Overlaying of Virginia Slave Children', 49, 3 (Fall, 1975).

H. Seibert, 'The Progress of Ideas Regarding the Causation and Control of Infant Mortality', 8, 4 (April 1940).

L. Stevenson, 'Science down the Drain: on the Hostility of Certain Sanitarians to Animal Experimentation, Bacteriology and Immunology', 29, 1 (January–February, 1955).

J. H. Warner, 'Physiological Theory and Therapeutic Explanation in the 1860s: the British Debate on the Medical Use of Alcohol', 54, 2 (Summer, 1980).

Bulletin of the Society of Medical History of Chicago

E. A. Underwood, 'The Field Workers in the English Public Health Movement', VI (October 1948).

Economic History Review

D. J. Oddy, 'Working-Class Diets in Late Nineteenth-Century Britain', XXIII, 2 (1970).

Feminist Studies

L. Oren, 'The Welfare of Women in Labouring Families: England, 1860–1950', I, 3–4 (Winter–Spring, 1973).

Journal of the History of Medicine and Allied Sciences

A. Beck, 'Some Aspects of the History of Anti-Pollution Legislation in England, 1819–1954', XIV (October 1959).

G. Behlmer, 'Deadly Method: Infanticide and Medical Opinion in Mid-Victorian England' XXXIV (October 1979).

V. Berridge, 'Opium in the Fens in Nineteenth-Century England', XXXIV (July 1979).

J. H. Cassedy, 'Hygeia. A Mid-Victorian Dream of a City of Health', XVII (April 1962).

C. B. Chapman, 'Edward Smith (?1818–1874), Physiologist, Human Ecologist, Reformer', XXII (January 1967).

A. Ciocco and D. Perrott, 'Statistics on Sickness as a Cause of Poverty. An Historical Review of U.S. and English Data', XII (January 1957).

J. M. Eyler, 'William Farr on the Cholera: the Sanitarian's Disease Theory and the Statistician's Method', XXVIII, (April 1973).

E. H. Gibson, 'Baths and Washhouses in the English Public Health Agitation, 1839–48', IX (October 1954).

R. M. MacLeod, 'The Edge of Hope: Social Policy and Chronic Alcoholism, 1870–1900', XXII (July 1967).

Bibliography

P. A. Richmond, 'Some Variant Theories in Opposition to the Germ Theory of Disease', IX (July 1954).

Journal of the Royal Institute of Public Health and Hygiene

D. E. Forsythe, 'The Evolution of the Child Welfare Services in England and Wales', 29 (January–December 1966).

Journal of the Royal Sanitary Institute

W. Stern, 'Water Supply in Britain: the Development of a Public Service', 74, 10 (October 1954).

Leicester Archaeological and Historical Society, Transactions

D. L. Ross, 'Leicester and the Anti-Vaccination Movement, 1853–1889', XLIII (1967–8).

Manchester Literary and Philosophical Society, Memoirs and Proceedings

A. Sharratt and K. R. Farrar, 'Sanitation and Public Health in Nineteenth-Century Manchester', 114 (1971–2).

Medical History

M. Barnet, 'The 1832 Cholera Epidemic in York', XVI (January 1972)
A. Beck, 'Issues in the Anti-Vaccination Movement in England', IV (October 1960).
T. Forbes, 'The Regulation of English Midwives in the Eighteenth and Nineteenth Centuries', XV (October 1971).
S. M. F. Fraser, 'Leicester and Smallpox: the Leicester Method', XXIV (July 1980).
R. E. Hughes, 'George Budd (1808–1882) and Nutritional Deficiency Diseases', XVII (April 1973).
W. E. Luckin, 'The Final Catastrophe-Cholera in London, 1866', XXI (January 1977).
T. McKeown, 'A Sociological Approach to the History of Medicine', XIV (October 1970).
R. MacLeod, 'Medico-Legal Issues in Victorian Medical Care', X (January 1966).
R. MacLeod, 'The Frustration of State Medicine, 1880–1899', XI (January 1967).
A. S. MacNalty, 'The Prevention of Smallpox: From Edward Jenner to Monckton Copeman', XII (January 1968).

New Society

A. Briggs, 'Public Health: "The Sanitary Idea" ', (15 February 1968).

A. Briggs, 'Public Health and the Health of the Nation', (22 February 1968).
H. J. Dyos, 'The Slum Observed' (1 February 1968).

Population Studies

D. V. Glass, 'Some Indications of Differences between Urban and Rural Mortality in England and Wales and Scotland', XVII, Part 3 (March 1964).
T. Ferguson, 'Public Health in Britain in the Climate of the Nineteenth Century', XVII, Part 3 (March 1964).
W. P. D. Logan, 'Mortality in England and Wales from 1848 to 1947', IV, Part 2 (September 1950).
T. McKeown and R. G. Record, 'Reasons for the Decline of Mortality in England and Wales during the Nineteenth Century', XVI, Part 2 (November 1962).

Proceedings of the Nutrition Society

D. J. Oddy 'Food in the Nineteenth Century: Nutrition in the first Urban Society', 29 (1970).
D. J. Oddy and J. Yudkin, 'An Evaluation of English Diets of the 1860s', 28 (1969).

Public Opinion

R. M. MacLeod, 'Law, Medicine and Public Opinion: the Resistance to Compulsory Health Legislation, 1870–1907, Part I', (Summer, 1967).
R. M. MacLeod, 'Law, Medicine and Public Opinion: the Resistance to Compulsory Health Legislation, Part II', (Autumn, 1967).

Social History

S. Novak, 'Professionalism and Bureaucracy: English Doctors and the Victorian Public Health Administration', 6, 4 (Summer, 1973).

The Pharos

C. B. Chapman, 'The Year of the Great Stink', 35 (July 1972).

Urban History Yearbook

W. E. Luckin, 'Death and Survival in the City: Approaches to the History of Disease', 1980.

Victorian Studies

R. M. MacLeod, 'The Alkali Acts Administration, 1863–84: the Emergence of the Civil Scientist', IX, 2 (December 1965).

Bibliography

Warwickshire History

R. I. Penny, 'The Board of Health and Victorian Stratford-upon-Avon. Aspects of Environmental Control', I, 6 (Autumn 1971).

Theses

A. J. Archer, *A Study of Local Sanitary Administration (1830–1875)*, MA., Bangor, 1967.

G. J. Barnsby, *Social Conditions in the Black Country in the Nineteenth Century* PhD., University of Birmingham, 1969.

J. Donnison, *The Development of the Profession of Midwife in England, from 1750 to 1902*, PhD., London University, 1974.

W. C. Dowling, *The Ladies' Sanitary Association and the Origins of the Health Visiting Service*, MA., University of London, 1963.

M. Elliott, *The Leicester Board of Health, 1849 to 1872. A Study of Progress in the Development of Local Government*, M.Phil, University of Nottingham, 1971.

H. Macdonald, *Public Health Legislation and Problems in Victorian Edinburgh, with Special Reference to the Work of Dr. Littlejohn as Medical Officer of Health*, PhD., University of Edinburgh, 1971.

F. McKichan, *Stirling, 1780–1880. The Response of Burgh Government to the Problems of Urban Growth*. M.Litt., University of Glasgow, 1972.

P. E. Malcolmson, *The Potteries of Kensington: a Study of Slum Development in Victorian London*, MPhil, University of Leicester, 1970.

J. Toft, *Public Health in Leeds in the Nineteenth Century. A Study of the Growth of Local Government Responsibility, c. 1815–1880*, MA., University of Manchester, 1966.

W. E. Townley, *Urban Administration and Health: A Case Study of Hanley in the mid-Nineteenth Century*, MA., University of Keele, 1969.

B. Wharton, *Aspects of Health in Victorian Dudley*, Diploma in History, University of London, 1975.

Index